M.R. Prince, T.M.Grist and J.F.Debatin
3D Contrast MR Angiography

D1297178

Springer

Berlin
Heidelberg
New York
Hong Kong
London
Milan
Paris
Tokyo

Martin R. Prince
Thomas M. Grist
Jörg F. Debatin

3D Contrast
MR Angiography

Third, Revised and Enlarged Edition

With 159 Figures in 305 Separate Illustrations and 24 Tables

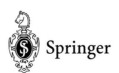

Springer

Jörg F. Debatin, M.D., M.B.A
Professor and Chairman
Department of Diagnostic and Interventional Radiology
University Hospital Essen
Hufelandstrasse 55, 45122 Essen, Germany

Thomas M. Grist, M.D.
Chief of Magnetic Resonance Imaging
Vice Chaiman for Research
Professor of Radiology and Medical Physics
Department of Radiology, University of Wisconsin – Madison
E3/311 600 Highland Ave. Madison, WI 53792-3252, USA

Martin R. Prince, M.D., Ph.D.
Chief of Magnetic Resonance Imaging, New York Hospital
Professor of Radiology
Columbia College of Physicians and Surgeons
Weill Medical College of Cornell University
416 East 55th Street, New York, NY 10022, USA

ISBN 3-540-42874-7 Springer-Verlag Berlin Heidelberg New York

Library of Congress Cataloging-in-Publication Data applied for

Bibliographic information published by Die Deutsche Bibliothek
Die Deutsche Bibliothek lists this publication in the Deutsche Nationalbibliografie;
detailed bibliographic data is available in the Internet at <http://dnb.ddb.de>.

Published in the medico-scientific book series of Schering

The book shop edition is published by Springer-Verlag Berlin Heidelberg New York Barcelona
Hong Kong London Milan Paris Tokyo

Where reference is made to the use of Schering products, the reader is advised to consult the latest
scientific information issued by the company.

All rights are reserved. No part of this publication may be translated into other languages, repro-
duced or utilized in any form or by any means, electronic or mechanical, including photocopying,
recording, microcopying, or by any information storage and retrieval system, without permission
in writing from Schering.

The subject matter of this book may be covered by one or more patents. This book and the information contained therein and conveyed thereby should not be construed as either explicity or
implicity granting any license; and no liability for patent infringement arising out of the use of the
information is assumed.

© 2003 by Schering
Printed in Germany

Cover-Design: Erich Kirchner, Heidelberg
Typesetting: Verlagsservice Teichmann, Mauer
SPIN: 11019473   21/3111 - 5 4 3 2 1 – Printed on acid-free paper

Acknowledgements

We gratefully acknowledge Hale Ersoy Erel, M.D. for compiling the Accuracy Data Tables and literature as well as many important contributions by colleagues at our respective institutions:

University Hospital Essen: Jörg Barkhausen, M.D., Andrea Borowski, R.T., Silke Bosk, R.T., Michael Forsting, M.D., Susanne Göhde, M.D., Mathias Goyen, M.D., Christoph Herborn, M.D., Peter Hunold, M.D., Mark E. Ladd, Ph.D., Sandra Massing, R.T., Harald Quick, Ph.D., Stephan Ruehm, M.D., Janine Smieja, R.T., Florian Vogt, M.D.

University of Wisconsin at Madison: Patti Brebrender RTR, Lynnette Frey RTR, Judy Fuller RTR, Sandra Fuller, Gina Greenwood RTR, Judy Imhoff, Tom Kerwin RTR, Tom McKinlay RTR, John McDermott, M.D. Kathy Robichaud RTR, Orhan Unal PhD, Myron Wojtowycz, M.D.

Cornell and Columbia Universities: Phil Alderson, M.D., Harry Bush, M.D., Maureen Carmody, Minh Chao, Linda Heier, M.D., Bernard Ho, Edna Hong, Helen Iwu, Ray Jean Buttiglieri, Craig Kent, M.D., Neil Khilnani, M.D., Joon Minn, M.D., Jim Powel, Tom Sos, M.D., H. Dirk Sostman, M.D., David Trost, M.D., Yi Wang, Ph.D., Richard Watts, Ph.D., Priscilla Winchester, M.D., Ramin Zabih, Ph.D., Bob Zimmerman, M.D.

We also acknowledge the vision of Luis E. Reimer-Hevia, Ph.D. and Thomas Balzer, M.D. of Schering AG to make this book possible, the contributions of Michelle Moore, our editors Ute Heilmann and Wilma McHugh, our production editor Kurt Teichmann, and also our colleagues who have contributed case studies (see List of Contributors).

List of Abbreviations

2D:	Two-dimensional
3D:	Three-dimensional
3D-TRICKS:	Three-dimensional Time Resolved Imaging on Contrast Kinetics
AAA:	Abdominal aortic aneurysm
AngioSURF:	Angiography system of unlimited rolling field-of-views
A/P:	Anterior to posterior
AVM:	Arterio-venous malformation
CE-MRA:	Contrast-enhanced magnetic resonance angiography
CNR:	Contrast-to-noise ratio
COPD:	Chronic obstructive pulmonary disease
CP:	Circularly Polarized
CT:	Computed tomography
CTA:	Computed tomography angiography
DSA:	Digital subtraction angiography
DUS:	Doppler ultrasound
ECG:	Electrocardiogram
EKG:	Electrocardiogram
ESCT:	European Symptomatic Carotid Trial
FIESTA:	Fast imaging employing steady state acquisition
FISP:	Fast imaging with steady state precession
FLASH:	Fast low angle shot
FMD:	Fibromuscular disease
FOV:	Field-of-view
FT:	Fourier transform
Gd:	Gadolinium
Gd-DTPA:	Gadolinium diethylenetriamine pentacetic acid
GRE:	Gradient recalled echo
HASTE:	Half-Fourier acquisition single-shot turbo spin-echo
IMA:	Inferior mesenteric artery
IMV:	Inferior mesenteric vein
IVC:	Inferior vena cava
kvo:	Keep vein open
MIP:	Maximum intensity projection
MOTSA:	Multiple overlapping thin slab acquisitions
MRA:	Magnetic resonance angiography

MRI:	Magnetic resonance imaging
ms:	milliseconds
MTF:	Modulation transfer function
NASCET:	North American Carotid Endarterectomy Trial
NEX:	Number of excitations
PAH:	Para amino hippurate
PE:	Pulmonary embolism
PR:	Projection reconstruction
PVD:	Peripheral vascular disease
R1:	T1 relaxivity
RF:	Radio frequency
ROI:	Region-of-interest
RVD:	Renovascular disease
s:	seconds
SAR:	Specific Absorption Rate
SE:	Spin echo
SENSE:	Sensitivity encoding
SFA:	Superficial femoral artery
SI:	Signal intensity
S/I:	Superior to inferior
SMA:	Superior mesenteric artery
SMASH:	Simultaneous acquisition of spatial harmonics
SMV:	Superior mesenteric vein
SNR:	Signal-to-noise ratio
SSFSE:	Single shot fast spin echo
SVC:	Superior vena cava
T:	Tesla
TASC:	TransAtlantic Inter-Society Consensus
TE:	Echo time
TIPS:	Transjugular intrahepatic porto-systemic shunt
TOF:	Time-of-flight
TR:	Repetition time
V/Q:	Ventilation/perfusion
VENC:	Velocity encoding value
VIE:	Virtual intravascular endoscopy
VIPR:	Vastly undersampled imaging with projection reconstruction
y-res:	Number of phase encoding steps in the y-axis
z-res:	Number of slices in the 3D volume

List of Contributors

Pelin Aksit, M.D.
Yoshimi Anzai, M.D.
J. Greg Baden, M.D.
Andrew Barger, M.D., Ph.D.
Matt A. Bernstein, Ph.D.
Gus Bis, M.D.
Wallter F. Block, Ph.D.
Georg Bongartz, M.D.
Matthias Boos, M.D.
Ruth C. Carlos, M.D.
James Carr, M.D.
Timothy J. Carroll, Ph.D.
Minh T. Chao
Thomas L. Chenevert, Ph.D.
Daisy Chien, Ph.D.
T.S. Chung, M.D.
Kevin Demarco, M.D.
Qian Dong, M.D.
Jiang Du, M.S.
Hale Ersoy Erel, M.D.
Sean Fain, Ph.D.
Helen M. Fenlon, M.D.
Tom Foo, Ph.D.
Jochen Gaa, M.D.
Mathias Goyen, M.D.
Brian H. Hamilton, M.D.
Thomas F. Hany, M.D.
Christoph Herborn, M.D.
Paul R. Hilfiker, M.D.
Bernard Ho
Kai Yiu Ho, M.D.
Vince Ho, M.D.
John Huston, M.D.
Lars Johanson, M.S.
Neil Khilnani, M.D.
Junhwan Kim, M.S.
Michael V. Knopp, M.D.
Lars Kopka, M.D.
Frank R. Korosec, Ph.D.
Glenn Krinsky, M.D.
Vivian Lee, M.D., Ph.D.

Tim Leiner, M.D.
Daniel A. Leung, M.D.
Debiao Li, Ph.D.
Jianqi Li, Ph.D.
Frank Londy, R.T. (R)
Jeffrey H. Maki, M.D., Ph.D.
James F.M. Meaney, M.D.
Charles Mistretta, Ph.D.
Mohammed Neimatallah, M.D.
Mathiys Oudkerk, M.D., Ph.D.
Dana C. Peters, Ph.D.
Kris Pillai, M.D.
Sanjay Rajagopalan, M.D.
Bernie Redd, M.D.
Jens Rodenwaldt, M.D.
Neil Rofsky, M.D.
Stephan G. Ruehm, M.D.
Stefan O. Schoenberg, M.D.
Anil Shetty, Ph.D.
Tom Sos, M.D.
David Stafford-Johnson, M.D.
Barry Stein, M.D.
Samer Suleiman, M.D.
J. Shannon Swan, M.D.
Frank Thornton, M.D.
David Trost, M.D.
Partick A. Turski, M.D.
John van Tassel, M.D.
Patrick Veit, M.D.
Karl Vigen, Ph.D.
Yi Wang, Ph.D.
Richard Watts, Ph.D.
Klaus U. Wentz, M.D.
Oliver Wieben, Ph.D.
Piotr Wielopolski, Ph.D.
Donald Willig, M.D.
Priscilla Winchester, M.D.
E. Kent Yucel, M.D.
Ramin Zabih, Ph.D.
Young Zhou, Ph.D.

Table of Contents

Introduction

Non-invasive, high-resolution contrast arteriography without arterial catheterization or nephrotoxicity is now a reality. It is accomplished using paramagnetic contrast (e.g., Gadolinium) and an MR scanner. Paramagnetic contrast media injected intravenously lights up arteries on MR images as the contrast bolus circulates through the vascular territory of interest. Vascular enhancement by paramagnetic contrast media is so strong that a small dose injected intravenously is sufficient to briefly enhance the entire arterial vascular tree. This allows large field-of-view imaging encompassing an extensive region of vascular anatomy. Using high performance gradient systems, high-resolution 3D volumes of image data can be acquired sufficiently rapidly to chase the bolus from thorax to ankles, thereby making whole body MRA possible with a single contrast injection. Subsequent post-processing allows an angiographic display of image data with multiple projections or 3D volume rendering.

The success of this technique is reflected by its incorporation into clinical practice in centers throughout the world. It has been applied to every vascular territory using various magnets and slightly differing imaging strategies. As is the case for all MR imaging techniques, a thorough understanding of underlying mechanisms and optimal technique are essential to fully exploit the diagnostic potential of this new form of angiography. Particularly important is the Fourier nature of MR data collection and the matching of low spatial frequency, central k-space data with the peak arterial phase.

This book will familiarize the reader with basic principles of 3D contrast MRA. All relevant technical aspects are addressed, imaging protocols are provided, and tailored imaging strategies are described for different vascular regions as well as for whole body MRA. The book also includes a glossary of relevant technical terms and an extensive bibliography.

CHAPTER 1

Basic Concepts

Why Use Paramagnetic Contrast?

Paramagnetic contrast agents enormously improve MR angiography image quality by increasing the signal-to-noise ratio reducing motion artifact by dramatically shortening scan times, eliminating flow artifacts and by providing the kind of "intuitive" contrast arteriogram image which clinicians automatically recognize and feel comfortable making decisions upon. Paramagnetic contrast agents shorten the T1 relaxation time of spins in the immediate vicinity of the paramagnetic molecules. Gadolinium is the most commonly used paramagnetic substance because of its high relaxivity and favorable safety profile when bound to a chelater. Additional paramagnetic contrast agents include iron oxide particles and manganese. Gadolinium chelates shorten the T1 relaxation time of blood in proportion to their concentration in the blood according to Equation 1.

$$\frac{1}{T1} = \frac{1}{1200ms} + R1\,[Gd] \tag{1}$$

where R1 = T1 relaxivity of the gadolinium chelate
and [Gd] = gadolinium concentration in the blood

By shortening the T1 relaxation time of blood, it is possible to acquire MR angiograms in which image contrast is based upon differences in the T1 relaxation between arterial blood, venous blood, and surrounding tissues (Figure 1.1). Unlike conventional MR angiography techniques, which rely on velocity-dependent inflow or phase shift effects, gadolinium contrast-enhanced MRA does not depend upon blood motion. As a result, motion and flow artifacts, seen with time-of-flight or phase contrast MR angiography, are largely eliminated with three-dimensional (3D) contrast MR angiography (Figure 1.2). In addition, the T1 shorten-

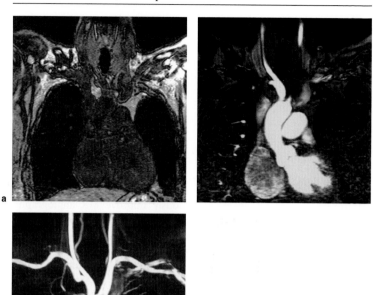

Fig. 1.1. 3D Contrast MRA of the Aortic Arch and Branch Vessels. (**a**) Pre-contrast source image, (**b**) source image during Gd-DTPA infusion, and (**c**) MIP display through all images demonstrates the aortic arch, proximal branch vessels, and pulmonary arteries.

ing effect of gadolinium allows in-plane imaging of vessels, thereby reducing the number of image sections required to display a large vascular territory. This, in turn, decreases image acquisition times.

Why Use A Three-Dimensional Imaging Pulse Sequence?

In contrast to computed tomography, where a 3D data set consists of multiple 2D slices acquired in rapid succession, the Fourier nature of 3D MR data acquisition involves collecting the entire 3D data set prior to reconstruction of any of the individual sections. Phase encoding is employed to spatially encode the y-axis as well as the z-axis position information. The resulting scan time is defined by Equation 2.

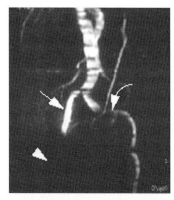

a

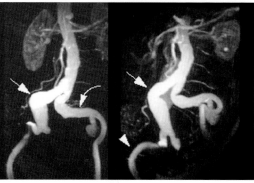

b

Fig. 1.2. Advantage of 3D Contrast MRA Compared to 2D Time-of-Flight (TOF). 2D TOF image of the distal aorta and iliac arteries (**a**) in a patient with aorto-iliac aneurysmal disease. Note the lumen of the right common iliac artery does not appear aneurysmal (*arrow*). This is because the 2D TOF sequence is sensitive to the more rapidly flowing protons, which are present only in the center of the lumen. Note also the apparent stenosis of the left iliac artery (*curved arrow*). This apparent stenosis is caused by saturation of protons moving in the same orientation as the acquisition slice, also known as in-plane flow suppression artifact. In addition, the 2D TOF exam shows complete signal loss in the region of the patient's right total hip prosthesis due to metal (susceptibility) artifact (*arrowhead*). There are also many areas of linear artifact in the aorta and left external and common femoral artery related to slice misregistration artifact. Two MIPs from the 3D contrast MRA sequence (**b**) in the same patient demonstrates the true size of the right iliac lumen (*arrow*) and shows that the left iliac artery is patent without stenosis (*curved arrow*). The 3D contrast MRA sequence is not sensitive to flow related artifacts observed in 2D TOF and 3D TOF methods. In addition, the 3D contrast MRA sequence shows signal in the vessels near the hip prosthesis (*arrowhead*). This is possible because 3D contrast MRA uses a shorter echo time (TE) than 2D TOF. Finally, note that the 3D contrast MRA images have no slice misregistration artifacts.

Scan Time = TR × Y-res × Z-res × NEX   (2)

where TR = repetition time

Y-res = number of phase encoding steps in the y-axis (= y resolution)

Z-res = number of phase encoding steps in the z-axis (= number of slices in the 3D volume), and

NEX = number of excitations averaged

Unlike 2D acquisitions (i.e. CTA), where a sudden motion by the patient will render one slice uninterpretable, in 3D MR, these artifacts are spread over the entire 3D data set. As long as they are not too numerous and do not occur during acquisition of central k-space data (more on k-space later), these artifacts will be averaged away. There may be minor degradation of the entire volume of image data, but individual slices will not be affected out of proportion to the rest of the data.

Three-dimensional gradient echo imaging provides a high-resolution volume of image data where every voxel is properly aligned relative to its neighbor, even if there is minor patient motion. This allows accurate post-processing of the data into different obliquities using a computer workstation. By comparison, 2D gradient echo techniques are corrupted by slice misregistration when there are minor patient motions. 3D data are also amenable to increasing reconstructed resolution by interpolation with zero filling.

With 3D acquisition, MR data for each voxel are accumulated over the entire scan, resulting in an improved signal-to-noise ratio as compared to a 2D strategy at the same section thickness. In addition, as compared to 2D imaging, 3D imaging minimizes stress on the gradients (with the same section thickness) and allows the use of shorter RF pulses. These factors allow shorter repetition times (TR), thinner sections, less dB/dt and a higher sampling efficiency. Section thickness can be reduced to less than 1 mm provided that there is sufficient signal-to-noise ratio. The shortened repetition and echo times make it possible to collect large 3D volumes of high resolution data or multiple successive lower resolution volumes in a 20–40 second breath-hold.

How Are Contrast Dose, Injection Rate, And Scan Time Related?

It is essential to inject sufficient paramagnetic contrast to reduce arterial blood T1 to well under the T1 of surrounding tissues. This will result in arterial blood appearing bright on the image compared to all other tissues. Shortening arterial blood T1 relaxation time also increases the image signal-to-noise ratio. With T1 relaxation time of 270 ms at 1.5 T, fat is the background tissue with the shortest T1. Thus, sufficient gadolinium should be injected at a sufficient rate of injection to reduce the T1 of blood to well under 270 ms.

T1 relaxivity is the property of paramagnetic compounds that indicates the amount of T1 shortening achieved for a given concentration of the paramagnetic compound. Currently available gadolinium chelates have a T1 relaxivity of around 4.5/mMolar · s. The relationship between blood T1 and gadolinium concentration is shown in Figure 1.3, which indicates that an arterial blood gadolinium concentration well in excess of 1 mMolar is required for MR angiography. To determine the appropriate dose and injection rate, however, it is necessary to understand what factors affect arterial gadolinium concentration. Arterial gadolinium concentration is proportional to the rate of intravenous injection and inversely proportional to the cardiac output as follows:

$$\text{Arterial Gd Concentration} = \text{Injection Rate/Cardiac Output} \qquad (3)$$

Equation 3 indicates that either increasing the injection rate or lowering cardiac output can increase arterial gadolinium concentration.

Generally, resting cardiac output ranges between 3-6 L/min. While it may be risky to be too aggressive about lowering cardiac output, it is useful to have the patient relax in a reclining position for about 30 minutes

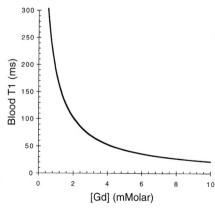

Fig. 1.3. Blood T1 versus gadolinium concentration calculated for relaxivity of 4.5/mMolar · s. Note that a blood [Gd] of at least 1 mMolar is required to achieve a T1 shorter than 270 ms, the T1 of fat.

prior to the 3D MR angiography examination. Cardiac output can also be minimized if the patient avoids eating or exercising immediately prior to the 3D MR angiography exam. Patients who are severely claustrophobic or anxious about the examination may benefit from a sedative, such as Diazepam (Valium 5–10 mg po) or Xanax (1–2 mg po), to help relieve the sympathetic stimulation related to anxiety. This, however, adds an element of risk to the procedure. Patients receiving diazepam or other sedatives must be accompanied by another adult and cannot be allowed to drive for at least 12 hours. Behavioral methods for promoting relaxation, including appropriate music and a video that prepares patients for the scan, may also be helpful.

Increasing injection rate increases Gd dose since the contrast dose is the product of injection rate and injection duration. To determine the optimum dose first consider injection duration of about the same as scan duration (more on shorter injection duration later). Figure 1.4 shows a computer simulation of the calculated arterial blood T1 relaxation time achieved at various gadolinium injection rates for a range of cardiac outputs. For a long, free breathing scan of around 3–4 minutes, an arterial blood T1 of approximately 150 ms provides adequate signal-to-noise ratio to resolve the aorta and the origins of the aortic branches. For a resting cardiac output of approximately 5 L/min, achieving an arterial blood T1 of less than 100 ms requires an injection rate of at least 0.2 ml/s (12 ml/min), and preferably greater than that. This injection rate (12 ml/min) sustained for a 3-minute scan duration translates into

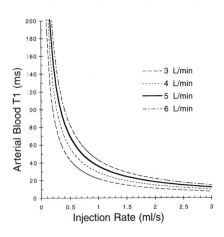

Fig. 1.4. Blood T1 versus gadolinium injection rate calculated for a relaxivity of 4.5/mMolar · s and a range of resting cardiac output. An injection rate of at least 0.2 ml/s to 0.3 ml/s is required to bring blood T1 down to around 150 ms (well below fat, 270 ms) for an average cardiac output of 5L/min (bold line).

a minimum gadolinium dose of 36 ml. Or for a faster scan, one could inject 36 ml of contrast at 2ml/s over 18 seconds and achieve a blood T1 of about 20 ms for even higher contrast between blood and background tissues. Faster scanning also has the advantage of reducing motion artifact by making breath-holding possible.

Shortening the scan time by reducing repetition time (TR) affects required contrast dose in two opposing ways. Shortening the TR 4-fold will reduce the scan duration 4-fold; thus, contrast injection will need to be only one fourth as long. This apparent reduction in contrast dose is offset by the requirement of an approximately 4-fold increase in the injection rate in order to recover the same amount of longitudinal magnetization in between pulses. Thus, there is no net effect on the contrast dose required if the signal-to-noise ratio is to remain unchanged. The shorter TR, however, with faster scanning improves background suppression, thereby enhancing the contrast-to-noise ratio. Since vessel visibility on 3D contrast MR angiography is determined by both the signal-to-noise and the contrast-to-noise ratios, shorter imaging times using a shorter TR do, in fact, permit use of less contrast while maintaining vessel visibility.

If TR is shortened by increasing the bandwidth, the effect is more complicated. Leaving all other factors unchanged, doubling the bandwidth reduces the signal-to-noise ratio by $1/\sqrt{2}$. To make up for this signal-to-noise loss, the injection rate must be increased by a $\sqrt{2}$ in addition to the increase required for the shorter repetition time. Thus, widening bandwidth is not the most contrast-efficient approach to shortening the scan although it may still be useful if it shortens the scan sufficiently to allow for breath-holding.

On the other hand, if the scan is shortened 2-fold by reducing the number of phase encoding steps by a factor of 2 without changing resolution, the signal-to-noise ratio is reduced by only $1/\sqrt{2}$ without any change in TR. For this 2-fold reduction in scan time, only a $\sqrt{2}$ increase in injection rate is required to maintain the signal-to-noise ratio. Thus, reducing phase encoding steps is a contrast-efficient approach to reducing scan times. Actually, there is a tendency to increase the voxel volume when the number of phase encoding steps is reduced; this contributes to an additional increase in signal-to-noise ratio at the expense of spatial resolution. One way to reduce phase encoding steps without affecting image resolution is to use partial Fourier imaging. This is sometimes referred to as a partial NEX or 0.5 NEX acquisition. Partial NEX is useful for 3D contrast-enhanced MR angiography when it does not lengthen the TE excessively, however, it may produce Fourier ringing artifacts. If partial NEX lengthens the echo time to where fat and water are out-of-phase then it may create artifacts at fat/tissue interfaces as well.

For extremely fast, time-resolved acquisitions, the contrast dose will have to be small because of the limit on how fast one can inject intravenously. Consider a scan duration of 3 seconds. It is difficult and probably not safe to inject faster than 5ml/second. Accordingly, the maximum possible contrast dose will be 15 ml. The maximum dose will be even less for faster scans.

Why Should The Data Acquisition Be As Fast As Possible?

As pointed out in the previous section, shortening scan time can enhance vessel visibility for a given contrast dose or provide the same image quality with a lower contrast dose. This is relevant for all vascular regions. A far more important benefit of shortening scan time is the ability to collect the entire 3D MR angiography data set in a single breath-hold. Generally, this becomes possible when scan time is shortened to under 45 seconds, and preferably to around 30 seconds in patients with normal pulmonary function or less than 15 seconds in dyspneic patients. By eliminating respiratory motion, breath-held data acquisition has vastly improved 3D contrast-enhanced MR angiography image quality in the abdomen and chest. It may be possible to resolve most pathology affecting the thoracic and abdominal aorta on non-breath hold 3D MR angiography acquisitions. But analysis of the pulmonary arteries and most aortic branch vessels requires data collection without respiratory motion artifact. Imaging systems that are not capable of acquiring 3D MR angiography data in a single breath-hold probably should not be used in the evaluation of vascular territories subject to respiratory motion, such as renal, mesenteric, or pulmonary arteries.

If the scan can be reduced to under 10 seconds, then it may be possible to acquire multiple, complete 3D acquisitions during a single breath-hold. This has the advantages of acquiring a data set prior to contrast arrival as well as during the different contrast phases (arterial, parenchymal, venous) within the same breath-hold. Digital subtractions can be performed isolating each vascular phase without misregistration. Multiple 3D acquisitions acquired in rapid succession demonstrate the time course of contrast-enhancement. Since at least one 3D acquisition in a series of several ultra fast (<<10 seconds) acquisitions acquired in rapid succession is likely to line up with the peak arterial phase of the bolus, this can simplify bolus timing. It is no longer necessary to perform a test injection or to use a gadolinium detection scheme to ensure optimal bolus timing. A refinement of this approach that makes rapid data acquisition possible, even on scanners with limited gradient performance, known as 3D TRICKS, is described in Chapter 2: Advanced Techniques.

Once data acquisition is sufficiently fast to complete the entire scan during a breath-hold, it may not always be better to further increase the data acquisition speed. If the echo time (TE) is short enough, the signal-to-noise ratio may improve with a narrower bandwidth. However, the echo time should not be allowed to increase beyond approximately 2 or 3 ms; otherwise, $T2^*$ and flow effects may begin to degrade image quality. Inevitably, shortening scan time requires limiting the number of phase encode steps which compromises spatial resolution. It is necessary to strike a balance between spatial and temporal resolution and the optimum will range from 2–3 seconds for test boluses and 2D projection MRA to 40–50 seconds for carotid or tibial arteries where high resolution is more important.

Breath-Holding: Inspiration Or Expiration?

Breath-holding is essential for achieving optimal 3D MR angiography image quality in the thorax and abdomen. It is important to determine how long a patient can suspend respiration prior to the examination because this defines the maximum possible scan duration without incurring respiratory motion artifacts. Examining the patient's respiratory pattern recorded by the magnet's respiratory bellows system is helpful. A patient breathing at a rate less than 20 breaths per minute with long pauses in between breaths can easily suspend breathing for 30 to 40 seconds. On the other hand, if the rate is greater than 25 breaths per minute with no pauses, breath-holding may be a struggle. If the rate exceeds 30 breaths per minute, the patient cannot breath-hold at all. A dry run of breath-holding before the patient is advanced into the gantry may also help determine how long the patient can suspend breathing.

Most patients find it easiest to hold their breath in maximum inspiration. However, if multiple breath-holds are required in succession, it is easier to reproduce the same degree of breath-holding by suspending breathing in expiration. Breath-holding in expiration is also better for EKG gated acquisitions, because it brings the heart closer to the skin to produce a stronger EKG signal at the skin surface. Oxygen administered by nasal cannula (2–4 liters) may improve the patient's breath-holding capacity. Oxygen can also be administered by affixing oxygen tubing to the roof of the scanner. This may simplify routine oxygen administration by eliminating the need to place a nasal cannula for each patient.

When using an automatic or MR fluoroscopic gadolinium detection scheme, the patient should be trained in advance to immediately begin breath-holding when given a signal. In addition to verbal cues, which may be difficult to hear, the patient can be signaled by touch or with the onset of a change in the gradient noise of the magnet.

How Do You Time The Intravenous Injection?

Optimal implementation of 3D contrast MR angiography requires accurate timing of the contrast bolus (Figure 1.5). Starting data acquisition too late relative to the contrast infusion leads to enhancement of venous structures; imaging too early results in severe artifacts that can render the examination non-diagnostic (Figure 1.5.b). Data collection needs to coincide with circulation of the gadolinium bolus through the vascular territory under investigation. The bolus must be of an appropriate duration and it must be timed to begin at the correct moment relative to the onset of data collection. In the ensuing discussion, it is important to differentiate between slower (free breathing) and fast (breath-hold) acquisitions.

First, consider the issue of how long to make the contrast injection. It is possible to take advantage of the Fourier nature of MR image data acquisition to avoid having to inject over the entire duration of scanning. MR data does not map pixel for pixel onto the image. Rather, the Fourier image data, generally referred to as k-space data, defines image features (Figure 1.6). High spatial frequency data, known as the periphery of k-space, determines image detail. Low spatial frequency data, known as central low spatial frequency k-space, dominates image contrast. By timing the injection for maximum arterial gadolinium concentration to occur during acquisition of central k-space data, it is possible to achieve the gadolinium contrast effect with a bolus lasting for only 1/2 to 2/3 of the scan. This reduces the total gadolinium dose. Alternatively, if the same amount of contrast is injected over this shorter period (1/2 to 2/3

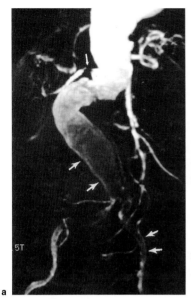

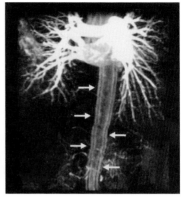

Fig. 1.5. Ringing Artifact on 3D Contrast MRA. Due to really slow flow in this patient with aortic aneurysmal disease (**a**), the gadolinium concentration in the infra-renal aorta and iliac arteries was still rising while the central k-space data were being acquired. The changing gadolinium concentration during acquisition of image data creates an edge, or ringing artifact. This artifact is characterized by bright (*arrows*) and dark lines paralleling the edges of blood vessels. In the suprarenal aorta, the gadolinium concentration had already reached a stable plateau level by the time central k-space data were being acquired and so there was no artifact. Also note a severe right renal artery stenosis (*small arrow*). On another example (**b**) of ringing artifact in a normal abdominal aorta (*arrow*), the contrast bolus timing is optimal for pulmonary arteries but the bolus is just beginning to arrive in the abdominal aorta when central k-space data are acquired.

Submitted by Jeffrey H. Maki, M.D., Ph.D. Seattle, and Martin R. Prince, M.D., Ph.D., New York.

of the scan), higher signal-to-noise and contrast-to-noise ratio data will lead to improved image quality. However, as the bolus becomes shorter, timing the bolus to perfectly coincide with central k-space data acquisition becomes more critical.

This leads to the issue of how to time the intravenous bolus relative to beginning the scan. The contrast travel time, i.e., the time required for the contrast bolus to travel from the injection site (typically in the antecubital vein) to the vascular territory under investigation is highly variable. It may be only 10 seconds in a young athlete with a proximal IV or as long as 50 seconds in an older patient with congestive heart failure and an IV in the hand.

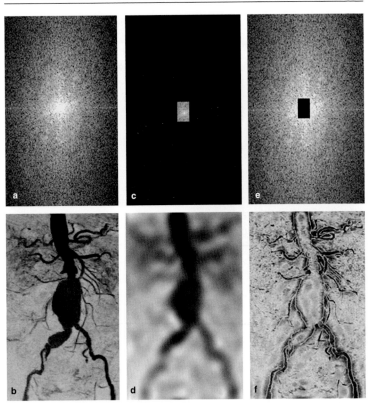

Fig. 1.6. Spatial Frequency Features of k-space. Images of an abdominal aortic aneurysm demonstrate the correspondence between k-space data used in reconstruction and image resolution. (**a**) The spatial frequency or "k-space" representation of the aorta is Fourier transformed to form an image (**b**). If only the central k-space is used in image formation (**c**), the resulting image (**d**) is a low resolution version of the original. The Fourier transformation of the high spatial frequencies (**e**), provides image detail (**f**) such as delineation of edges. Submitted by Oliver Wieben, Ph.D. and Frank Korosec, Ph.D., Madison.

For slow scans lasting more than 1–2 minutes, timing is easy because errors of 10-15 seconds are small compared to the total scan duration. Since central k-space data for most pulse sequences are collected during the middle of the scan (sequential mapping of k-space), it is important to time the bolus to assure a contrast presence in the vascular territory under investigation during the middle of the scan. Thus, for slower scans, it is appropriate to begin injecting a few seconds after starting the scan and finish the injection just after the middle of the acquisition. Once the gadolinium injection is complete, a second syringe with saline is used to flush the remaining contrast out of the iv tubing and arm vein into the central circulation. The contrast travel time will naturally result in the arterial phase of the bolus lining up approximately with the middle of the acquisition.

It is also important to assure a consistent paramagnetic contrast concentration during acquisition of central k-space data. Large changes in arterial T1 relaxation during collection of central k-space create severe ringing (Maki) artifacts (Figure 1.5). For this reason, the contrast bolus should cover at least half the scan time. This way the leading and trailing edges of the bolus occur during the periphery of k-space.

For faster scans lasting less than 40 seconds, timing of the contrast bolus is considerably more important and challenging. Bolus timing errors of 10-15 seconds can ruin the scan. Thus, it is essential to determine the appropriate scan delay between beginning the injection and beginning the scan. Again, assuming that k-space is mapped sequentially (as is the default for most scans), this can be accomplished using Equation 4.

$$\text{Scan Delay} = \text{Contrast Travel Time} + \frac{\text{Injection Time}}{2} - \frac{\text{Scan Time}}{2} \quad (4)$$

Note that if injection time equals scan time, scan delay is equal to contrast travel time. If infusion time is shorter than imaging time, scan delay will be less than contrast travel time. If k-space is mapped centrically or elliptically (i.e., central k-space data are acquired at the beginning of the scan), scan delay should equal contrast travel time plus an extra 5 or 6 seconds so that data collection does not begin on the leading edge of the bolus. The crucial aspect lies in accurate determination of contrast travel time from the peripheral vein where it is injected to the vascular territory under consideration. For this purpose, several different strategies can be employed.

The easiest, but least successful of these strategies, is known somewhat whimsically as the "best guess" technique. The contrast travel time is estimated based upon the patient's age and history, including cardiac status and the artery to be imaged. For Pulmonary arteries a typical contrast travel time is 5–10 seconds. It is longer for the Abdominal Aorta.

A proposed formula for estimating contrast travel time to the common femoral artery is $10.6 + 0.143 \times$ age $+ 4.8$ (if aneurysm present) $+ 3.8$ (if male) and 2.8 (if there is a history of myocardial infarction).

Failure rate of this "best guess" technique is related to the distance the contrast bolus needs to travel and scan duration. While it often works for imaging pulmonary arteries, it frequently results in sub-optimal image quality when imaging the systemic arterial system. It is much more likely to work for 40–50 second scans than for 20–30 second scans. We, therefore, strongly recommend using one of the following approaches for fast arterial scans.

Test Bolus Technique

A bolus-timing acquisition can be performed prior to acquisition of 3D MR angiography data set using a small gadolinium contrast dose of 1–2 ml. This test bolus is flushed with a sufficient volume of saline to advance the contrast into the superior vena cava. Fast GRE (turboflash) images are acquired at fixed time intervals (every 1–2 seconds) through the vessels of interest for approximately 40 seconds. To avoid inflow signal changes throughout different phases of the cardiac cycle, a thick section (15–20 mm) should be acquired through the aorta in a sagittal or sagittal oblique plane.

Alternatively, rapid sequential imaging can be performed in the axial plane if a non-selective preparatory inversion pulse is used to null blood signal (TI=100 ms). With this preparatory pulse, the test bolus dose can be reduced. The disadvantage of this approach lies in the extra time required for the preparatory pulse, which reduces the rate of image updating. It thereby slightly compromises temporal resolution of the contrast travel time determination. However, adequate temporal resolution is usually obtained even while using preparatory pulses since measurement of contrast arrival needs only to be within 2 to 4 seconds of the actual arrival time.

Contrast travel time can be determined by visual inspection (Figure 1.7) or may be based on sequential signal intensity measurements in a region-of-interest placed within the aorta at the appropriate level. Be sure to identify time to peak arterial contrast, not arrival time. Most often, visual inspection is satisfactory, however, signal intensity measurements can be useful when variations in signal due to pulsatility within the aorta obscure contrast enhancement. In this manner, image acquisition can be timed such

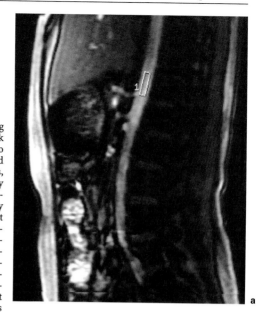

a

Fig. 1.7. Test Dose Timing Scan Data. A 20 mm thick sagittal 2D gradient echo acquisition (**a**) was obtained repeatedly at 2 s intervals, beginning simultaneously with injection of a 2 ml Gd-DTPA test bolus followed by a saline flush. The contrast travel time to the mid-abdominal aorta is determined by placing a region-of-interest (ROI) (box number 1) over the mid-abdominal aorta on each successive image in order to plot the change in aorta signal as a function of time after initiating the test bolus. Graph of aorta signal intensity as a function of time following the test bolus (**b**). The contrast travel time can usually be determined by visually inspecting the images for the onset of signal enhancement. The graph also shows the moment of arrival of the contrast in the aorta. The scan delay in this patient was 14 seconds.

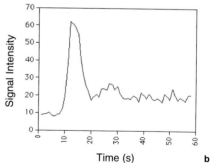

b

that the presence of the contrast bolus peak coincides exactly with the sampling of central k-space lines.

An alternative method of performing a test bolus that is particularly useful for extremities, and aortic arch, is known as 2D projection MR Angiography. With this technique a slightly larger dose of 5 ml can provide a DSA-like series of time-resolved images from which bolus timing information can be obtained (see Chapter 2 and Figure 2.5).

Automatic Triggering

Another approach to bolus timing uses a pulse sequence that can automatically detect contrast arrival in the aorta (Figure 1.8). This pulse sequence automatically synchronizes 3D MR angiography data acquisition with the arterial phase of the contrast bolus. The operator selects a region of aorta to be sampled at 20 ms intervals. As contrast arrives in the aorta, the signal within the sampling region increases several-fold. A trigger threshold of typically 20% signal increase will detect the leading edge of the contrast bolus. This gives the patient time to take in a deep breath and suspend respiration before the actual scan commences 6–8 seconds later. By beginning the scan with the center of k-space, i.e., centric or elliptical centric encoding, there is synchronization between the arterial phase of the bolus and elliptical centric acquisition of central k-space data. Commercial versions of this pulse sequence are unfortunately only available for a limited number of magnets. For a 1.5 Tesla Horizon magnet, it is know as "SmartPrep" (GE Medical Systems), or Care Bolus (Siemens Medical Systems). A recent refinement is to recess the absolute center of k-space a few seconds in from the beginning to avoid leading edge ringing artifact.

Fluoroscopic Triggering

Another triggering approach is to use MR fluoroscopy in order to rapidly obtain and reconstruct 2D gradient echo images of the aorta while injecting a paramagnetic contrast agent (Figure 1.9). When the agent is seen arriving in the aorta, the operator initiates switching from 2D gradient echo imaging to 3D spoiled gradient echo gadolinium MR angiography imaging sequence beginning with acquisition of central k-space data. This provides a potentially more reliable way of ensuring acquisition of central k-space data during the moment of peak arterial phase gadolinium concentration. 2D gradient echo imaging using MR fluoroscopy can include complex subtraction of an early pre-contrast, mask image in order to more clearly show early arrival of the contrast bolus.

If triggering is too early, there may be ringing artifacts from acquiring the absolute center of k-space on the leading edge of the bolus (Figure 1-5b). This can be eliminated by recessing the absolute center of k-space a few seconds into the scan.

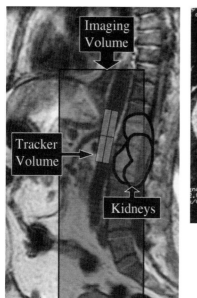

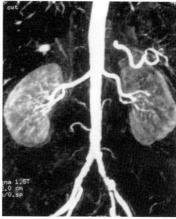

a

c

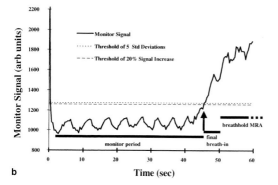

b

Fig. 1.8. Example of Bolus Timing by Automatic Contrast Detection. For abdominal MRA, (**a**) a single "tracker" voxel is prescribed in the mid-abdominal aorta. Typically, the tracker voxel is $4 \times 4 \times 10$ cm. The contrast-detection algorithm automatically initiates the transition from monitor-mode to image acquisition-mode when the signal from the tracker volume exceeds specified thresholds. In this example (**b**), the arrow depicts the transition point at five standard deviations and 20 percent signal increase. At this point, the patient is instructed to suspend breathing in inspiration and the 3D imaging volume data is acquired (**c**).

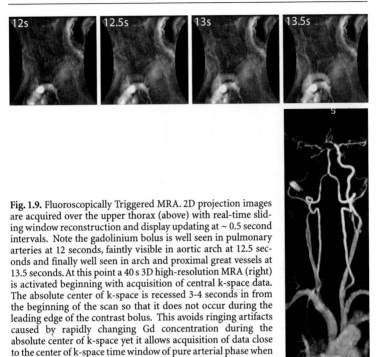

Fig. 1.9. Fluoroscopically Triggered MRA. 2D projection images are acquired over the upper thorax (above) with real-time sliding window reconstruction and display updating at ~ 0.5 second intervals. Note the gadolinium bolus is well seen in pulmonary arteries at 12 seconds, faintly visible in aortic arch at 12.5 seconds and finally well seen in arch and proximal great vessels at 13.5 seconds. At this point a 40 s 3D high-resolution MRA (right) is activated beginning with acquisition of central k-space data. The absolute center of k-space is recessed 3-4 seconds in from the beginning of the scan so that it does not occur during the leading edge of the contrast bolus. This avoids ringing artifacts caused by rapidly changing Gd concentration during the absolute center of k-space yet it allows acquisition of data close to the center of k-space time window of pure arterial phase when venous enhancement has not yet occurred.

Submitted by Richard Watts, Ph.D., New York.

Multiphase: Time-Resolved 3D MRA

An approach that is virtually independent of the exact contrast travel time is to collect multiple sets of 3D image data so rapidly that at least one 3D data acquisition lines up with the arterial phase of the gadolinium bolus (Figure 1.10). This requires an acquisition time for the entire 3D volume on the order of 10 seconds or less. In addition to simplifying contrast bolus timing, this multiphase technique also provides temporal information about relative rates of enhancement of various structures within the field-of-view. This can help assess the hemodynamic significance of any visualized stenoses. It can also be used to help characterize other pathology, such as parenchymal lesions in the liver or other organs. An image data set acquired prior to contrast administration can

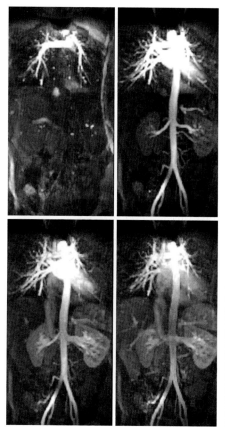

Fig. 1.10. 3D TRICKS: Normal Aorta and Pulmonary Arteries. A series of MIP displays through a time-resolved 3D Contrast MRA exam is shown. Sequential 3D data sets were acquired at 5 second intervals following rapid injection of a 34 ml bolus of Gd-DTPA. The first phase demonstrates pulmonary arterial enhancement, followed by aortic then venous signal enhancement. A pre-contrast image was used as a mask to subtract the non-enhanced images from the contrast-enhanced images, thereby reducing background signal. The 3D MR DSA method eliminates the need for timing the contrast bolus. Submitted by Thomas M. Grist, M.D., Madison.

be subtracted from a data set acquired during the arterial phase to improve image contrast-to-noise ratio. Subtraction of arterial phase images from equilibrium phase images will highlight the veins. For very fast scans, running a continuous subtraction will show regions of increasing and decreasing contrast concentration.

The frame rate of 3D MR DSA determines the fidelity of image subtraction and the ability to isolate selective arterial, parenchymal, and venous phases of contrast enhancement. For optimal results, it is essential to maximize the frame rate. With the fastest scanners that have the most state of the art gradient performance, the minimum data acquisition time for a full 3D data set is approximately 2–3 seconds. This frame rate (1 data set every 2–3 seconds) is adequate temporal resolution to isolate arterial and venous phases in virtually all vascular territories including chest, abdomen, peripheral circulation and even carotid arteries and cerebral vascular circulation.

Most older scanners require at least 15–20 seconds for a full 3D data set acquisition. This is inadequate temporal resolution for multiphase imaging. It would require too long a breath-hold for obtaining both a mask and contrast-enhanced image data within a single breath-hold. To enhance the frame rate, clever post-processing schemes have been proposed which can provide very high frame rates, even with standard gradient performance. For more details, see Chapter 2 on Advanced Techniques.

What Is The Optimum Contrast Dose?

From an image quality point of view, generally the more contrast the better. However, it is also important to consider safety, practicability, and cost. While doses of up to 0.5 mmol/kg have been used at some centers, smaller doses have been shown to provide adequate image quality. In a breath-held 3D MR angiography study of renal arteries in 10 volunteers, four doses of Gd-DTPA were compared: 0.05, 0.1, 0.2, and 0.3 mmol/kg. While measurement of signal-to-noise ratio in the proximal and distal renal arteries revealed a direct relationship to contrast dose, analysis of qualitative visibility data revealed continuous improvement up to a dose of only 0.2 mmol/kg. The benefit from further increasing the dose to 0.3 mmol/kg was not statistically significant.

It is important to note, however, that patients with cardiovascular disease may require higher doses of contrast than normal volunteers to optimally visualize vascular pathology. This is because higher signal-to-noise ratio is required to resolve fine details of severe stenoses and atherosclerotic irregularities. For patients with large aortic aneurysms or dissections, it takes more Gd contrast to fill the aneurysm or false lumen. It is also more difficult to optimally time the contrast injection in sick patients and higher doses help to compensate for errors in bolus timing. Higher doses may also be required for the portal vein because of the dilution and extraction of contrast that occurs en route to the portal circulation. The dose must also be increased when performing the stepping table method that rapidly images several successive stations marching down the patient's legs during a single long contrast bolus.

Contrast dose can be selected by following the pattern used in conventional angiography where all patients receive the same volume of contrast for a given run. There may be some dose adjustment for extremely large or small patients. Following this strategy, every patient receives 30 ml of gadolinium (the contents of two bottles, each containing 15 or 20 ml). Extremely large patients weighing more than 100 kg receive 40-60 ml and small patients weighing less than 50 kg receive 20 ml. Using 30 ml for most patients allows the operator to get used to a standard volume of contrast and injection rate for every case. As the operator becomes more skillful at properly timing the injection and selecting optimal imaging parameters, it becomes possible to obtain the same image quality with smaller doses of gadolinium.

While most investigators propose doses ranging from 0.1 to 0.3 mmol/kg, it is important to note that these guidelines may be modified to meet special circumstances. If higher resolution is needed, higher doses may be required. Shorter acquisition strategies and more sophisticated pulse sequences may use substantially lower contrast dosages. For example, using mask subtraction or with a time-resolved MR DSA acquisition method where 3D MR angiography images are acquired every 5–10 seconds, early experience suggests that the doses of contrast can be reduced to 0.05–0.1 mmol/kg. Furthermore, the optimal contrast dose is dependent upon the vascular territory being imaged. Aspects of how to optimize dosage for each vascular territory are discussed in Chapters 3–11.

How Much Contrast Media Is Safe?

Extracellular gadolinium chelates currently available with FDA approval all have excellent safety profiles. Although most agents have been tested in human subjects at doses considerably exceeding regulatory guidelines without a significant incidence of adverse events, the user should strive to limit the administered dose to lie within regulatory limits. Since different agents have different regulatory approvals in different countries, manufacturers should be asked about relevant circumstances.

Gadolinium chelates are among the safest contrast agents. Serious idiosyncratic reactions are rare; one study reports a rate of serious reactions of 1:20,000. Only one death has been reported in the literature that has been directly attributed to gadolinium contrast. Gadolinium compounds have no clinically detectable nephrotoxicity. They can be used safely at the maximum dose in patients with renal failure. For these reasons, 3D contrast-enhanced MR angiography is particularly useful in patients with renal insufficiency or a history of allergic reaction to iodinated contrast. Note that because extracellular gadolinium chelates are predominantly excreted via a renal route, patients who are anuric or with profound renal insufficiency (serum creatinine greater than 6 ml/dl) may benefit from dialysis following 3D contrast MR angiography in order to speed gadolinium elimination from the circulation. There is also anecdotal evidence that idiosyncratic reactions to gadolinium contrast agents may be more common in patients with a history of allergic reaction to iodinated contrast. Also note that Gd-DTPA is ionic, hyper-osmolar and irritating to tissues. Venous thrombosis at the injection site has been reported. The potential for venous thrombosis may be minimized by ensuring that gadolinium is flushed from the vein using a 20-30 ml saline flush with every large dose injection. Gd-DTPA has been reported to have cardiac depressant effect when administered as a fast bolus via central line due to DTPA affinity for calcium.

Finally it is important to recognize that linear gadolinium chelates, gadodiamide and gadoversetamide may interfere with serum calcium measurements. Although calcium levels in the patient are unaffected, the standard colorimetric laboratory test for serum calcium yields spuriously low results directly proportional to the concentration of gadodiamide in the serum sample.

How Many Times Can 3D Contrast MR Angiography Be Repeated?

As 3D contrast MR angiography methods become faster, it is possible to reduce the contrast dose necessary for a satisfactory examination. Therefore, it becomes possible to perform examinations at multiple stations or to repeat the exam at a single station and still stay within regulatory guidelines for the maximum allowed dose. For example, if a dose of 0.1 mmol/kg is administered at each station, three separate injections with 3D MR angiography data acquisitions at three separate locations can be performed without exceeding current regulatory guidelines for a total dose of 0.3 mmol/kg. However, when multiple stations are examined, it becomes necessary to remove bright signal from contrast accumulation in the background tissues and veins. This can be accomplished by subtraction of images acquired immediately prior to the arrival of contrast agent from images that are acquired during contrast injection. When using digital subtraction, it is helpful to escalate the dose with each successive injection.

This helps to offset effects of residual gadolinium contrast in the arteries, which can lower arterial signal following subtraction. For example, with a three station MR DSA exam, doses of 0.75, 0.1, and 0.125 mmol/kg are recommended. Some centers have reported repeating 3D contrast MR angiography multiple times using 0.2–0.3 mmol/kg for each acquisition.

What Is The Optimum Injection Rate?

Peripheral intravenous contrast injection should be modulated to assure a homogeneous contrast presence in the arterial system under investigation during central k-space data collection. Due to contrast dilution at the leading and trailing edges of the bolus as well as variable transit times through different portions of the pulmonary circulation, the contrast bolus tends to lengthen as it travels from the cubital vein through the heart and lungs to the arteries being imaged. This bolus dispersion increases with the distance the bolus must travel. In one volunteer study, a 10 second bolus of 25 ml Gd-DTPA lengthened to an average bolus length of 17 seconds in the aorta at the level of the renal arteries. This contrast dispersion is less relevant for slower 3D MR angiography acquisitions that may last two or more minutes, but it has an important effect on ultrafast breath-hold and especially time-resolved acquisition strategies. While contrast dispersion depends on individual cardiovascular parameters, which are difficult to predict, it is safe to assume that a minimum of 5–7 seconds of bolus prolongation will occur in most individuals. Longer dispersion times can be expected for peripheral vasculature and less dispersion can be expected for pulmonary arteries. For fast breath-held acquisitions of the systemic arterial system, the total dose of contrast should be administered at a rate that results in an injection time that is at least 5–7 seconds shorter than the data acquisition time. For most individuals, this translates into a contrast injection rate ranging between 2 and 3 ml/s. A saline flush should be injected at the same rate immediately following the contrast injection.

Do You Need A Power Injector?

Use of a power injector (Figure 1.11) is helpful as it allows precise infusion of paramagnetic contrast using predefined weight-adjusted rates and volumes. Saline flush is available not only to keep the venous access open (KVO-mode), but also to advance the contrast column through the

Fig. 1.11. MR Compatible Power Injector (Spectris, Medrad, www.medrad.com). The power injector has two syringes, one for delivering the contrast and a second for injecting a saline flush. Typically, the dead space in the intravenous line is 5 cc, therefore the saline flush is useful to clear the line following contrast injection. The injector has the capability to accurately deliver contrast at precisely defined rates and can be programmed to provide many different contrast injection schedules depending upon the application and the total dose used. Use of the injector allows for the test bolus and the contrast injection to be performed by an operator who does not enter the magnet room. In addition, the MR-compatible injector allows a single scanner operator to perform the injection and image acquisition sequence.

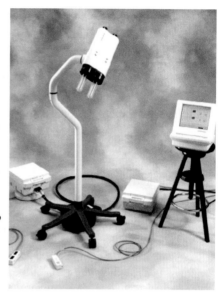

veins of the arm into the superior vena cava without any delay following the contrast bolus. These features are useful for fast breath-hold data acquisition strategies.

How Do I Optimize A Hand Injection?

Most centers do not have a power injector; thus, contrast must be injected by hand. In addition, hand injection is required for pediatric patients, patients with central lines and PICC lines, and for tenuous IVs in the hand or wrist. For hand injections, a standardized, hand-infusion tubing set should be used. An example is shown in Figure 1.12. This example (SmartSet, Topspins, Inc.) was designed to allow simultaneous attachment of two syringes with check valves that allow the operator to inject the contrast agent and then immediately follow with a saline flush. The switch from gadolinium to saline flush occurs automatically and instantaneously. This is particularly important for fast breath-hold scans, where it is essential to inject and flush rapidly with no gap in the bolus. Ideally, the tubing set will be attached to the same size intravenous catheter in every patient so the operator will always feel the same resist-

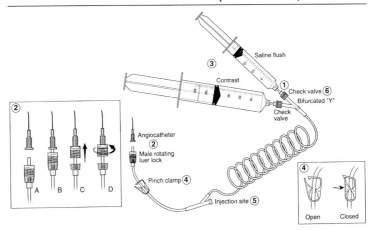

Fig. 1.12. Hand Tubing Set for Intravenous Infusions (SmartSet, Topspins, www.topspins.com). A 2 meter length of coiled tubing has two injection sites with check valves (6) to permit simultaneous attachment of a 60 ml contrast syringe and a 20 or 30 ml saline flush syringe (3). The automatic check-flow valve system allows immediate switching from the contrast infusion to saline flush. This avoids having a gap in the middle of the bolus, which can degrade image quality. A spin-lock (2) simplifies attachment to angiocatheters and pinch clamp (4) prevents fluid dripping when IV is removed. A sideport (5) close to angiocatheter allows IV testing/flushing or administration of medications close to IV site in the event of a contrast reaction. The tubing has a thick-wall and high durometer to prevent occlusion if the tubing is inadvertently pinched or kinked when advancing the patient into the magnet.

ance to flow. Either 20 or 22 gauge angiocatheters are acceptable. If 22 gauge is used, however, it may be necessary to warm the gadolinium to body temperature in order to lower its viscosity in preparation for injecting. Otherwise, the resistance to flow may be too great for a hand injection at the high rate required for fast breath-hold scans.

Injecting by hand has some important advantages. It is easier to detect problems with the IV site by sensing the resistance to injection. This makes it easier to detect extravasation before the entire dose of gadolinium has been administered. It may also be easier to ensure perfect breath-holding when the operator is standing next to the patient during the scan. Hand injection may allow a faster injection than is possible with a power injector, because the operator knows how fast is safe. This is especially important when using tenuous IVs in the hand or wrist.

To set up for hand injection, the tubing is initially primed with saline and attached to the angiocatheter. This is done prior to putting the patient into the magnet so there will be no delay between the pre-contrast and dynamic contrast-enhanced images. Immediately prior to initiating the scan, the tubing is primed with gadolinium such that once the injection begins, there is no delay to fill the tubing. Once the contrast injection and saline flush are completed, a clamp on the tubing is engaged so that it can be removed without dripping fluid.

Regardless of the injection method used, IV access should be maintained for at least 5–10 minutes after performing the injection since most allergic reactions occur during this time.

What Happens If Gadolinium Extravasates?

Extravasation of extracellular gadolinium contrast agents has been studied in animal experiments. Extravasation is well tolerated without causing significant inflammatory reactions. This has also been our experience in patients as well. The osmolality of available gadolinium chelates is lower than that of most iodinated contrast agents. In addition, the volume administered is significantly lower than when iodinated contrast is used for CT angiography. Under any circumstance, it is less than 60 ml, which is considered safe to extravasate, even with iodinated contrast agents. Thus, the risk of incurring harm due to extravasation of even large portions of the contrast bolus appears negligible. Still, the proper functioning of the venous access should be ascertained prior to contrast bolus administration by injecting a small amount of saline or by aspirating blood. With tenuous or fragile IV lines, hand injection will be safer and is preferred.

Why Use Gradient Echo Imaging With Spoiling?

Gradient echo pulse sequences are used for 3D contrast-enhanced MR angiography because of their high speed, short echo times and T1 weighting. Gradient echo imaging can be performed in a steady state mode or with spoiling of the residual magnetization after each echo before giving the next pulse. Spoiling is useful because it accentuates T1 contrast and thus magnifies the effect of T1 relaxation contrast agents such as gadolinium chelates. By suppressing signal from background tissues, spoiling enhances image contrast without incurring any time penalty. Note that some suppression of blood signal occurs as well, although not as much as background tissue, because motion of blood spoils some of its residual signal. Additional background tissue suppression can also be achieved with subtraction of a pre-contrast mask acquisition (Figure 1.13), fat saturation pulses or inversion pulses but at the expense of an increase in scan time. A way to achieve some fat suppression without requiring extra time for extra pulses is to adjust the bandwidth and echo fraction to obtain an echo time where fat and water are out-of-phase. At 1.5 Tesla, an echo time of 2–2.5 ms is appropriate to maximize this chemical shift effect. Out-of-phase echo times should be used with caution, though, because of the potential for introducing India ink artifacts at fat tissue borders.

Scanners with extremely high gradient performance and TRs less than 3-4 ms may obtain real arterial SNR increases from steady state gradient echo sequences. These techniques, known as trueFISP, FIESTA or balanced FFE are particularly useful for imaging the slower flow of veins

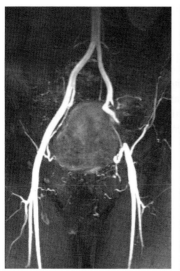 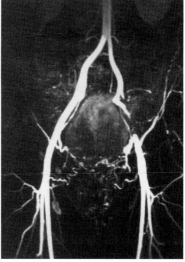

a   b

Fig. 1.13. Benefit of Image Subtraction. Image subtraction may be used to reduce background signal, and thereby improve vessel-to-background contrast-to-noise ratio: MIP through the unsubtracted source images (**a**) and MIP through the images obtained after subtracting the pre-contrast source images from the contrast-enhanced source images (**b**). Note the improved demonstration of small vessel detail in the MIP through the subtracted images.

and also for perfusion imaging where simultaneous visualization of vessels and background tissue is desirable.

What Is The Best Echo Time (TE)?

Echo time should be short enough to eliminate dephasing artifacts and to minimize T2* signal decay. This requires an echo time less than about 3 ms. Further reductions in echo time can shorten the TR and further reduce flow and susceptibility artifacts. This can be particularly helpful in the lung, where suppression of susceptibility artifacts at air-tissue interfaces with a very short TE can permit imaging of pulmonary perfusion. It is also helpful to have the shortest possible TE when imaging patients who have surgical clips to minimize metallic susceptibility artifacts. Imaging highly concentrated gadolinium during direct MR venography (see Chapter 11) also benefits from using the shortest possible echo times (preferably < 1 ms). Keep in mind, however, that shortening echo time by widening the bandwidth substantially reduces the image signal-to-noise ratio.

What Is The Best Repetition Time (TR)?

Shorter TR translates directly into shorter data acquisition times. This allows for either a shorter overall scanning time, multi-phase imaging, or higher resolution. The decrease in the signal-to-noise ratio associated with a reduction in TR can be compensated by concentrating the contrast bolus with a faster injection rate. Thus, the TR should be made as short as possible without excessively widening the bandwidth. Most manufacturers have developed special 3D gradient echo pulse sequences using fast radio frequency (rf) pulses for 3D contrast MRA. These allow repetition times that are substantially shorter than what is achieved with standard 3D gradient echo pulse sequences. These optimized pulse sequences with the shortest possible repetition times often make it possible to complete high-resolution, 512 matrix data acquisition within a breath-hold, but they may not be as useful for applications outside of MR angiography because the short rf pulses result in more aliasing (wrap-around artifact) in the slice direction.

What Is The Best Flip Angle?

Gradient echo imaging requires selection of the flip angle (sometimes known as tip angle). Theoretical and phantom experiments (Figure 1.14) suggest that the technique is not very flip angle dependent. Any flip angle in the range of 20°–60° is acceptable. We routinely use a 45° flip angle for arterial phase imaging when the injection rate is 2 ml/s and the TR > 6 ms. It may be useful to reduce the flip angle to 30° for venous and equilibrium phases to compensate for reduced T1 relaxation when the contrast dilutes into the entire blood pool. However, there will be some loss of image contrast at this lower flip angle. For lower contrast doses, slower injection rates, or imaging with very short TR (TR < 5 ms), a lower flip angle is optimal. At a TR of 2–3 ms, a flip angle of 20°-30° is better. In any case, it is necessary to reduce the flip angle at very short TR (<5 ms) due to SAR limitations. For higher doses and imaging with a longer TR, a higher flip angle is more appropriate.

In patients who have metallic stents, a higher flip angle is useful to improve visualization of blood inside the stent. A small increase in flip angle is acceptable for large diameter nitinol or titanium aortic stents. A larger increase in flip angle is necessary for smaller stents with a tighter mesh. Reports of 3D Gd:MRA with flip angles as high as 150° have shown promise in renal and iliac artery stents for eliminating the Faraday Cage effect which attenuates delivery of rf energy inside metal stents. In our own experience, 75° is acceptable for platinum renal artery stents.

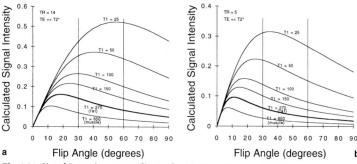

Fig. 1.14. Signal Intensity versus Flip Angle. (**a**) TR = 14 ms and (**b**) TR = 5 ms, assuming that T2<<T2*. For a wide range of blood T1, a flip in the range of 30° to 60° provides substantial contrast between fat (T1 = 270 ms) and fluids with T1 < 150 ms. A flip angle at the higher end of this range is optimum for fast injection rates (lower T1) and longer TR, while a lower flip is better for slower injection rates (higher T1) and shorter TR.

What Receiver Bandwidth Should Be Used?

Adjusting receiver bandwidth is one of the principle mechanisms for manipulating TR, TE, and signal-to-noise ratio. A wider bandwidth allows shorter TE and shorter TR for faster scanning but at the expense of signal-to-noise ratio. On the other hand, increased signal-to-noise ratio is achieved by using narrower bandwidth but at the expense of a longer TE and TR, and thus a slower scan. Using a narrow bandwidth also increases the severity of chemical shift artifact, although this is generally not a problem with 3D contrast-enhanced MR angiography because background tissues are so dark. To avoid sacrificing signal-to-noise ratio, the bandwidth should be as narrow as possible without causing echo time to exceed 2.5 ms, or at most 3 ms. Unfortunately, this still often requires a fairly wide bandwidth of approximately 32 kHz.

How Can Acquisition Time Be Shortened?

The time to acquire a 3D volume of image data can be reduced by decreasing the TR. Depending upon the MR scanner, this may require purchasing high performance gradients and optimized pulse sequences with shorter rf pulses. Beyond reduction in TR, there are several additional options for reducing the acquisition time. One is to use a wider bandwidth, although this causes a reduction in signal-to-noise ratio. Another is to reduce scan resolution or coverage. Finally, there are several k-space tricks that shorten acquisition time by reducing the number of phase encoding steps without sacrificing resolution.

One of the simplest ways to shorten scan time is to reduce the matrix size along phase encode or slice select spatial directions. For example, the number of slices that are acquired may be reduced at the expense of spatial coverage or resolution in the slice direction. Likewise, the number of phase encode steps can be reduced at the expense of resolution in the phase encoding direction. Reducing resolution in the frequency encoding direction has only a small effect on scan time reflecting only minor reductions in TR due to gradient and receiver sample time effects.

The sacrifice in acquired spatial resolution may be avoided by implementation of a rectangular or asymmetric field-of-view. Be careful not to make the field-of-view too narrow in the left-right (L-R) direction when scanning in the coronal plane as this can cause wraparound artifact. A small amount of wraparound artifact may be acceptable since the vasculature of interest is generally close to the mid-line while wraparound corrupts the periphery of the image. It may also be possible to minimize wraparound effects by using a phased array coil, which has the strongest signal centrally and for which the signal fades out more peripherally. Thus, using a narrow coil, any wraparound tends to be faint (Figure 1.15).

Partial Fourier techniques (also called fractional or partial NEX) represent another approach to reducing acquisition time without sacrificing resolution or affecting TR. These techniques enable a 3D volume of image data to be reconstructed without having a complete set of Fourier image data. For example, reducing the NEX to 0.5 reduces the acquisition time by almost one-half. On most MR systems it may be necessary to select a "full echo" or nearly full echo in order to implement the fractional NEX option. This prolongs the echo time slightly and may give rise to more flow related artifacts. However, with high performance gradients, acceptable echo times of less than 3 ms are generally possible if the band width is not too narrow. Although partial NEX is recommended as

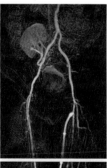
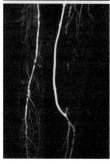

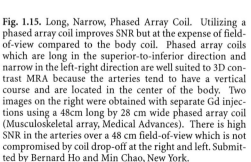

Fig. 1.15. Long, Narrow, Phased Array Coil. Utilizing a phased array coil improves SNR but at the expense of field-of-view compared to the body coil. Phased array coils which are long in the superior-to-inferior direction and narrow in the left-right direction are well suited to 3D contrast MRA because the arteries tend to have a vertical course and are located in the center of the body. Two images on the right were obtained with separate Gd injections using a 48cm long by 28 cm wide phased array coil (Musculoskeletal array, Medical Advances). There is high SNR in the arteries over a 48 cm field-of-view which is not compromised by coil drop-off at the right and left. Submitted by Bernard Ho and Min Chao, New York.

a way of efficiently reducing scan time, it may also create k-space ringing artifacts if the pulse sequence is not optimized. When it lengthens the TE to where fat and water are out-of-phase, ~2.1 ms at 1.5 Tesla, it may introduce India ink artifact at fat-tissue boundaries.

What Is Zero-Filling,
And How Does This Effect Reconstructed Spatial Resolution?

The apparent, or reconstructed, spatial resolution can be improved by interpolation schemes. One of the best interpolation methods commonly used for MR angiography is a method known as zero-filling. Interpolation by zero-filling is performed by expanding k-space with zeros at its periphery prior to performing the Fourier transform to reconstruct the image. If the original matrix size is 128, zero-filling can be used to reconstruct additional intermediate pixels so that the image is reconstructed with 256 pixels. This approach is particularly useful for increasing the number of apparent slices in the 3D contrast MR angiography data set. Two-fold, zero filling in the slice select direction doubles the number of reconstructed sections by creating overlapping sections. It is important to realize, however, that zero filling does not affect coverage or section thickness. Rather, by overlapping, it increases the number of reconstructed sections, which improves the quality of reformations and MIPs, particularly in oblique planes. In addition, zero filling reduces partial volume averaging errors.

Is Image Subtraction Helpful? How Is It Done?

Digital image subtraction is used to eliminate background signal in 3D contrast MRA. Enhanced contrast-to-noise translates into better visualization of small vessels and a reduction in the required contrast dose. Subtraction also helps to eliminate wraparound artifacts, although artifact from enhancement of vessels occuring outside of the field-of-view will not be removed by subtraction. Another important benefit of subtraction, which can be used in time-resolved examinations, relates to the ability to selectively image vessels on the "up slope" or "down slope" of contrast enhancement. This can be helpful in separating arteries from veins.

Subtraction is typically performed on an independent computer workstation. It is important to use source images, or better yet, Fourier image data, for the subtraction process. Subtraction of MIP images is not useful. If subtraction of successive breath-held scans is performed, it is important to coach the patient before the study so that the degree of inspiration for each 3D data acquisition is similar. Breath-holding in expiration has been recommended to maximize reproducibility of diaphragm position between mask and arterial phase images. As in all subtractions, motion between mask and enhanced images can lead to artifacts. Therefore, it is desirable to obtain the mask immediately before injecting the contrast. This is best accomplished with techniques that acquire sequential data sets, like the time-resolved method. However, the misregistration artifacts associated with motion are generally less severe on Gd:MRA compared to x-ray DSA because subtraction for DSA is performed on a pixel-by-pixel basis rather than over a thick volume of data for MRA.

How Should 3D MRA Data Sets Be Interpreted?

3D MR angiography image data are best interpreted on an independent computer workstation with 3D reconstruction capabilities. Image analysis should always include careful scrutiny of individual source images as well as thin multiplanar reformations of the underlying 3D data set in multiple planes oriented for each vessel of interest. In this way, venous overlap can be eliminated and the course of tortuous vessels can be unfolded. Indeed, this represents a significant advantage of 3D MR angiography over conventional angiography. Maximum intensity projection images can also be performed in order to see vessels over longer distances on a single image. Other rendering techniques, such as exoscopic surface rendering or endoscopic "virtual" surface rendering, minimum intensity and average intensity projections, and curved planar reformations, may also be useful at times. Valuable diagnostic information may be lost if the interpretation does not take advantage of these capabilities.

Maximum Intensity Projection

Maximum intensity projection images are produced with a ray tracing algorithm. The maximum intensity encountered along any predefined direction of parallel rays is assigned to the displayed pixel. In this way, 3-dimensional data can be collapsed into a 2-dimensional image. MIP reconstructions emphasize Gd-enhancing vessels and thereby resemble conventional contrast angiographic images. For this reason, they tend to be well received by referring physicians and are particularly useful for surgical planning.

The procedure for performing subvolume maximum intensity projections is illustrated in Figure 1.16. After collecting a large coronal 3D volume of image data encompassing the abdominal aorta and its branches, an MIP can be performed to show the celiac, superior mesenteric artery, and inferior mesenteric artery to best advantage. This is

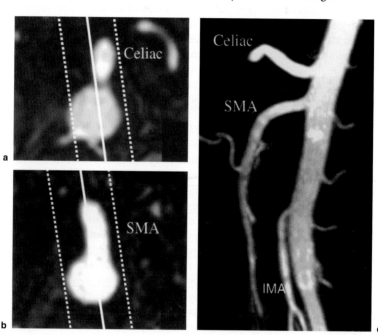

Fig. 1.16. Subvolume Maximum Intensity Projection (MIP). Subvolume MIPs are generally performed on a separate computer workstation. After loading the 3D volume of data into the computer workstation, the individual vessels can be examined using reformations to scroll through the 3D data set. In evaluating the abdominal aorta, an axial reformation shows that the celiac axis (**a**) arising from the aorta and a more inferior axial reformation shows the superior mesenteric artery (SMA) arising from the aorta (**b**). Using these reformations (a and b) as a guide, selective volume angled with the SMA and thick enough to encompass the celiac SMA and abdominal aorta in order to obtain a sagittal oblique subvolume MIP (**c**) encompassing the entire abdominal aorta. Submitted by Qian Dong, M.D., Ann Arbor.

done by first scrolling through the data with axial reformations in order to identify the celiac, the superior mesenteric artery, and the inferior mesenteric artery. These reformations will show the angle at which these vessels arise from the aorta. A subvolume that is oriented at this angle with sufficient thickness to include the celiac, superior mesenteric artery, inferior mesenteric artery, and abdominal aorta can then be positioned using these axial reformations as a guide. The subvolume MIP should be thick enough to include the vessels of interest. However, it should not be too thick as this will include excess background tissue signal which degrades image quality. Then, the maximum intensity projection images acquired through this subvolume of data will show the anterior and posterior margins of the aorta as well as the origins of the celiac, superior mesenteric artery, and inferior mesenteric artery in profile for evaluation of atherosclerotic disease. This procedure of using reformations as a guide to performing subvolume MIPs can be used to optimize demonstration of any artery or vein of interest.

Exoscopic Surface Rendering

Images can be rendered using a ray casting algorithm that selects visible voxels by tracing rays from an instantaneous viewing position (Figure 1.17). The surfaces (opaque voxels) are identified by a thresholding technique. For exoscopic viewing, sometimes referred to as volume rendering, a virtual light source and observer are positioned outside the vessel. While the images provide a more three-dimensional appreciation of the arterial anatomy, the diagnostic value of this postprocessing method remains limited to description of pathologies and demonstration of outer shape or topographic arrangement of the vasculature. Little information is provided about the vessel lumen. However, the ability to demonstrate complicated three-dimensional relationships, such as tortuous arteries and especially a tortuous aorta, have made volume rendering well-received in the evaluation of aortic aneurysmal disease.

Volume rendering may be improved using a soft surface or ramped surface and some translucency. These methods allow more information about the lumen to be incorporated into the final reconstruction and generally more accurately reflect the true vascular pathology.

Endoscopic "Virtual" Surface Rendering

A newer technique combining 3D contrast MRA with a post-processing software, known as Virtual Intravascular Endoscopy (VIE), allows the viewer to interactively navigate inside a vessel. By positioning the virtual light source and the observer inside the vessel, the vascular walls are illuminated from the inside (Figure 1.17). The threshold can be set arbitrarily to choose the surface for viewing. Pre-processing the image data is not required. The diagnostic utility of endoscopic arterial viewing is very limited. In a study encompassing 3D MRA examinations of the abdominal arterial system from 20 patients, the availability of virtual endoscopic views did not enhance diagnostic accuracy and improved diagnostic confidence in only a few cases. Thus, the additional reconstruction effort cannot be justified.

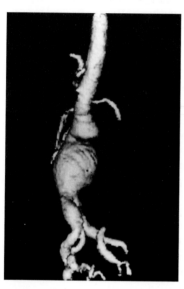
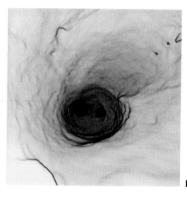

a

b

Fig. 1.17. Shaded Surface Display (SSD) and Virtual Intraluminal Endoscopic (VIE) of AAA. 3D MR angiogram acquired in a patient with an infrarenal bilobed abdominal aneurysm extending into both iliac arteries. The surface-rendered display (**a**) provides a more three-dimensional view of the underlying morphology. This is most helpful for demonstration purposes, and in our experience also aids the surgeons in planning the operation. The data can be further post-processed to provide a virtual endoluminal view (**b**). The virtual observer's position is within the aortic aneurysm looking down onto to aortic bifurcation into the two common iliac arteries.

There may be a role for virtual endoscopic viewing in patients considered for percutaneous endoluminal stenting of aortic aneurysms. Endoscopic 3D views allow measurement and characterization of the aortic lumen proximal, within, and distal to the aneurysm. The aneurysmal neck as well as the luminal morphology of the iliac arteries can be assessed.

Are Blood Pool Contrast Agents Needed For MR Angiography?

Currently, 3D contrast MRA is performed with gadolinium chelates that have regulatory approval for use in humans. These compounds are referred to as extracellular agents because their small size allows them to leak out of capillaries and redistribute into the extracellular fluid compartment. Since 3D contrast MRA is performed during the arterial phase of the first pass of a bolus, the redistribution at the capillary level does not affect the MR angiogram.

Many additional MR contrast agents are under development. Some new agents have higher relaxivity and different routes of excretion but still distribute into the extracellular spaces. Others are large enough or bind to large serum molecules so that they do not leak out of the capillaries (Figures 1.18 and 1.19). They stay within the intravascular compartment. These agents are referred to as blood pool or intravascular contrast agents.

Many of these new compounds will likely be available for bolus application. Thus, first pass, arterial phase imaging will also be possible (Figure 1.18a). The longer intravascular half-life of these agents may allow imaging longer for higher resolution or imaging additional vascular territories during the equilibrium, blood pool phase. These advantages may be tempered by problems associated with venous overlap and safety related dose limitations. Nevertheless, a number of applications are likely to benefit from the introduction of blood pool contrast agents. Among them, pulmonary and coronary 3D MRA may feature prominently. For example, pulmonary arteries and pulmonary perfusion defects of PE can be imaged during the first pass, arterial phase. Then peripheral veins can be imaged during the blood pool phase. Other uses relate to venous imaging and "road map" imaging for monitoring vascular interventions. Blood pool agents may also be useful for identifying GI bleeding using delays in a manner analogous to labeled red cells. Similarly, they can be used to detect slow or intermittent stent graft leaks. (Fig. 1.20).

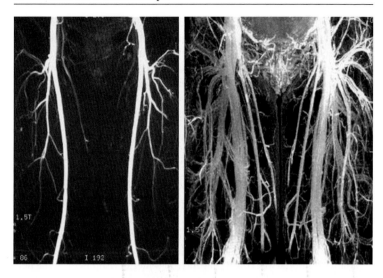

Fig. 1.18. Peripheral MRA Using Blood Pool Contrast Agent. Early (arterial) and late (steady state arterial/venous) images were acquired during and immediately following the IV injection of 0.05 mmol/kg ms-325 Gd contrast agent. The intravascular contrast agent binds transiently and reversibly to human serum albumin, therefore prolonging the half-life of the agent in the blood. The early images demonstrate excellent and selective vascular enhancement despite a lower dose than typically used for extracellular gadolinium chelates. Torso Phase Array Coil, Coronal Acquisition, TR/TE/flip = 8/2.1/60°, Field-of-View = 360 × 270 × 88 mm, Matrix = 512 × 256 × 44, 1 NEX, zero filling interpolation of slices, Sequential Phase Encoding Order, Acquisition Time = 50 s. The blood pool agent also allows the acquisition of high resolution images in the steady state. Torso Phase Array Coil, Coronal Acquisition, TR/TE/flip = 20/2.1/30°, Field-of-View = 440 × 330 × 128 mm, Matrix = 512 × 512 × 128, 1 NEX, zero filling interpolation of slices, Sequential Phase Encoding Order, Fat Saturation, Acquisition Time = 8 min. Reprinted with permission from Grist et al., Radiology 1998; 207:539-544.

Clearly, however, 3D contrast MRA can be performed well without blood pool agents. Extracellular agents not only provide excellent image quality, but, as indicated previously, they also have an outstanding safety profile, which will be difficult to match with any new agent.

Can Stents Be Imaged with 3D Contrast MRA?

Intravascular stents are being widely used to improve vessel patency rates following balloon angioplasty. Citing stent-related artifacts associated with various 2D spin echo and gradient echo sequences, MR imag-

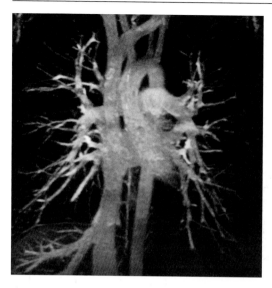

Fig. 1.19. Blood Pool Agents: Iron Oxide. Pulmonary angiogram acquired in a volunteer as part of a phase 1B study using an intravascular contrast agent. The 3D MRA data set (4.0/1.6/40°) was acquired breath-held over 30 s. The intravascular contrast agent had been administered intravenously, approximately 3 hours prior to the acquisition of this data set. There is homogeneous enhancement of all vascular structures. The data set permits exquisite visualization of the pulmonary arteries and pulmonary veins, as well as the systemic arterial and systemic venous circulation. The hepatic veins are visualized in great detail. NC 100150 is a colloidal preparation of ultrasmall, superparamagnetic iron oxide crystals with an oxidized starch coding developed by Amerham Health. The vascular half-life is thus dependent on ranges between 3 and 4 hours. Submitted by Jörg F. Debatin, M.D., Essen.

ing is generally not used for the assessment of stent patency. Recent data documented the imaging characteristics of various plain and covered stents regarding depiction of the stent-contained lumen with fast 3D MRA acquisitions (Figure 1.21). Employing 3D sequences with short TE's (1.4 ms and 2.1 ms), and higher flip angles, the results were more promising for MRA than previously thought.

Magnetic resonance artifacts associated with endoprostheses are related to both stent geometry and the underlying metal composing the stent. The effect of the metal dominates when imaging the stainless steel Palmaz Stent or the cobalt-based alloy Wallstent. Both prostheses caused

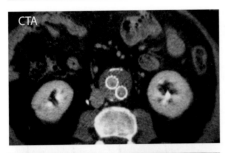

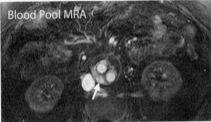

Fig. 1.20. Blood Pool MRA Shows Aortic Stent Graft Leak. CTA (top) fails to identify endoleak in patient with nitinol stent graft for abdominal aortic aneurysm. Endoleak is suspected because the aneurysm did not contract post stenting. Blood pool agent 3D MRA (below) at 24 hours post injection of iron oxide (AMI code 7228) shows large collection of contrast agent (*arrow*) outside of the stent graft. The leak is still contained within the aneurysmal abdominal aorta. MRA data are collected with an axial 3D spoiled gradient echo volume using an inversion pulse for fat suppression. Submitted by Hale Ersoy Erel, M.D., Ankara.

large signal voids on 3D MRA images, rendering assessment of the stent lumen, and thus stent patency, impossible. The covered Corvita Stent is constructed from the same cobalt-based alloy as the Wallstent. However, it contains a tantalum core, which reduced the susceptibility artifact. Although the artifact was less pronounced on images acquired with a shorter TE, it was too extensive to exclude the presence of stenosis. On the other hand, stents made of nitinol (Cragg Stent, Cragg EndoPro System 1 Stent, Passager Stent) caused only minor artifacts. The nitinol frame filaments of the stent-grafts were identifiable on the individual sections and reformations as distinct areas of signal void, allowing for a detailed assessment of stent structure. The stented lumen could be assessed sufficiently to exclude the presence of a hemodynamically significant (>50% luminal narrowing) stenosis. Similarly, no artifact was seen with the Vanguard AAA Stents. Platinum stents are also relatively free of MR artifact.

Luminal patency of selected commercially available plain and covered stents can indeed be assessed with 3D contrast MRA. Sometimes the stent wire creates a Faraday cage effect even though the metal is non-magnetic. This Faraday cage effect reduces the rf penetration into the stent decreasing the effective MR signal within the stent. One way to overcome this

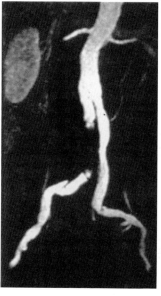

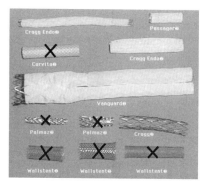

Figure 1.21. Intravascular Stents. Three-dimensional MRA of the abdominal aorta (**a**) containing a covered abdominal aortic aneurysm (AAA), bifurcated AAA stent, as well as a Wallstent in the right iliac leg. The Wallstent had been placed to stabilize the right iliac leg for correction of a Vanguard stent deformity. While the bifurcated Vanguard stent does not obscure the arterial lumen of the infrarenal aorta or the left iliac leg, the Wallstent causes a complete signal void. Covered and non-covered stents that have been evaluated for 3D MRA imaging (**b**). Several stents cause complete obliteration of the vascular lumen (crossed out) while others permit full assessment of the lumen. Submitted by Paul Hilfiker, M.D., Zurich.

problem is to use a higher flip angle. Flip angles of 75–150° have been shown to effectively increase the signal of blood within stents.

How Does 3D Contrast MR Angiography Compare to 3D CTA?

In principle, 3D contrast-enhanced MR angiography is similar to contrast-enhanced helical computed tomography angiography (CTA). It does, however, have several advantages:

1. Compared to iodinated contrast, gadolinium contrast agents have a far more favorable safety profile. Anaphylactic reactions are rare. In addition, paramagnetic agents are not nephrotoxic and are routinely used in patients with renal failure. This is of particular benefit in the evaluation of renal arterial disease, which is often associated with

impaired renal function. Even at the higher dose of 0.3 mmol/kg, the MR contrast volume is still less than half of the iodinated contrast required for CTA and only one tenth the iodinated contrast dose on a molar basis.

2. The imaging plane of 3D MR angiography acquisitions can be adjusted to fit the anatomy of the vascular territory under consideration. The ability to acquire data in coronal or sagittal planes provides greater vessel coverage at high resolution with fewer slices. This is of particular relevance in the assessment of aortic disease, such as dissections, where it is important to determine the extent of vessel involvement within the chest and abdomen.

3. Reconstruction of projection images from a 3D contrast-enhanced MR angiography data set is considerably simpler than from 3D CT data sets. On 3D contrast-enhanced MR angiography images, only arterial vessels contain bright signal. There is no signal emanating from surrounding structures. Bone, as well as calcium, remains dark. Unlike CTA, no effort is required to segment image data to eliminate bone, calcified plaques and other structures, which might obscure the reconstructed vascular anatomy. With 3D contrast-enhanced MR angiography, vascular projection images can be reconstructed automatically.

4. MR angiography images are acquired without ionizing radiation. This is of great advantage in the assessment of young patients. Since very thin images are required for adequate depiction of the vascular anatomy, the radiation dose associated with CTA is considerable, especially in critical areas such as the neck or pelvis. 3D MR angiography acquisitions can be repeated multiple times before, during, and post contrast to evaluate temporal patterns of enhancement without any concern for radiation exposure.

5. While CTA is based on a slice-by-slice acquisition of image data in the axial plane, the 3D MR angiography technique uses a 3D Fourier technique. This permits selective refreshing of select portions of k-space, resulting in a substantial improvement in temporal resolution. With MR-DSA, new 3D data sets can be collected every 1 to 5 seconds. Thus, 3D MR-DSA techniques are much better suited for time-resolved exams, e.g., similar to those obtained with conventional angiography. This has important ramifications because it allows for the possibility of separating arterial and venous phases, obtaining mask images for digital subtraction, and assessing the physiologic significance of arterial lesions by evaluating organ perfusion.

CHAPTER 2

Advanced Techniques

Background

Advances in magnet technology, gradient performance, pulse sequence design and MR contrast agents continue to improve contrast MRA image quality. These advances allow imaging with higher resolution, with increased anatomic coverage, with higher SNR and sufficient speed to temporally resolve passage of contrast from arterial to venous to equilibrium phases. Contrast MRA is also fast enough to follow a bolus as it passes through the thorax and down the body to perform whole body 3D MRA. These more advanced techniques are described in greater detail in this chapter organized according to strategies for increased signal to noise, for time-resolved imaging, for higher resolution and finally for increased anatomic coverage.

Increased SNR

FIELD STRENGTH: As the magnet field strength increases, there are more protons oriented with the main magnetic field, known as B_0-field. The increased number of protons leads to an increase in signal which scales roughly linearly with B_0-field strength. If electronic noise can be maintained at a low level, then the signal-to-noise ratio will double as the B_0-field increases from 1.5 to 3 Tesla.

In addition, tissue T1 relaxation times are prolonged at 3 Tesla compared to 1.5 Tesla which leads to greater background tissue suppression. Relaxivity of currently available gadolinium chelates is not significantly different between 1.5 and 3 Tesla.

One limitation of higher field imaging is increased power deposition in tissue associated with the higher frequency excitations. This issue of higher absorption at 3T compared to 1.5T which can restrict the high SAR pulse sequences is generally not an issue for 3D contrast MRA, because 3D gradient echo imaging uses only a partial flip angle with minimal SAR. One disadvantage of imaging at higher field strength is the associated increase in susceptibility artifact. Indeed this is accentuated with the use of gradient echo technique. However, in practice (see Figure 2.1), susceptibility has not been a problem for 3D MRA with very short echo times.

CONTRAST AGENTS: Since the paramagnetic contrast agent and arterial blood concentration is directly related to the intravenous injection rate, higher SNR is achieved by injecting faster. But there is a limit to how fast contrast can be injected safely, typically 3–4 ml/second for a

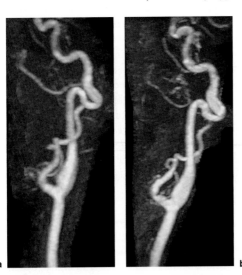

a   b

Fig. 2.1. Comparison of 1.5T and 3.0T MRA of the extracranial carotid arteries.
Clinical Scenario: 54-year-old female with suspected carotid occlusive disease.
Technique: TR/TE/Flip = 6/7/1/5/30°, Field-of-View = 220 × 154 × 67 mm, Matrix = 276 × 155 × 48 reconstructed to 416 × 224 at 70% rectangular Field-of-View. For the 1.5T MRA image matrix was 256 × 224 × 48. 25 ml gadolinium injected at 2 ml/s, time with a test bolus.
Interpretation: The 3.0T MRA shows improved vessel edge definition relative to the 1.5T MRA. The improved signal-to-noise ratio at higher field strengths allows for higher spatial resolution. Relative voxel volume is 0.62 mm^3 for 3T MRA, compared to 1.15mm^3 for 1.5T MRA, before zero- filling.
Diagnosis: Patent tortuous internal carotid artery.
Submitted by Matt A. Bernstein, Ph.D., and John Huston, M.D., Mayo Clinic, Rochester.

peripheral intravenous line. One way to instantly double the injection rate is to utilize a gadolinium chelate preparation with double the standard concentration. Gadobutrol (Gadovist, Schering AG) is now available in Europe in a 1.0 Molar preparation which is twice the standard 0.5 Molar concentration of all other gadolinium contrast agents. Initial experience has shown that based on same dose and injection times Gadobutrol is associated with 70% more signal in the arterial phase of the peripheral vasculature compared to Magnevist. The cause for this observation remains unclear at this time, but may reflect higher relaxation of Gadovist compared to Magnevist. The effect of Gadovist on 3D MRA is illustrated in Figure 2.2.

Another contrast agent improvement is to increase the relaxivity. Doubling the relaxivity is equivalent to doubling the concentration.

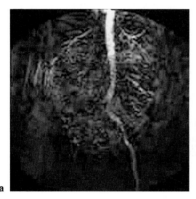

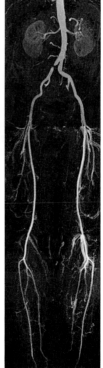

Fig. 2.2. MRA with Gadobutrol.
Clinical Scenario: Right buttock and lower limb claudication.
Technique: Coronal acquisition, TR/TE/flip =5.1/2.3/40, Field-of-View = 400 × 320 × 64mm, Matrix = 512 × 160 × 16 with zero interpolation to 32 slices, elliptical centric ordering of k-space following injection of 10 ml Gadovist at 0.4ml/s, timed using fluoroscopic triggering.
Diagnosis: Focal severe right common iliac stenosis, good distal run-off vessels.
Submitted by James F. M. Meaney, M.D., St. James's Hospital, Dublin.

Relaxivity is affected by the contrast agent rotational correlation time. At 1.5T, relaxivity increases for larger Gd-chelate complexes that rotate more slowly. One way to make the Gd-chelate complex larger is to add a side group with affinity for albumin so the gadolinium chelate attaches to albumin upon contact with blood. Gd-BOPTA has a weak interaction with albumin which approximately doubles its relaxivity (Figure 2.3). MS 325 interacts even more strongly with albumin and has a ~4-fold increase in relaxivity (Figure 1.18) compared to standard Gd-chelates. Blood pool or intravascular contrast agents are large enough (or bind to large enough molecules when injected) to prevent leaking out of capillaries such that they stay within the intravascular compartment.

In view of the rapid progress of MRA techniques based on the use of extracellular agents, the future of intravascular contrast agents for morphologic imaging of the arterial vascular tree outside the coronary arteries remains questionable. With regard to whole-body MRA, intravascular contrast agents might be advantageous in allowing an initial, first-pass whole-body MRA-exam, followed by steady-state phase focused, high-resolution MRA to further assess lesions identified on whole-body MRA.

Time Resolved Imaging

2D PROJECTION MR ANGIOGRAPHY: Two dimensional imaging has been largely supplanted by higher resolution 3D volume imaging because 3D has a single center of k-space for defining image contrast, high SNR, reduced motion artifact, thinner slices with very short echo time, ability to reconstruct at multiple obliquities and spectacular volume rendering. However 2D imaging has the advantage of being faster than 3D because there is no phase encoding in the 3rd direction, the slice select direction. With projection imaging, a single, thick 2D slice can image a volume of tissue as large as in a 3D acquisition. Although it provides only a single projection per injection, the high temporal resolution enables following the contrast bolus passage through vascular anatomy at sub-second temporal resolution (Figure 2.4). It also detects early enhancement in tumors, vascular malformations and inflamed tissues. In diabetic patients, time-resolved imaging can detect the enhancement associated with charcot joints, cellulitis and impending ulceration (Figure 2.5).

2D MR DSA is performed by prescribing a single 2D slice of sufficient thickness to encompass the entire region of interest. The same 2D image is acquired repeatedly while injecting a small dose of Gadolinium contrast.

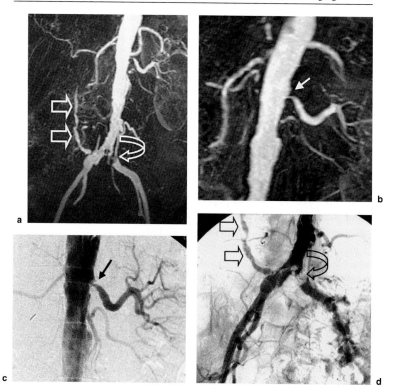

Fig. 2.3. Renal MRA with Gd-BOPTA.

Clinical Scenario: CREST Syndrome with history of right renal artery bypass for occlusive arteritis.

Technique: Phased array coil, coronal acquisition TR/TE/flip = 7/1.3/30, Field-of-View = 320 × 320 × 78, matrix = 512 × 160 × 26 with zero filling to 512 × 512 × 52, 14 ml Bopta (0.1mmol/kg) infused at 1 ml/s timed with Smartprep using elliptical centric ordering of k-space. (**a**) MIP and (**b**) subvolume MIP of left renal artery with (**c** and **d**) angiography correlation for left renal artery stent placement.

Interpretation: Severe left renal artery stenosis (solid arrow) and occluded right renal artery. Severe and heavily calcified left iliac artery stenosis (*curved arrow*). Right renal artery bypass graft (*open arrows*) is severely diseased and requires a separate contrast injection (**d**) at conventional angiography to visualize.

Diagnosis: Severe left renal artery stenosis, occluded right renal artery with severely diseased aorto-renal bypass graft.

Submitted by Patrick Veit, M.D., Essen.

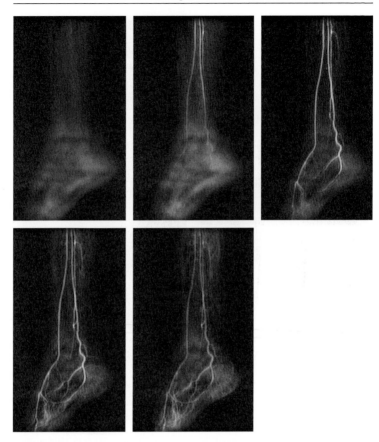

Fig. 2.4. 2D Projection MRA of Normal Foot. A single 2D spoiled gradient echo slice is acquired in the sagittal plane. The 2D image is sufficiently thick (typically 6–10 cm) to encompass the entire foot. It is acquired repeatedly at 1–2 second intervals for 1 minute beginning simultaneously with injection of 5–6 ml Gd. One of the early, pre-contrast images is used as a mask for subtraction from later images to obtain a digital subtraction angiography effect. The series of subtracted images provide a movie of contrast passage through the foot. Vector subtraction is performed on Fourier data to take advantage of phase and magnitude effects of the gadolinium contrast agent. Submitted by Yi Wang, Ph.D., and Martin Prince, M.D., New York.

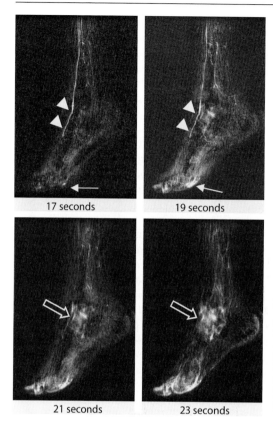

17 seconds

19 seconds

21 seconds

23 seconds

Fig. 2.5. 2D Projection MRA of Diabetic Foot. Sequential 2D images following injection of 5ml Gd and subtraction of pre-contrast mask show the dorsalis pedis artery (*arrowheads*) at 17 seconds but the posterior tibial artery and plantar arch are occluded. At 19 seconds, early enhancement under the great toe indicates a site of impending ulceration. At 21 and 23 seconds enhancement in the LisFranc joint indicates early Charcot changes. Submitted by Martin R. Prince, M.D., Ph.D., New York.

Typically 5–6 ml of contrast is sufficient as long as it is injected rapidly as a bolus. By hand injecting, it is generally possible to inject the entire dose in about 1 second. Using an automatic valve system (Smartset, Topspins, Inc.) facilitates immediately flushing Gd through IV tubing and arm veins with 20 ml saline. Normally the images are relatively featureless but by subtracting a pre-contrast mask image from the images acquired during contrast arrival in the arteries, a DSA-like series of time-resolved images is produced. It is critical to perform a vector subtraction either in Fourier space or from the phase and magnitude data in order to take advantage of both phase and magnitude effects of gadolinium in creating the subtracted image.

Subtracted images can often be improved by standard post-processing techniques used with conventional DSA. For example, one can try different masks to find the one that best supresses background signal. Alternatively, multiple masks can be averaged to enhance SNR (Figure 2.6). Multiple arterial phase images can be combined as well. A program for post-processing 2D projection MRA data is available from Cornell University *www.pcmri.com*. Because of the small Gd dose required, this is a useful technique for use as a test bolus. The time to Gd arrival in the 2D projection MRA images can be used as the contrast travel time for calculating Gd infusion timing for subsequent higher resolution 3D MRA. Alternatively, several time-resolved views at different obliquities of the vessels of interest can be obtained with several quick runs by injecting 5 or 6 ml of Gd contrast for each run.

MR FLUOROSCOPY: If 2D projection MRA is reconstructed and displayed immediately after the data are acquired, near real time observation of Gd contrast passage through vascular anatomy is possible. This enables an operator to watch the arrival and passage of a contrast bolus through vessels and tissues. Normally a 2D image with a 10ms TR and 100 phase encoded steps will require 1 second to acquire the data. This results in an MR Fluoroscopic rate of 1 image per second. There is also a delay between when contrast arrives in an artery and when it shows up on the MR Fluoroscopy related to the 1 second data acquisition time and additional time for image reconstruction. This lag time can be reduced by reconstructing with a sliding window technique that updates more frequently than once per second. Furthermore, by oversampling the center of k-space and using thick slabs that allow shorter TR, the frame rate can be further accelerated.

In regions of large diameter arteries and minimal background tissue, i.e. the thorax, mask subtraction is unnecessary. Eliminating subtraction of background tissue speeds reconstruction and further reduces lag time. MR Fluoroscopy has been advocated for 3D contrast MRA bolus timing (Figure 1.9) and also for surveying vascular anatomy by sliding the patient through the magnet on a moving table during a test bolus injection.

3D TRICKS: An alternative method for acquiring angiograms is to rapidly acquire multiple 3D volumes. By acquiring images throughout the passage of the bolus of contrast agent, multiphase techniques are inherently insensitive to inter-patient variability of contrast arrival. An additional benefit

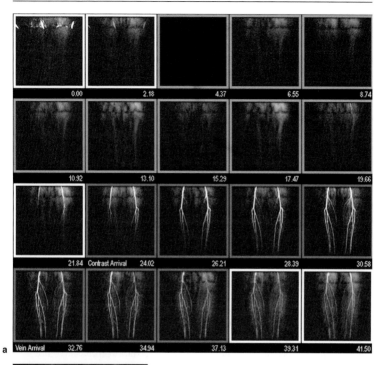

0.00	2.18	4.37	6.55	8.74
10.92	13.10	15.29	17.47	19.66
21.84 Contrast Arrival 24.02		26.21	28.39	30.58
Vein Arrival 32.76	34.94	37.13	39.31	41.50

a

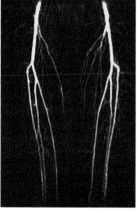

b

Fig. 2.6. AutoDSA. Time-resolved 2D Projection MRA of the trifurcation shown in (**a**) has several time frames preceding contrast arrival (masks) and several arterial frames. By averaging multiple masks and averaging multiple arterial phase images, a composite image (**b**) is created with higher SNR. The composite image also has better depiction of small vessel detail. The numbers under each time frame in (**a**) correspond to seconds elapsed since initiation of contrast injection. This allows bolus timing for subsequent 3D MRA.

Submitted by Junhwan Kim, M.S. and Ramin Zabih, Ph.D., Ithaca.

of time-resolved acquisitions is the ability to depict pathologically delayed vessel filling. But one important limitation to time-resolved imaging is that spatial resolution must be sacrificed to provide temporal resolution.

Another approach to time resolved image acquisition that reduces loss of spatial resolution relies on the fact that much of the information to form an MR image is present in the central region of k-space. By acquiring a multiphase exam in which the central phase encoding values are acquired more often than the outer regions of k-space, a faster time-series of 3D images may be reconstructed. This technique, Time Resolved Imaging of Contrast Kinetics (TRICKS), retrospectively combines the central phase encoding values with high-spatial frequency data acquired later in time (Figure 2.7). In effect, TRICKS oversamples the

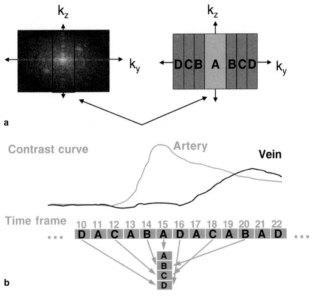

Fig. 2.7. 3D-TRICKS acquisition technique. (a) K-space data from acquisition may be segmented into independent regions, labeled A through D. The region demarcated "A" reflects the center k-space data, while B-D represent the edges of k-space. (b) The center k-space data of Segment A is required repeatedly throughout the acquisition, alternating with higher spatial frequency data acquired at the edges of k-space (b). An image may be reconstructed by combining center k-space values with adjacent values of the periphery of k-space. In this fashion, sequential time-resolved images may be reconstructed at fixed intervals.

Submitted by Charles A. Mistretta, Ph.D. and Thomas M. Grist, M.D., Madison.

central region of k-space relative to the sampling rate of the outer regions. In this way TRICKS is able to consistently capture an arterial time frame, free of venous overlay even in regions of rapid venous return, such as the carotid arteries. In the distal extremities, where bolus chase techniques have been shown to be sensitive to contrast arrival time and venous overlay, TRICKS has been successful in acquiring diagnostic images in patients with severe vascular pathology (Figure 2.8).

A logical extension of the oversampling of the central phase encodes is to acquire the highest spatial frequencies only at the end of the contrast-enhanced scan, as in a "keyhole" acquisition. By acquiring the k-space points that contribute to edge depiction only once at the end of the scan, the frame rate during the arterial phase is not compromised. Since recirculation of the initial bolus of contrast prolongs intravascular T1-shortening, sampling the highest k-space lines up to 3–4 minutes after first pass of the contrast is possible. The extended sampling of the data

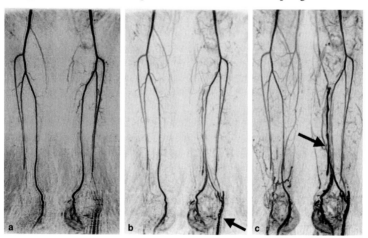

Fig. 2.8. Time-resolved MRA of arterio-venous malformation. 3D TRICKS sequence of left foot arterio-venous malformation. (a) Demonstrates simultaneous enhancement of runoff arteries bilaterally, with early enhancement of the left dorsalis pedis artery. (b) Shows a tangle of vessels in the anterior foot (*arrow*) with early enhancement of the tibialis posterior vein. (c) Confirms early filling of the venous system on the left, due to the short transit time in this arterio-venous malformation. Sequence parameters were selected to reconstruct each time frame at 5 second intervals. Gadolinium dose 12 ml at 1.0 ml/s. The time-resolved exam allows investigation of differential filling patterns in the lower extremity.

Submitted by Young Zhou, Ph.D. and Thomas M. Grist, M.D., Madison.

leads to improved SNR and resolution (Figure 2.9). Some venous enhancement may occur, however, as manifested by edge enhancement of the venous system. One limitation of this approach is a tendency for ringing artifacts from edge enhancement if the temporal separation between central and peripheral k-space data acquisition is long compared to the bolus duration.

NON-CARTESIAN MRA STRATEGIES: Despite recent advances in rapid image acquisitions spelled out in the preceding sections, the use of conventional Fourier spin-warp imaging is limited in its ability to meet the

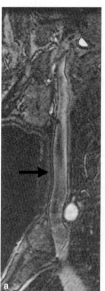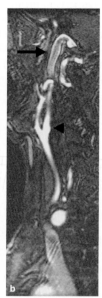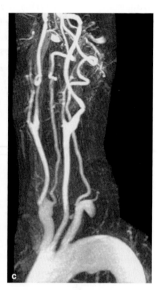

Fig. 2.9. Carotid MRA with extended acquisition. The exam demonstrates a one-minute acquisition using an elliptical-centric acquisition technique, with extended duration to acquire higher spatial resolution. Because the center of k-space is acquired at the onset of the acquisition, it is possible to extend the image acquisition to acquire higher spatial frequencies later, following the arrival of contrast in the arterial and venous systems. (**a, b**) Source images from the acquisition demonstrate strong carotid arterial enhancement (*arrowhead*), and weaker edge enhancement of the jugular vein (*arrows*). (**b**) Despite the fact that image data are acquired during the presence of venous enhancement, the heavily centrically encoded acquisition allows satisfactory venous suppression (**c**), while making it possible to achieve high resolution.

Submitted by Thomas M. Grist, M.D., Madison.

demands of high resolution MRA. The dependence of spatial resolution on image acquisition time will ultimately limit the image detail that may be achieved. However, novel alternate approaches to MR image acquisitions are beginning to show promise as a means to address some of the technical challenges facing the development of conventional MRA. Traditional Fourier encoded techniques generally involve "Cartesian" or "Rectilinear" sampling methods because they sample k-space in a rectilinear fashion. New methods typically sample Fourier-Data in a non-rectilinear fashion; therefore, they are classified as "Non-Cartesian".

UNDER SAMPLED PR: Radial projection reconstruction (PR) k-space trajectories were introduced as the first technique for performing spatial localization in MRI by Lauterbur. Rather than sampling k-space on a rectilinear grid as is done with conventional MR acquisitions, PR acquisitions sample k-space on radial trajectories. An example of radial k-space sampling is shown in Fig. 2.10. Unlike conventional MRA acqui-

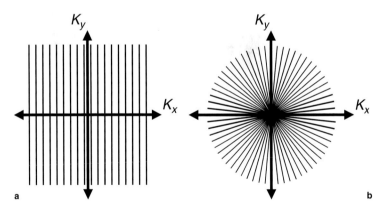

Fig. 2.10. Comparison of Cartesian k-space sampling (**a**) with radial sampling (**b**). Conventional Cartesian k-space acquisition strategies sample the k-space representation of an image on a rectilinear grid as shown in (**a**). Projection reconstruction algorithms use radial sampling techniques, which sample the center of k-space during every echo, similar to the spokes of a wheel (**b**). Therefore, the radial sampling approach obtains information from low spatial frequencies (image contrast) as well as high spatial frequencies (image detail) from every echo. Under-sampling (reducing the number of projections) in the radial dimension does not cause wrap-around artifact or reduce spatial resolution as in Cartesian sampling, but does create streak artifact in the image. Submitted by Tim Carroll, Ph.D. and Karl Vigen, Ph.D.

sitions, radial k-space trajectories sample both the center and periphery of k-space on each echo.

We have seen that reducing the image acquisition time with Fourier encoding can be achieved by undersampling, or acquiring fewer phase encoding values. Undersampling in Fourier encoded MRI usually requires the acquisition of low spatial resolution images, small fields of view or highly anisotropic spatial resolution. Undersampling in PR acquisitions is achieved by decreasing the number of angular samples. This does not decrease spatial resolution or field of view. Decreasing the number of radial samples results in a streak artifact, similar to those seen in CT exams from bone or metal. The PR undersampling artifact has proven to be less problematic in CE-MRA because blood vessels are the dominant signal source, which creates streaks over unimportant background tissues. But in CT, artifact from bone, the dominant signal source, can confound diagnosis of important adjacent organs.

Figure 2.11 shows a comparison between a conventional Fourier and undersampled PR contrast enhanced exam. In the PR image, small structures are visualized with greater resolution than the Fourier

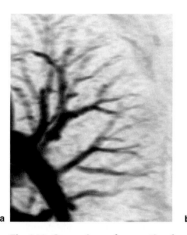
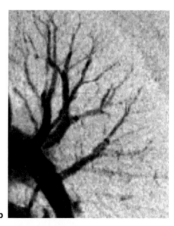

a   b

Fig. 2.11. Comparison of conventional rectilinear Fourier encoding with projection reconstruction. (a) A Fourier encoded examination of the pulmonary vascular tree is compared with (b), an under-sampled projection reconstruction (PR) examination in the same patient. The examination time was the same for both studies. However, in-plane spatial resolution for the under-sampled projection reconstruction image (0.7×0.7 mm) is greater than the Cartesian acquisition (0.7×2.0 mm). (b) The smaller voxel size results in lower signal-to-noise ratio, however. Submitted by Dana C. Peters, Ph.D.

encoded image acquired in the same time. In order for Fourier encoding to acquire the same spatial resolution, a longer imaging time is required.

PR-TRICKS : As described above, TRICKS encoding is able to increase the frame rate over the normal multi-phase exam by re-sampling the center of k-space at a higher rate than the higher spatial frequencies. However, the re-sampling of the center of k-space results in TRICKS exams having lower spatial resolution than single-image acquisitions acquired in the same time. The short imaging times that are possible with undersampled PR acquisitions are ideal for time-resolved exams. By combining an under-sampled PR k-space trajectory to sample k-space in the kx-ky plane with a TRICKS encoding in the slice direction, the frame rate of TRICKS exams may be increased. Using a combined PR–TRICKS acquisition, it is possible to acquire high resolution (0.7 mm $\times$ 0.7mm $\times$ 1.0 mm) 3D volumes with a frame rate = 2s/frame). An example of multiple time frames from a PR-TRICKS exam of the lower leg vessels is shown in Figure 2.12.

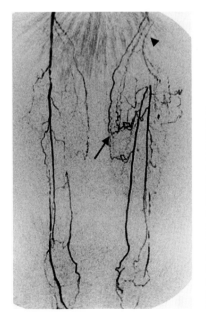

Fig. 2.12. PR-TRICKS exam of lower extremity occlusive disease. Coronal projection from the arterial phase of a PR-TRICKS exam of the leg using radial sampling in the R/L and S/I direction, and conventional Cartesian encoding in the slice direction. Images were reconstructed at 2 second intervals, with an in-plane resolution of 0.7 $\times$ 0.7 mm. The images demonstrate occlusion of the left tibio-peroneal trunk (*arrowhead*) with reconstitution of the posterior tibial artery via collateral circulation (*arrow*). Severe disease is also seen on the right.
Submitted by Jiang Du, M.S. and Kris Pillai, M.D., Madison.

VIPR : Motivated by the scan time reductions achieved with under-sampled PR, radial under-sampling has been extended into three dimensions. Previous implementations of under-sampling relied on traditional Fourier encoding in the slice direction. The VIPR (Vastly under-sampled Isotropic Projection Reconstruction) acquisition samples k-space using 3D radial trajectories (Figure 2.13).

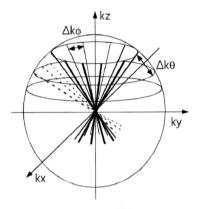

Fig. 2.13. Diagram of the k-space trajectory for a 3D projection acquisition. Each readout goes through the center of k-space and is defined by the angle θ relative to the k_z-axis and by the angle φ relative to the k_y-axis. Every projection samples out to the same maximum k-space value, k_{max}.

There are several advantages to the VIPR sampling strategy. First, because radial sampling is performed in 3D, the spatial resolution and coverage of these exams is isotropic. This aspect is particularly useful because it largely eliminates the need for scan volumetric localization. In addition, reprojection at any angle of obliquity does not degrade spatial resolution. The ability to undersample in 3D without a loss in coverage or spatial resolution allows for high spatial resolution images to be acquired in a comfortable breath-hold.

By interleaving sets of projection angles, it becomes possible to acquire high spatial resolution, isotropic 3D volumes. Time resolved VIPR acquisition of $256 \times 256 \times 256$ volumes in under 4 seconds is possible. Figure 2.14 shows a coronal view of several time frames that depict the pulmonary arteries. A later frame in the same acquisition demonstrates the aorta. The large coverage and isotropic spatial resolution allow reprojection of these time-resolved acquisitions in any plane, and facillitates volume rendering (Figure 2.15).

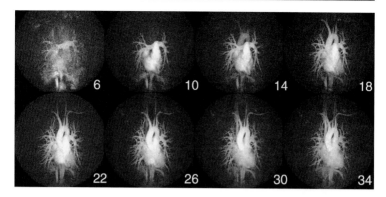

Fig. 2.14. Temporal processing of the VIPR projections generates a set of time-resolved image volumes. Coronal MIPs of these volumes are annotated with the time after contrast injection. The frames depict passage of the contrast from the arterial vessels, through the pulmonary veins and into the aorta and great vessels. (Reprinted with permission from Barger AV, Block WF, Toropov Y, Grist TM, Mistretta CA. Time-resolved contrast-enhanced imaging with isotropic resolution and broad coverage using an under-sampled 3D projection trajectory. Magn Reson Med 2002;48:297-305).

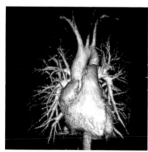

a

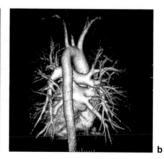

b

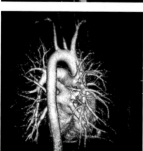

c

Fig. 2.15. The Isotropic resolution provided by VIPR facilitates volume rendering. Here all the projections from a breath-hold are combined with equal weighting to display a combination of arterial and venous vessels in the (**a**) AP view, (**b**) PA view, and (**c**) oblique view. (Reprinted with permission from Barger AV, Block WF, Toropov Y, Grist TM, Mistretta CA. Time-resolved contrast-enhanced imaging with isotropic resolution and broad coverage using an under-sampled 3D projection trajectory. Magn Reson Med 2002; 48:297–305.)

Higher Resolution

PARALLEL IMAGING (SENSE and SMASH):   Generally, higher spatial resolution requires longer imaging times in order to collect additional k-space coefficients. However, a family of techniques for collecting multiple k-space coefficients simultaneously utilizing coil arrays has emerged. This allows either higher resolution with no time penalty or faster scanning at the same resolution. Although there is a loss in SNR, in the event of faster imaging, this may be partially compensated for by

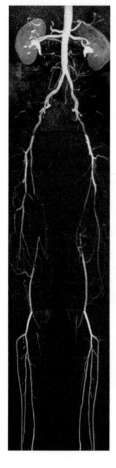

injecting the same dose of gadolinium faster to match the shorter scan duration and achieve higher arterial Gd concentrations.

SENSE refers to a technique in which FOV is reduced in the phase direction by sampling only every other phase encode step. This normally results in aliasing. However if multiple coils are used, then the aliasing can be unwrapped by determining how close the signal is to each of the coils. The potential increase in speed is directly proportional to the number of coils in the coil array. There is a time penalty for acquiring a coil sensitivity map. However, this can be performed prior to or after the contrast-enhanced MRA and does not interfere with or prolong the actual 3D contrast MRA data collection during the arterial phase of the bolus (see Figure 2.16).

SMASH refers to a technique in which coil geometry allows for simultaneous acquisition of multiple spatial frequency modes.

Fig. 2.16. Parallel Imaging with SENSE. Parallel imaging with SENSE utilizing a phased array body coil accelerates data acquisition in the first station (abdomen-pelvis) to 10 seconds so that the bolus chase exam can keep up with the flow of contrast down the legs. After rapid table motion, the thigh station is acquired with the body coil using centric encoding. Then after a final rapid table movement, the calf station is acquired with centric encoding and extended duration (77 seconds) for high-resolution imaging of the smaller infra-popliteal arteries. Submitted by Jeffrey H. Maki, M.D., Ph.D., Seattle.

SPIRAL IMAGING: Another way to image faster and at higher resolution, is to acquire more than one line of k-space coefficients in longer spirals, instead of using the traditional shorter, rectilinear k-space trajectories. In this way, more k-space coefficients are acquired per TR for either faster imaging or higher resolution. Since this technique begins each line of k-space data at the center, there is an inherent over-sampling of the center k-space. This lends itself well to time-resolved imaging at high temporal resolution with sliding window reconstructions. Spiral imaging has a short echo time because each spiral begins at the center of k-space. However it requires a longer sampling time such that in case of fast turbulent flow, the end of each spiral may not be collecting useful data. For this reason, very high bandwidth is critical. There can also be image distortion from off-resonance effects. These can be partly corrected with phase maps acquired prior to or after gadolinium injection. Spiral MRA is illustrated in Figure 2.17.

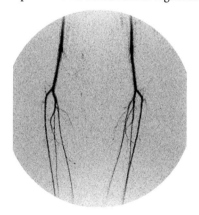

Fig. 2.17. Spiral Gd:MRA. 2D projection image of the trifurcation obtained in just under 1 second with 5ml Gd injected at 5ml/s using spiral k-space trajectories. Submitted by Yi Wang, Ph.D. and Jiangi Li, Ph.D., Pittsburgh.

Whole-Body MRA

Since atherosclerotic disease affects the entire arterial system, extended coverage allowing concomitant assessment of the arterial system from carotid arteries to the distal runoff vessels is desirable. Parenchymal enhancement and contrast dose regulations had initially limited contrast-enhanced 3D MRA to the display of the arterial territory contained within a single field-of-view extending over 40–48 cm. The implementation of "bolus chase" techniques extended coverage to encompass the entire run-off vasculature, including the pelvic, femoral, popliteal and trifurcation arteries. The implementation of faster gradient systems has laid the foundation for a further extension of the bolus chase technique: whole-body coverage extending from the carotid arteries to the run-off vessels with 3D MRA has become possible in merely 72 seconds.

The whole-body MRA concept is based on the acquisition of five overlapping 3D data sets acquired in immediate succession. The first data set covers the aortic arch, supra-aortic branch arteries and the thoracic aorta; the second data set covers the abdominal aorta with its major branches including the renal arteries; the third data set displays the pelvic arteries; the last two data sets cover thigh and calf arteries, respectively.

After planning the 3D acquisitions using a "TrueFISP moving vessel scout" and determining contrast arrival time to mid-aorta using test-bolus technique, a commercially-available fast spoiled gradient echo, FLASH-3D-sequence is employed (Magnetom Sonata, Siemens, Erlangen/Germany: TR/TE: 2.1 ms/ 0.7 ms, flip angle: 25°, 40 partitions interpolated by zero-filling to 64, slab thickness: 120 mm, slice thickness: 3.0 mm interpolated to 1.9 mm, FOV: 390 × 390 mm, matrix: 256 × 225 interpolated by zero-filling to 512 × 512, read-out bandwidth = 863 Hz/pixel, acquisition time: 12 s). To avoid any gaps, the 3D data sets are overlapped by 3 cm, resulting in a cranio-caudal coverage of 176 cm. Each 3D data set is collected over 12 seconds.

A weight-adjusted dosage of 0.2 mmol/kg body weight Gd-BOPTA (diluted with 0.9% of normal saline to a total volume of 60 ml) Gd-BOPTA or Gadovist is injected using a biphasic protocol: the first half is injected at a rate of 1.3 ml/s, while the second half is administered at a rate of 0.7 ml/s. The contrast is flushed with 30 ml of saline injected at 1.3 ml/s.

Correlation with a limited number of regional DSA exams revealed the diagnostic performance of whole-body MRA to be sufficient to warrant use as a noninvasive alternative to DSA. Compared with conventional catheter angiography, according to the findings of two independent, blinded readers, whole-body MRA had overall sensitivities of 91% (95% CI 0.76-0.98) and 94% (0.8-0.99), and specificities of 93% (0.85–0.97) and 90% (0.82-0.96) for the detection of substantial vascular disease (luminal narrowing >50%). Interobserver agreement for assessment of whole-body magnetic angiograms was very good (kappa=0.94; 95% CI 0.9-0.98).

The performance of whole-body 3D MRA can be further improved by using the AngioSURF-system (Figure 2.18), which integrates the torso-

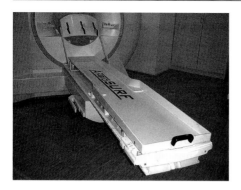

Fig. 2.18. AngioSURF, Angiographic System for Unlimited Rolling Field-of-views (MR-Innovation GmbH, Essen/Germany), is a manually-driven table platform for the acquisition of high-resolution contrast-enhanced whole-body 3D MR angiography. The AngioSURF-system can be installed on top of the original table of a SIEMENS MR scanner. It enables the patient to be manually moved between the circular polarized (CP) CP Spine and the CP BodyArray surface coils. This technique allows for whole-body 3D data acquisition thanks to the stepwise movement of the volunteer/patient relative to the surface coils. With this approach, the achievable signal-to-noise-ratio (SNR) is significantly enhanced as compared to data acquisition with the body coil of the scanner. A high-resolution whole-body MR angiogram, for example, can be acquired in 72 seconds with the administration of a single contrast bolus.

surface coil for signal reception thereby improving SNR and spatial resolution. Using the surface coil resulted in higher SNR and CNR values translating into sensitivity and specificity values of 95.3% and 95.2%, respectively, for detection of significant stenoses (luminal narrowing > 50%) in lower extremity peripheral vascular disease.

For the AngioSURF-exam all patients are placed feet first within the bore of the magnet and examined in the supine position on the fully MR-compatible AngioSURF platform, which is placed on the existing table top (Figure 2.18). The AngioSURF platform (MR-Innovation GmbH, Essen/Germany) fits on most standard MR systems manufactured by Siemens, Erlangen/Germany. The platform, at 240 cm in length, is placed on 7 pairs of roller bearings anchored within the existing patient table. Up to six 400mm 3D data sets can be acquired in succession. Markers permit adjustment of the desired field-of-view. Signal reception is accomplished using posteriorly located spine coils and an anteriorly located torso phased array coil, which remains stationary within the bore. While the two utilized elements of the spine coil integrated in the patient table are utilized with the standard torso phased array coil, the torso array coil is anchored in a height-adjustable holder that remains fixed to the stationary patient table. Thus, data for all stations are collected with the same stationary coil set positioned in the isocenter of the magnet.

Atherosclerosis is a systemic disease, affecting the entire arterial system. But the diagnostic approach to atherosclerosis has remained segmental, largely due to limitations inherent to X-ray angiography, including radiation exposure, iodinated contrast dose risks, invasiveness and economic factors. Magnetic resonance imaging can provide images of the vascular system by virtue of the fact that moving blood looks bright compared with non-moving tissues using certain special acquisition modes. Many of the limitations of non-enhanced MR angiographic studies have been overcome by administering gadolinium-based magnetic resonance contrast media. If dynamically infused during data acquisition, Gd-based contrast agents shorten the T1 relaxation time of the flowing blood resulting in a selective display of the arterial system.

Using the latest high performance scanner and gradients, the acquisition time for a complete 3D data set can significantly be reduced. By shortening the repetition time to 2.1 ms, a 3D data set of adequate resolution can be collected in merely 12 s. Thus, up to five 3D data sets can be collected within the short intra-arterial contrast phase of slightly more than 60 seconds (Figure 2.19). To assure maximal arterial enhancement, Gd-BOPTA, a paramagnetic contrast agent with high intravascular relaxivity owing to weak albumin binding is employed. Alternatively Gadovist can be employed. Improved signal within the arterial system using a phased-array torso surface coil directly translates into an increase in achievable spatial resolution, which amounts to 0.8x0.8x2 mm (post-interpolation pixel size) in the applied protocol. This enables better delineation of smaller vessels, especially tibial vessels.

In patients with peripheral vascular disease, it is desirable to localize and gauge the severity of occlusive arterial lesions to assist planning interventions (Figure 2.20). The TransAtlantic Inter-Society Consensus (TASC) on Management of Peripheral Arterial Disease recommends that – depending on local availability, experience, and cost - duplex scanning or magnetic resonance angiography can be used as a preliminary, noninvasive examination before angiography.

In a series of 100 consecutive patients with PVD who were initially referred for the MR-based assessment of the peripheral vasculature, the

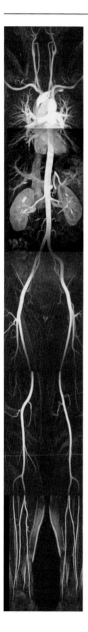

applied AngioSURF-exam revealed additional clinically relevant disease in 25 patients (33 segments): renal artery narrowing (15) (Figure 2.21), carotid arterial stenosis (12), subclavian artery stenosis (2), and AAA (4).

The high degree of concomitant arterial disease in patients with peripheral vascular disease is not surprising. It merely underscores the systemic nature of atherosclerosis. Patients with intermittent claudication are at particularly high risk of atherosclerotic disease affecting other parts of the circulation. PVD, due as it is to atherosclerosis, is rarely an isolated disease process.

Fig. 2.19. AngioSURF –based 3D whole-body MR-angiogram consisting of five 3D data sets collected over 72 seconds. The acquisition time for each 3D data set amounts to 12 seconds. During a 3 second acquisition break the table was manually repositioned to the center of the subsequent image volume. With 5 successive acquisitions craniocaudal coverage thus extended over 180 cm, while the total data acquisition time amounted to 72 s. Multihance® (Bracco, Milan/Italy) was administered at a dose of 0.2 mmol/kg BW at a rate of 1.3 ml/s for the first half and 0.7 ml/s for the second half of the contrast volume, followed by a 30 ml saline flush using an automated injector (MR Spectris, Medrad).The scan delay was determined with a 2ml test bolus at the level of the descending aorta. The quality of the whole body MR-angiogram is sufficient to assess the arterial system from the supra-aortic arteries to the run-off vessels. Submitted by Stephan Ruehm, M.D., Ph.D. and Jörg F. Debatin, M.D., Essen.

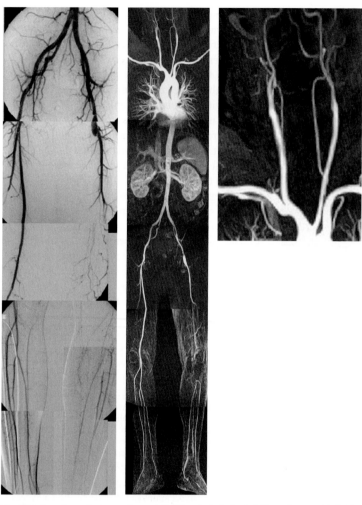

Fig. 2.20. Invasive catheter angiogram (left) and whole-body MR angiogram (right) in a 54-year-old male patient with PVD, history of bypass-graft left leg. The catheter angiogram shows a high-grade stenosis of the proximal anastomosis of the bypass-graft and an occlusion of the superficial femoral artery/popliteal artery on the left. The whole-body MR angiogram reveals these pathologic findings to same advantage. In addition, due to the extended coverage of the anatomy, a high-grade stenosis of the right internal carotid artery was detected which was clinically unsuspected. Submitted by Mathias Goyen, M.D. and Christoph Herborn, M.D., Essen.

The extent of coexisting cardiovascular disease needs to be appreciated to ensure that clinicians will treat PVD in an appropriate context. Studies on the prevalence of coronary artery disease (CAD) in patients with PVD show that history, clinical examination, and electrocardiography typically indicate the presence of CAD in 40% to 60% of such patients, although this may often be asymptomatic as it is masked by exercise restrictions in these patients. The link between PVD and cerebrovascular disease (CVD) seems to be weaker than that with CAD. Using duplex sonography, carotid disease has been found in 26% to 50% of patients with PVD. Most of these patients will have a history of cerebral events or a carotid bruit and are at increased risk of further events.

The fact that in our series twelve unsuspected carotid lesions in ten (10) patients were identified highlights the often too symptom-focused means of patient questioning. Since all studied patients presented with symptoms suggestive of peripheral vascular disease, the patients' histories were focused on that region. Only very direct questioning revealed additional symptoms suggesting carotid disease in three patients.

Approximately one fourth of PVD patients have hypertension, and in these patients consideration should be given to the possibility of renal artery narrowing. In our cohort, 13 patients (13%) showed renal artery disease with a luminal narrowing greater than 50% (Figure 2.21).

There is ongoing controversy about the value of screening all patients with PVD, symptomatic or not, for carotid disease and aortic aneurysms. There is no doubt that claudicant patients are more likely to have significant asymptomatic disease in these areas than the general population, but the treatment of asymptomatic carotid disease is still controversial, and there is the issue of yield versus cost of such screening tests.

It has to be mentioned that our approach – although referred to as a whole-body MRA exam - does not cover the intracranial or coronary arteries, which still require a dedicated approach for diagnostic assessment.

However, noninvasiveness, three-dimensionality, extended coverage and high contrast conspicuity are the characteristics of whole body MR angiography that combine to allow a quick, risk-free, and comprehensive evaluation of the arterial system in patients with atherosclerosis. It is essential for patients with extra-anatomic axillary-to-femoral bypass grafts and is useful as a screening tool in patients with peripheral vascular disease.

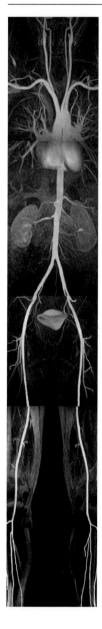

Fig. 2.21. Angio*SURF*-based whole-body 3D MR-angiogram of a 42 year-old male patient with hyptertension.

The exam consists of five slightly overlapping 3D data sets collected over 72 seconds. The acquisition time for each 3D data set amounts to 12 seconds. During a 3 second acquisition break the table is manually repositioned to the center of the subsequent image volume. With five successive acquisitions craniocaudal coverage thus extends over 176 cm, while the total data acquisition time amounted to 72 s. Gd-BOPTA was administered at a dose of 0.2 mmol/kg BW at a rate of 1.3 ml/s for the first half and 0.7 ml/s for the second half of the contrast volume, followed by a 30 ml saline flush using an automated injector (MR Spectris, Medrad).The scan delay was determined with a 2ml test bolus at the level of the descending aorta.

Sequence parameters: FLASH 3D: TR/TE 2.1/ 0.7 ms, flip angle: 25°, 40 partitions interpolated by zero-filling to 64, slab thickness: 120 mm, slice thickness: 3.0 mm interpolated to 1.9 mm, FOV: 390 × 390 mm, matrix: 256 × 225 interpolated by zero-filling to 512 × 512, acq. time: 12 s per station.

Findings: high-grade stenosis of the right renal artery, no signs of peripheral vascular or carotid artery disease.

Submitted by Mathias Goyen, M.D., Essen

Chapter 3

Pulmonary MRA

Background

Pulmonary MR angiography has faced the challenges of overcoming respiratory motion, cardiac pulsation, and susceptibility artifact at air-tissue interfaces while still being able to resolve small sub-segmental pulmonary arteries. Early development of pulmonary MRA techniques focused on black blood and time-of-flight approaches. Neither of these has proven reliable. Three-dimensional (3D) contrast MRA now offers several advantages that make pulmonary MRA possible. The 3D spoiled gradient echo technique has an intrinsically short echo time (TE). With high performance gradients, echo times under 3 ms and even 1–2 ms are available. These are sufficient to eliminate pulmonary susceptibility artifact. Enhancement with paramagnetic contrast eliminates inflow variations that create pulsation artifact on time-of-flight and phase contrast imaging. Breath-holding eliminates respiratory motion artifact. The net result is that it is now possible to depict smaller, more distal pulmonary arteries, comparable to spiral CTA (computed tomographic angiography) without incurring the risks associated with intravenous administration of a large bolus of iodinated contrast (Figure 3.1).

Technique

There are two fundamentally different approaches to performing 3D contrast MRA of the pulmonary arteries. One approach is to acquire a single coronal 3D volume encompassing both lungs. This is performed with a single large dose of paramagnetic contrast (typically 0.2–0.3 mmol/kg or 40 ml). A large FOV is required to encompass both lungs and to avoid excessive wraparound artifact from arms and shoulders. While wraparound can be somewhat reduced by elevating the arms over the

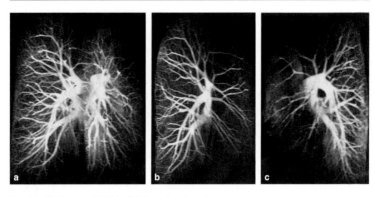

Fig. 3.1. 3D Contrast MRA of Pulmonary Arteries.

Clinical Scenario: Patient with abnormal ventilation/perfusion (V/Q) scan.

Technique: Two sagittal acquisitions (one for each lung), TR/TE/Flip =6.5/1.6/25°, Rectangular Field-of-View = 340 mm in S/I Direction, Matrix = 512 × 106 × 44 with zero filling to reconstruct 96 sections, Acquisition Time = 17 s, two separate injections of 20 ml gadolinium contrast at 2 ml/s for each lung, and timed for the arterial phase using a test dose of 5 ml.

Interpretation: Composite coronal MIPs of both right and left lungs (**a**), sagittal oblique MIP of right lung (**b**), and sagittal oblique MIP of left lung (**c**) shows normal pulmonary arteries with no pulmonary embolism. Absence of pulmonary embolism was confirmed by conventional pulmonary arteriography.

Diagnosis: Normal pulmonary arteries, no embolism.

Submitted by Piotr Wielopolski, Ph.D., and Matthijs Oudkerk, M.D., Ph.D., Rotterdam.

head, it is virtually impossible to completely eliminate wraparound from the shoulders. Thus, generally a FOV of 40 cm–48 cm is required. It may be possible to have a smaller FOV with a tolerable amount of wraparound if a phased array coil with limited sensitivity in the left-to-right direction is employed. In this case, wraparound from the distant edges of the arms and shoulders will be depicted as a faint shadow projected on top of the brighter image of the lungs.

The second approach is to perform two separate sagittal acquisitions, each with a separate injection of paramagnetic contrast. By frequency encoding in the S/I (superior-to-inferior) direction, phase encoding in the A-P direction, and using the slice encoding gradient to limit the left-right dimension of the volume, the problem of wraparound artifact is eliminated. In this way, a far smaller FOV can be used to obtain high resolution images within a shorter breath-hold interval. The advantages associated with higher resolution, elimination of tissue wraparound artifacts and shorter data acquisition times are offset to some degree by the necessity to acquire two data sets with two injections as well as a more complex data analysis. Indeed, the sagittal approach tends to miss the central pulmonary circulation, which can be a problem if the patient has an abnormality involving the main pulmonary artery. Since paramagnetic contrast is injected twice, it is necessary to reduce the volume of each injection to avoid exceeding the FDA-approved limit of 0.3 mmol/kg. Using a smaller volume of gadolinium contrast may require more precise timing of the bolus in order to assure that central k-space data are acquired during the pulmonary arterial phase of the bolus.

There are a number of important general rules that apply to both approaches. For diagnostic image quality, it is essential to acquire the data in apnea. Acquiring image data in a breath-hold eliminates the need for respiratory triggering or for navigator echoes. This limits the application of 3D contrast MRA to those patients who have sufficient cardiopulmonary reserve to be able to suspend breathing. One advantage of the sagittal acquisition is that the duration of breath-holding can be reduced without sacrificing spatial resolution. Breath-holding can also be shortened by using magnet systems with the highest available gradient performance. With such systems, a single lung can be imaged in less than 10 seconds. It is also important that the echo time be well under 3 ms in order to minimize susceptibility artifact from air-tissue interfaces throughout the lungs. Acquisition of multiple signal averages is counterproductive but multiphase imaging can be very useful to see arterial, venous and parenchymal phases of contrast enhancement.

Because of the importance of breath-holding, it is important to adjust the imaging time to the needs of each individual patient. Some patients with respiratory distress can barely hold their breath for 10 or 15 seconds, whereas others may easily suspend breathing for 30-40 seconds. Prior to finalizing imaging parameters, a test breath-hold may be performed outside the gantry in order to determine appropriate scan duration. If the patient is intubated, pharmacological muscular relaxation may be useful to prevent spontaneous breathing during suspension of ventilation. It is essential to have a respiratory therapist present to run the ventilator during breath-holding.

After acquiring pulmonary arterial phase image data, equilibrium phase data should be collected during another breath-hold. It may be useful to acquire several sets of equilibrium phase data to ensure that at least one of them is obtained during complete suspension of respiration.

This equilibrium phase data may be useful in the event that the pulmonary arterial phase acquisition was not timed properly or has motion artifact. It is also useful for identifying metastases, atelectasis, or other enhancing abnormalities, which may create symptoms causing suspicion of pulmonary embolism. Equilibrium phase data may also provide the best assessment of the pulmonary veins.

After acquiring the arterial and equilibrium phase 3D data sets, it is essential to interactively analyze the data on a dedicated workstation that is capable of performing reformations, overlapping and sub-volume maximum intensity projections, and image averaging. Data should be reformatted to systematically identify each pulmonary arterial vessel down to the segmental level; otherwise, emboli may be overlooked. When a relatively high dose of gadolinium is used, it may be possible to identify regions of greater suspicion for emboli by the presence of a perfusion defect. It is also important to recognize that the maximum intensity projection algorithm may not depict an embolus that is only partially occluding flow in a vessel. This potential pitfall can be overcome by interactively scrolling through data sets using source images and multiplanar reformats.

Complimentary Sequences

Following 3D contrast MRA, it may be useful to acquire thick axial 2D time-of-flight images with respiratory gating or phase reordering with respiration. This may provide another chance to visualize the pulmonary arteries in cases where breath-holding for 3D contrast MRA was unsuccessful. If EKG gating, navigator echoes, and phase reordering with respiration become available for 3D spoiled gradient echo imaging, they may represent opportunities for further improvement of the technique. It has been suggested that thrombus may show up as T1-bright on spin echo images. In our experience, however, this is an unreliable approach to identifying emboli within the pulmonary arteries. However, axial T1 and T2-weighted spin echo sequences obtained pre Gd are useful for patients with mediastinal masses.

Following pulmonary imaging, it may be useful to image deep veins of the pelvis and thighs in order to make a complete evaluation for venous thrombo-embolic disease. This can be performed post Gd either as two large FOV coronal 2D or 3D gradient echo volumes encompassing deep veins of the pelvis and then the thighs. Alternatively, if the Gd effect is beginning to diminish, axial time-of-flight images can be acquired from the inferior vena cava down to just below the knee. These need not be contiguous slices if time is limited. An axial gradient echo acquisition with 3–5 mm thick slices and a 5–10 mm gap will not miss the clot since deep venous thrombus is always longer than 1 cm.

Clinical Applications

Three-dimensional contrast MRA is increasingly used for imaging pulmonary arteries. Its use still falls far short of CTA, which has emerged as the modality of choice for the evaluation of patients with suspected pulmonary embolism. Data from multiple studies (Table 3.1) shows credible evidence that 3D contrast MRA will supplant CTA in the near future for patients with renal insufficiency or a history of severe allergic reaction to iodinated contrast.

Table 3.1. Accuracy of 3D contrast MRA for Pulmonary Embolism

Author	Year	Journal	# of Patients	Sensitivity	Specificity
Isoda	1995	JCAT	18	80 %	95 %
Wolff	1996	Acad Rad	34 (18*)	68 – 76 %	93 – 95 %
Meaney	1997	NEJM	30	75–100 %	95–100 %
Gupta	1999	Radiology	36	85 %	96 %
Kreitner	2000	RFGRNBV	20	87 %	100 %
Kruger	2001	Chest	50 (15*)	100 %	
Goyen	2001	JMRI	8	100 %	75 %
Oudkerk	2002	Lancet	118	77 %	98 %

* Correlation available

Pulmonary Embolism

Classically, the diagnosis of pulmonary embolism (PE) is established by ventilation/perfusion (V/Q) isotope lung scanning, with arteriographic validation in patients with indeterminate scan results or in patients with discordance between the V/Q scan results and the clinical impression. V/Q scanning, however, provides only indirect evidence of PE since it is based upon unmatched ventilation-perfusion defects. For intermediate probability or indeterminate V/Q scans, further imaging is warranted. Since there is significant cost and some morbidity associated with pulmonary arteriography, physicians are reluctant to use this test. As a result, treatment for pulmonary embolism is often undertaken without the benefit of a definitive diagnosis.

A major impetus for using a cross-sectional imaging technique for the diagnostic workup of patients suspected of PE is based on the desire to image the pulmonary arteries directly, without incurring high cost, and, of course, patient morbidity. Initially, spiral CTA had a distinct advantage over MR angiography in evaluating suspected PE. Recent advances in 3D contrast MRA, however, show considerable promise because MRA has developed into an inexpensive, fast, accurate, and reliable test for the assessment of PE.

A major advantage of the MR angiography approach may lie in its ability to examine the lower extremity veins for deep venous thrombosis and conduct 3D contrast-enhanced pulmonary MR angiography as a single comprehensive exam lasting less than 60 minutes. Neither venography nor pulmonary angiography, if performed alone, is capable of identifying all patients with thrombo-embolic disease. A technique capable of quickly screening the lower extremity veins as well as pulmonary arteries may be of significant benefit in definitively establishing the diagnosis of venous thrombo-embolic disease.

Analysis of the 3D contrast MRA image data should include reformations in axial and several oblique planes in order to identify pulmonary arteries down to the segmental level. Sometimes the right middle lobe segmental artery is excluded because of its anterior course. Emboli are identified as intraluminal filling defects just as on conventional catheter pulmonary arteriography (Figure 3.2). There may also be an associated wedge shaped perfusion defect distal to the embolus. Data from six studies (Table 3.1) indicate the sensitivity and specificity for diagnosing pulmonary embolism are in the 75–100% range, which is superior to ventilation-perfusion imaging and comparable to CTA.

Pulmonary Hypertension

Secondary causes of pulmonary hypertension, such as chronic obstructive pulmonary disease, pulmonary fibrosis, and intracardiac shunts, can be assessed by plain radiographs, high-resolution computed tomography, and echocardiography. Pulmonary arteriography is employed to either exclude a diagnosis of chronic thrombo-embolic hypertension or, in the case of known thrombo-embolic hypertension, to prepare for surgical endarterectomy. Conventional arteriography is only performed as a last resort in these patients with pulmonary hypertension because of the four-fold increased procedural mortality. In this setting, 3D contrast

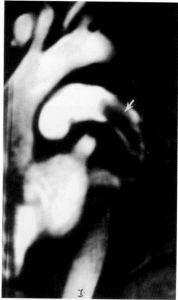

a

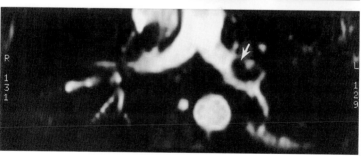

b

Fig. 3.2. Pulmonary Embolism.

Clinical Scenario: 49-year-old male with right ilio-femoral DVT and new shortness of breath.

Technique: Coronal Acquisition, TR/TE/ Flip = 7/2.1/45 °, 1 NEX, Field-of-View = 360 × 360 × 98, Matrix = 256 × 128 × 28, Sequential Ordering of k-space, Acquisition Time = 28 s, 40 ml gadolinium contrast infused at 2 ml/s and timed empirically.

Interpretation: Sagittal oblique (**a**) and axial (**b**) MIPs show a large filling defect in the left descending pulmonary artery.

Diagnosis: Pulmonary embolism.

Submitted by James F.M. Meaney, M.D. and Martin R. Prince, M.D. Ph.D., New York.

MRA should be performed in the coronal plane to demonstrate the central pulmonary arterial anatomy (Figure 3.3). The 3D nature of the contrast MRA data actually provides a better delineation of the central pulmonary arteries than conventional angiography, where the catheter may be advanced into the pulmonary arteries beyond significant pathology. Pulmonary artery hypertension is diagnosed when the right pulmonary

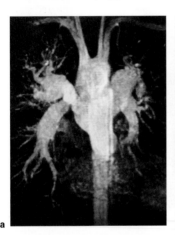

a

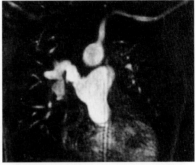

b

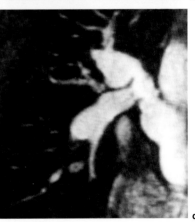

c

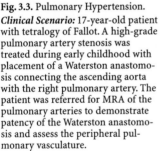

Fig. 3.3. Pulmonary Hypertension.
Clinical Scenario: 17-year-old patient with tetralogy of Fallot. A high-grade pulmonary artery stenosis was treated during early childhood with placement of a Waterston anastomosis connecting the ascending aorta with the right pulmonary artery. The patient was referred for MRA of the pulmonary arteries to demonstrate patency of the Waterston anastomosis and assess the peripheral pulmonary vasculature.
Technique: 3D MRA 4.0/1.8/40°, 0.5 NEX.
Interpretation: The MIP image of the 3D MRA data set (a) reveals evidence of severe pulmonary arterial hypertension with dilatation of the central pulmonary arteries and a dramatic change in caliber towards the periphery. Selective coronal-targeted MIP demonstrates the Waterston anastomosis arising from the ascending aorta and connecting to the right pulmonary artery. The anatomy is even displayed to better advantage on an oblique reformatted image (c).
Diagnosis: Pulmonary arterial hypertension due to Waterston anastomosis.
Submitted by Jörg F. Debatin, M.D., Essen.

artery is greater than 28 mm in diameter and there is rapid proximal to distal tapering of the pulmonary arteries. One study found these criteria on 3D Gd MRA to be 89% sensitive and 100% specific for diagnosing pulmonary artery hypertension in 18 of 50 patients. In addition, 3D contrast MRA can accurately diagnose chronic pulmonary embolism, which is one of the few correctable causes of pulmonary arterial hypertension. MRA shows the central stenosis caused by old organized pulmonary embolism. MRA can also diagnose pulmonary arterial involvement with Takayasu's arteritis.

Table 3.2. Pulmonary Artery Hypertension (Right PA>28 mm + rapid tapering)

Author	Year	Journal	# of Patients	Sensitivity	Specificity
Kruger	2001	Chest	50	89 %	100 %
Greil	2002	JACC	61 (25*)	100 %	100 %

* Correlation available

Table 3.3. Pulmonary Involvement with Takayasu Arteritis

Author	Year	Journal	# of Patients	Sensitivity	Specificity
Yamada	2000	JMRI	30 (20*)	100 %	100 %

* Correlation available

Arterio-Venous Malformations (AVM)

In most instances, 3D contrast MRA can demonstrate vascular pathways in patients with pulmonary AVMs because of the large size of the supplying artery and draining vein (Figure 3.4). Small AVMs, less than 5 mm, may be missed. Mapping out the anatomy prior to embolization helps to facilitate procedural planning, including coil sizing or embolization balloon sizing. It also reduces procedure time. Following coil embolization, however, the metal artifact makes it difficult to visualize the region of AVM by MRI.

Table 3.4. 3D Contrast MRA for detecting Arteriovenous Malformation or Fistula

Author	Year	Journal	# of Patients	Sensitivity	Specificity
Vrachliotis	1997	JMRI	1		
Bertezene	1998	ER	1		
Khalil	2000	Chest	5 (38**)	78 %	100 %
Maki	2001	Radiology	8 (6*)	80 %	
Goyen	2001	JMRI	1		
Ohno	2002	Radiology	8 (15**)	93 %	

* Correlation available   ** Number of lesions

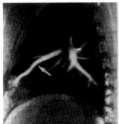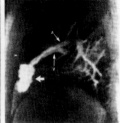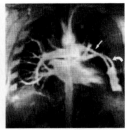

Fig. 3.4. Arteriovenous Malformation.

Clinical Scenario: 29-year-old male with shortness of breath and cyanosis.

Technique: ECG-triggered with 70 percent Acquisition Window, Sagittal Acquisition, TR/TE/Flip = 5/2/14°, Field-of-View = $350 \times 263 \times 75$, Matrix = $256 \times 96 \times 30$, Acquisition Time = 24 s, 0.2 mmol/kg gadolinium contrast infused at 2 ml/s and timed empirically with a 5 s delay, followed by a Coronal Acquisition, Field-of-View = $460 \times 403 \times 55$, Matrix $256 \times 112 \times 22$, Acquisition Time = 19 s, 0.1 mmol/kg injected at 2 ml/s and timed empirically with an 8 s delay.

Interpretation: Sagittal arterial phase MIP (**a**) shows a large arterial feeder to an arterio-venous malformation that is better seen during the equilibrium phase (**b**). There is a large nidus (*fat arrow*), a single feeder artery (*arrow* – a), and a single draining vein (*arrow* – v). Coronal acquisition during the equilibrium phase also shows the nidus with enlarged feeding artery (*straight arrow*) and draining vein (*curved arrow*).

Diagnosis: Pulmonary arterio-venous malformation.

Submitted by Gus Bis M.D., and Anil Shetty, Ph.D., Royal Oak. Reprinted with permission from Journal of Magnetic Resonance Imaging 1997;7:434-436.

Lung Tumors

Although the accuracy of 3D contrast MRA for staging lung tumors remains undetermined, our experience suggests this technique may be useful for staging tumor patients who cannot tolerate iodinated contrast. In one study, lung tumors were identified by the technique with a sensitivity and specificity of 100 % compared to computed tomography. MR angiography demonstrates the relationship of central tumors to the main pulmonary arteries and provides similar or superior information to computed tomography for preoperative surgical planning. A more comprehensive study by Ohno, et al., in 50 patients, 20 with surgical correlation, showed 3D contrast MRA to be superior to CTA in detecting vascular invasion. Obtaining delayed, equilibrium phase images is important as mediastinal tumors and metastases may take a few minutes to enhance following Gd injection (Figure 3.5).

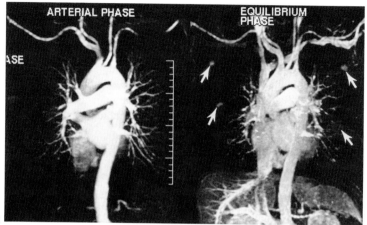

a   b

Fig. 3.5. Lung Metastases.
Clinical Scenario: 65-year-old male with prostate cancer and new shortness of breath.
Technique: Sagittal Acquisition, TR/TE/Flip = 6.9/1.2/45 °, Field-of-View = 360 × 360 × 98 mm, Matrix = 256 × 128 × 28, Sequential Ordering of k-space, Acquisition Time = 27 s, 40 ml gadolinium contrast infused at 2 ml/s and timed empirically.
Interpretation: Arterial phase (a) coronal MIP shows normal aorta and pulmonary arteries; no pulmonary embolism identified. Equilibrium phase MIP (b) shows multiple enhancing lung nodules (*arrows*).
Diagnosis: Lung metastases.
Submitted by Martin R. Prince, M.D., Ph.D., New York.

Table 3.5. Accuracy of 3D Contrast MRA for Tumor Vascular Invasion

Author	Year	Journal	# of Patients	Sensitivity	Specificity
Ohno	2001	JMRI	50 (20*)	78 %	73 %

* Correlation available

Pediatric Pulmonary MRA of Congenital Abnormalities and Anomalies

Pulmonary arterial anomalies tend to present early in life because of their effect on oxygenation and their common association with congenital heart disease. In pediatric patients, 3D contrast MRA is often not necessary because the fast flow in children tends to produce diagnostic black blood, time-of-flight and cine images. However, when these flow-based techniques are not sufficient to map out the pulmonary vascular anatomy, 3D contrast MRA represents an additional useful technique for sorting out the vascular anomalies (Figure 3.6 and 3.7) without requiring radiation exposure. A major study by Kondo, et al., in 73 patients was highly accurate using breath-holding in patients greater than 10 years of age but allowing free breathing in younger, sedated patients. Even greater accuracy (100%) was achieved by Greil, et al., using general anesthesia and breath-holding in all young patients. Greil found that 46% of 3D MRA examinations provided clinically important information not available from other sources. For example, in 8 patients MRA showed both the compression of pulmonary veins and the mechanism of compression (dilated atria post Fontan, scoliosis or compression between descending aorta and atria).

Fast multiphase imaging is recommended in babies and toddlers to eliminate the complexities of bolus timing because of the fast transit time and small contrast volumes. To achieve short 3D acquisition time, slice thickness as large as 3–4 mm is acceptable, even in babies. With

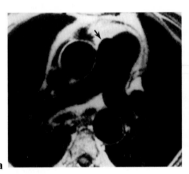
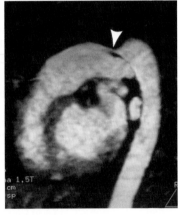

Fig. 3.6. Ductus Arteriosus.

Clinical Scenario: 46-year-old female with a machinery murmur.

Technique: Sagittal Acquisition, TR/TE/Flip = 6.7/1.8/45°, Field-of-View = 320 × 240 × 90 mm, Matrix = 256 × 128 × 28, Sequential Ordering of k-space, Acquisition Time = 21 seconds, 40 ml gadolinium contrast infused at 2 ml/s and timed empirically.

Interpretation: Axial spin echo image (**a**) shows a bulge in the main pulmonary artery contour. A sagittal oblique subvolume MIP (**b**) reveals a small communication between the aorta and main pulmonary artery at the site of the ductus arteriosus.

Diagnosis: Patent Ductus Arteriosus.

Submitted by Martin R. Prince, M.D., Ph.D., New York.

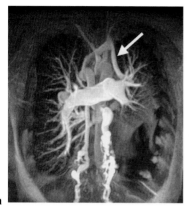 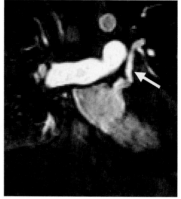

a   b

Fig. 3.7. Partial Anomalous Pulmonary Venous Return.

Clinical Scenario: 58-year-old male with shortness of breath. History of remote ASD repair.

Technique: Phased array coil, Coronal Acquisition, TR/TE/Flip = 4.7/1/30, Field-of-view = 400 × 400 × 120 mm, Matrix 320 × 192 × 42. Fluoroscopically triggered exam, 30 ml gadolinium contrast agent injected at 2.0 ml/s.

Interpretation: (**a**) Pre-operation MIP display, Anterior view. Enlarged pulmonary arteries due to chronic pulmonary hypertension. Anomalous left upper lobe pulmonary vein drains to the left brachiocephalic vein (*arrow*). The extensive azygous collaterals are due to the venous hypertension and increased venous flow in this patient with an associated SVC stenosis. (**b**) Post-operative exam following connection of anomalous vein to left atrium (*arrow*).

Diagnosis: Partial anomalous pulmonary venous return from left upper lobe.

Submitted by Frank Thornton, M.D., and Samer Suleiman, M.D., Madison.

babies, it is also essential to use the smallest possible coil that they can fit into (e.g. knee coil for neonates and head coil for larger babies).

Sequestration (Figure 3.8) may also be diagnosed by 3D contrast MRA. The sequestered lobe is identified by its T2 bright signal on SSFSE. The arterial supply and venous drainage is identified on 3D contrast MRA in order to assist with surgical resection and to discriminate intralobar from extralobar sequestration. Intralobar sequestrations commonly drain via pulmonary veins while the extralobar have anomalous venous drainage.

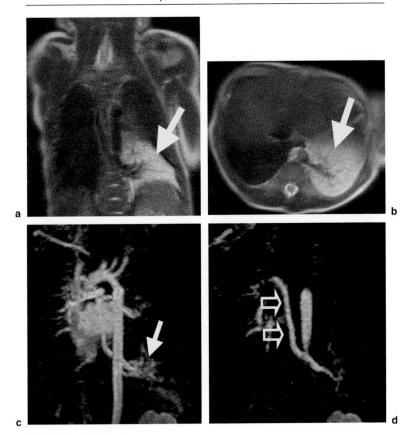

a
b
c
d

Fig. 3.8. Newborn MRA.

Clinical Scenario: 4 day-old-male with left thoracic mass discovered on prenatal ultrasound.

Technique: Coronal acquisition in knee coil during free breathing, TR/TE/flip = 7/1.5/30, Field-of-View: $60 \times 160 \times 44$, Matrix = $256 \times 128 \times 22$ with 2-fold zero interpolation in the slice direction, sequential ordering of k-space, 3ml Gd injected slowly by hand over 10 seconds beginning simultaneously with initiating the 30 second scan.

Interpretation: SSFSE in Coronal (a) and Axial (b) planes shows a T2 bright mass (*arrow*) with central flow void in the left thorax just above the diaphragm. 3D Contrast MRA with whole volume MIP (c) shows two arterial feeders into the mass (*arrow*) arising from descending thoracic aorta. Subvolume MIP (d) demonstrates venous drainage via azygos vein (*open arrows*).

Diagnosis: Sequestration.

Submitted by Martin R. Prince, M.D., Ph.D., New York.

Table 3.6. Pediatric Pulmonary MRA of Congenital Abnormalities and Anomalies

Author	Year	Journal	# of Patients	Sensitivity	Specificity
Pulmonary Venous and other Anomalies					
Bertezene	1998	ER	1		
Masui	2000	JMRI	23	96 %	100 %
Ferrari	2001	JACC	20 (19*)	80 %	50 %
Godart	2001	Heart	6	100 %	
Greil	2002	JACC	61 (25*)	100 %	100 %
Congenital Pulmonary Artery or Shunt Stenosis					
Masui	2000	JMRI	15 (31**)	75 %	100 %
Kondo	2001	AJC	73	92.7 %	96.2 %
Geva	2002	Preprint	32	100 %	100 %
Sequestration					
Au	1999	BrJR	1		
Gilkeson	2002	Tex Heart J	1		

* Correlation available

** Number of lesions

Pitfalls

There are several important potential pitfalls to be aware of when imaging the pulmonary arteries with the 3D MRA.

Susceptibility Artifacts

These occur at air-tissue interfaces and can obscure image detail. The echo time should be chosen sufficiently short (< 3 ms) to avoid these artifacts.

Motion Artifacts

The presence of respiratory motion may cause blurring, which can easily obscure subtle findings of a segmental or sub-segmental embolus. When the data is corrupted by respiratory motion, it is better to make no effort to interpret the study rather than provide false assurances that no embolus is identified.

Partial Voluming

When emboli are only partially obstructing flow, they may be missed on thick MIP images. Thus, it is important to interpret the data interactively in multiple planes. Reconstructing with interpolation by zero-filling also helps to maximize the chance of spotting emboli.

Misinterpretation of Perfusion

Although perfusion defects are a marker of embolism, they can be seen with other pathologies, including bullae, emphysema, and tumor encasement of a vessel. They may also be positional due to the tendency for greater perfusion of the dependent portion of the lung.

Atelectasis

Atelectatic lung enhances dramatically. Although lung may be atelectatic as a result of pulmonary emboli, atelectasis is common in many clinical settings. It may also be rounded and simulate a mass.

Chapter 4

Thoracic Aorta

Background

The thoracic aorta is a frequent focus of atherosclerotic disease, which can result in acute life threatening as well as in chronic conditions. Less commonly, the thoracic aorta is affected by congenital malformations, trauma or inflammatory processes. Speed and ease of patient management favours CT for the assessment of acute conditions such as aortic trauma or acute thoracic dissections. For all other pathology, MRI has been established as the imaging modality of choice for evaluating the thoracic aorta.

3D contrast MRA should be an integral part of any comprehensive imaging protocol of the thoracic aorta. The technique is fast, does not require EKG gating, and provides a detailed 3D data set of the thoracic aorta, which can be reformatted into any desired obliquity. Beyond eliminating the risks of arterial catheterization, iodinated contrast, and ionizing radiation, 3D contrast MRA combines the advantages of arterial contrast with a cross-sectional format. Since image quality is not affected by slow flow, differentiation of thrombus from slow flow is never a problem. Multiplanar reformation of the image data aids in the display of the often-complex aortic anatomy. Vessel diameters can be accurately determined, and the origins of arch vessels are depicted in detail (Figure 4.1).

While 3D contrast MRA is unsurpassed for assessing the aortic lumen, it should be complemented by a black blood spin echo sequence for depiction of the aortic wall and, at least in some cases, a cine-type bright blood sequence for the evaluation of functional flow dynamics. The latter can be particularly useful in assessing aortic valvular disease and aortic dissections in which entry and re-entry sites may only become visible during part of the cardiac cycle. Note, however that the

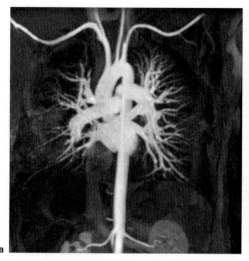
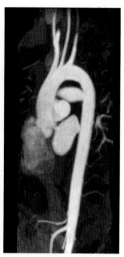

a   b

Fig. 4.1. Normal Aorta.

Clinical Scenario: 42-year-old male with chest pain referred for MRA of the thoracic aorta.

Technique: Phased Array Torso Coil, Coronal Acquisition, TR/TE/ Flip = 6.8/2.1/45°, 0.75 NEX, Field-of-View = 380 × 380 × 120 mm, Matrix = 256 × 160 × 40 with zero filling interpolation in the slice direction to create 80 slices, centric ordering of k-space, Acquisition Time = 37 s, 40 ml gadolinium contrast infused at 2 ml/s, timed empirically.

Interpretation: Coronal MIP (a) demonstrates a normal thoracic aorta with normal great vessel. Targeted MIP (b) reconstructed in the sagittal plane provides even better delineation of the arch vessel origins.

Diagnosis: Normal thoracic aorta.

Submitted by Martin R. Prince, M.D., Ph.D., New York.

slow flow artifact and lack of detail on Black Blood MRA can sometimes be confusing (Figure 4.2).

Technique

Patients are imaged in the supine position. The arms should be placed above the head to avoid aliasing and to ensure a downhill path for venous return. This aids in maintaining a compact contrast bolus. While the body coil generally provides sufficient signal, a phased array torso coil renders superior image quality as long as the patient is not too large. In placing the phased array coil, it is important to include the lower por-

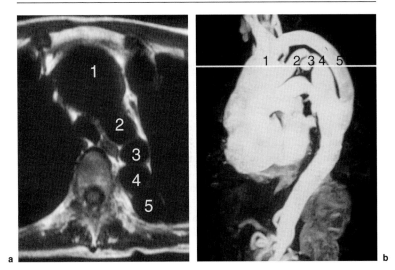

Fig. 4.2. Black blood versus Gd-MRA.

Clinical Scenario: Coarctation follow-up.

Technique: Oblique sagittal acquisition, TR/TE/Flip = 21/6/30°, Field-of-View = 400 × 300 × 90 mm, Matrix = 512 × 160 × 32. Sequential ordering of k-space following injection of 40ml Magnevist pushed slowly by hand over the first 2/3 of the acquisition.

Interpretation: Black Blood MRA (**a**) is confusing and difficult to interpret because of the multitude of vascular structures. Sagittal oblique MIP of 3D Gd-MRA (**b**) shows the aortic coarctation bypass repair and identifies all the vascular structures: 1 = ascending, 2 = arch coarct segment, 3 = pseudoaneurysm, 4 = post arch segment leading to descending aorta, 5 = extra-anatomic bypass.

Diagnosis: Widely patent coarctation repair with intact proximal and distal anastomoses. Submitted by Neil Rofsky, M.D., and Glenn Krinsky, M.D, New York.

tion of the neck within the coil field-of-view if depiction of the arch vessels is desired. If the entire aorta is to be evaluated, the coil can be placed lower so that the abdominal aorta, along with its important branches, can be included. For some phased array coils (most Torso Array coils), the superior-to-inferior coverage is improved by rotating the coil 90° so that the longer dimension of the coil is oriented superior-to-inferior and the shorter dimension is left-to-right. Alternatively, newly developed phased array coils offer a full 48 cm of superior-to-inferior coverage (musculo skeletal array, ICG Medical Advances).

The morphology of the aorta can be complex. Congenital anomalies, aortic valvular disease, aneurysms and dissections, as well as generalized atherosclerotic disease, can alter its normal course. Thus, an extensive localizer should be acquired prior to the prescription of the 3D MRA volume acquisition. Any fast 2D gradient recalled echo acquisition is suitable. It is possible to resolve most thoracic aortic pathology on non-breath-held 3D contrast MRA acquisitions. This is particularly true for pathology involving the descending aorta, such as aortic coarctations. Due to its stable paravertebral course, the descending thoracic aorta does not move much with respiration. Small children with suspected coarctation can thus be examined without breath-holding. Breath-holding does, however, improve image quality in the ascending aorta and aortic arch. If assessment of arch vessel origins is desired, the data must be collected during apnea. To assure proper positioning, the patient should be instructed to take a similar depth of inspiration for the localizer as well as the 3D contrast MRA acquisition. The simplest approach to reproducible breath-holding positions is to instruct the patient to suspend breathing in expiration.

As in other vascular territories, the fast, breath-held 3D MRA acquisition technique requires timing the contrast bolus with either an automatic trigger or a test bolus. For imaging aortic aneurysms, which contain particularly slow flow, it is important to anticipate a long contrast travel time to fill the entire aorta. It may take another 8–10 seconds after contrast arrives in the aorta before it reaches peak concentration. In addition, slow flow in the false lumen of a dissection also needs to be considered. The need for timing sequences can be eliminated if very fast time-resolved techniques are employed. These can be particularly helpful in the setting of an aortic dissection with delayed filling of the false lumen.

Yet another strategy is to perform two contrast MRA studies of the aorta. First, a low-resolution, time-resolved MRA of the aorta is acquired with a small test dose. Then a high resolution 3D MRA is performed with a larger dose using bolus timing information from the initial time-resolved test scan.

Based on the localizing images, the 3D MRA volume acquisition can be planned in either the coronal or sagittal plane. The coronal plane covers more anatomy but requires more sections, and thus may not be fast enough to be completed in a breath-hold on slower scanners. Coronal acquisitions also require a larger FOV to avoid wrap-around artifact from the shoulders. This in turn lowers resolution. A sagittal acquisition may make it possible to evaluate the entire thoracic aorta with fewer or thinner sections. Obviously, the choice of imaging plane depends on the aortic anatomy as displayed on the localizer images. If display of the subclavian arteries is desired, data sets should be collected in the coronal imaging plane.

To assure coverage of the desired anatomy without aliasing artifacts, a preliminary 3D data set should be collected prior to the administration of the contrast bolus. These images can subsequently also be used as a baseline for image subtractions. To compensate for slow flow, two 3D contrast MRA data sets can be collected. The first is timed for optimal aortic contrast opacification; a second set is acquired following a short 10 second breathing interval.

Different contrast doses are currently employed for imaging the thoracic aorta. A dose of 0.2 mmol/kg can be considered sufficient. Good image quality has also been achieved with a dose of 0.1 mmol/kg, but this requires a fast scanner with more perfect bolus timing. Alternatively one can give every patient the same volume of Gd, 1 bottle containing 20 ml.

Complimentary Sequences

The diagnostic value of 3D contrast MRA is limited to assessing the aortic lumen. Characterization of the vessel wall and perivascular tissues may also be necessary, for example, in the evaluation of inflammatory diseases (aortitis). Increasingly, intramural hemorrhage is also recognized as an early form of dissection. This can be accomplished by including a T2-weighted sequence prior to and a delayed T1-weighted sequence following the 3D contrast MRA acquisition. In the presence of aortitis, T2-weighted images will demonstrate thickening and increased signal within the aortic wall. For delayed T1-weighted imaging, the 3D contrast MRA sequence can be repeated 2 minutes following the contrast administration. Use of a lower flip (about 20°–30°) improves visualization of surrounding tissues. Alternatively, T1-weighted GRE or Spin Echo images more analogous to CTA can be acquired in the axial plane with 8 to 10 mm thick 2D sections. Flow compensation and phase reordering with respiration (respiratory compensation), need to be employed. ECG gating is optional. Axial gradient echo images obtained post-contrast should be collected with a large flip angle of 60° or higher to take advantage of the combination of inflow effects and gadolinium-induced T1 shortening. If gating is not used, multiple excitations (4 NEX) may be employed to average out cardiac motion and pulsatility artifacts.

Additional functional information can be gathered with the use of cine-type imaging. Cine phase contrast acquisitions permit measurement of flow velocities, as well as flow volume, at any desired level of the thoracic aorta as long as the imaging plane is chosen perpendicular to the aorta. More commonly TrueFISP Cine sequences are collected. Short acquisition times permit data collection within the confines of a single short breath-hold. This type of imaging is particularly useful in the evaluation of dissections. The movement of the intimal membrane can be readily mapped over the cardiac cycle. Entry and re-entry sites, which may be evident only at systole, can be confirmed with this technique. Turbulent flowjets at the site of stenosis or coarctation are a sign that the stenosis is hemodynamically significant.

Clinical Applications

3D contrast MRA has emerged as the foundation of any MR-based imaging protocol for assessment of the thoracic aorta. While careful attention to technique is required, 3D contrast MRA provides sufficient data for a comprehensive analysis of the thoracic aorta. (Figure 4.1). In addition to atherosclerotic irregularity (Figure 4.3), all relevant disease processes can be fully depicted.

Aortic Dissection

Separation of the intima and adventitia is the underlying anatomic abnormality in an aortic dissection (Figures 4.4, 4.5 and 4.6). It usually occurs at the junction between the middle and outer third of the media. The dissection may involve a localized area or the entire circumference of the aorta. The Stanford classification of aortic dissections separates those affecting the ascending aorta (type A), which require emergency surgery, from those affecting only the descending aorta (type B), which can be managed medically. In the DeBakey classification, the "A" dissections are further divided into a "type I" affecting both the ascending and descending aorta and a "type II" affecting only the ascending aorta. Dissections limited to the ascending aorta may be associated with cystic medial necrosis (with or without Marfan's syndrome).

After diagnosing an aortic dissection, the extent and relationship to branch vessels should be determined, and the true lumen must be separated from the false lumen. Generally, the true lumen is smaller, oval, hugs the inner curve of the aorta, and contains faster flowing blood. The false lumen is generally larger, crescent shaped, and on the outer curve

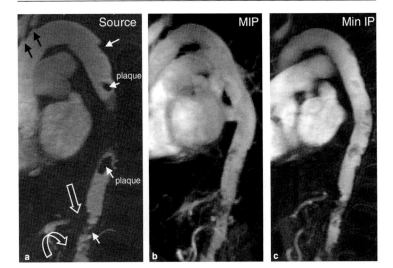

Fig. 4.3. Atherosclerotic Aorta.

Clinical Scenario: Blue toe Syndrome – Question embolic source in aorta.

Technique: Sagittal acquisition, TR/TE/flip = 6/1.2/40, Field-of-View = 440 × 360 × 90, Matrix = 256 × 160 × 30 with 2-fold zero filling to 60 slices. 30 ml Gd injected by hand over 15 seconds and timed with SmartPrep.

Interpretation: Source image (**a**) shows multiple large atheromata (*white arrows*) projecting into the lumen of the thoracic and abdominal aorta which may represent a source of distal emboli. Atheromata are not as well seen on the MIP (**b**) because the plaques are surrounded by bright signal in blood. The average intensity projection (**c**) is better for detecting atheromata but still not as good as the source images. Innominate and subclavian artery origins are stenotic (*black arrows*). Large atherosclerotic plaques occlude the origins of Celiac (*open arrow*) and SMA (*curved arrow*).

Diagnosis: Atherosclerotic Aorta with occlusive disease of great vessel origins, celiac and SMA.

Submitted by Martin Prince, M.D., Ph.D., New York.

of the aorta containing slower flow. Sometimes aortic cobwebs, representing fragments of media, can be seen in the false lumen. High pressures within the false lumen can increase its size and cause compression of the true lumen.

What the clinician wants to know in the setting of an aortic dissection:

- Extent of aortic dissection
- Entry and re-entry locations
- Side branch involvement (particularly mesenteric and renal arteries)
- Classification of aortic dissection

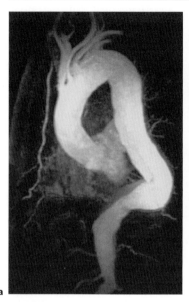

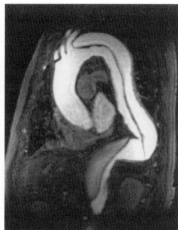

a

b

Fig. 4.4. Aortic Dissection.

Clinical Scenario: 57-year-old male with sudden onset of chest pain resulted in a urgent admission to the hospital to rule out myocardial infarction. Based on ECG and laboratory findings, an aortic dissection was suspected. The patient was referred for an MRA for confirmation.

Technique: Phased Array Torso Coil, Sagittal Acquisition, TR/TE/Flip = 3.8/1.5/50°, 1.5 mm isotropic resolution following zero interpolation in the slice and phase encoded direction, centric phase encoding order, Acquisition Time = 30 s. Intravenous injection of 20 ml paramagnetic contrast bolus at 1 ml/s without timing scan.

Interpretation: Sagittal MIP image (**a**) of the data set does not permit full delineation of the intima within the aortic lumen. Rather, the exact extent of the type B dissection, originating directly distal to the left subclavian artery take-off is well depicted on a sagittal source image (**b**). The false lumen is seen arching along the outside of the aortic arch. The delayed perfusion of the compressed "true" aortic lumen results in slightly reduced signal.

Diagnosis: Acute aortic dissection (type B) involving the thoracic aorta.

Submitted by Georg Bongartz, M.D., Basel.

3D contrast MRA is the basis for answering most of these questions. Multiplanar reformations provide a detailed appreciation of whether branch vessel origins emerge from the true or false lumen. Furthermore, extension of the dissection into branch vessels is depicted. It is also possible to locate the sites of communication between true and false lumen,

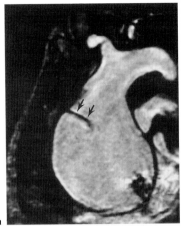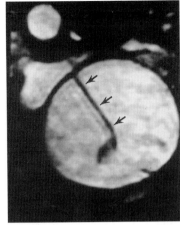

a   b

Fig. 4.5. Aortic Dissection.
Clinical Scenario: 73-year-old patient with back pain was referred for MRA to rule out a dissection.

Technique: Body Coil, Sagittal Acquisition, TR/TE/Flip = 12/3/60°, Field-of-View = 380 $\times$ 280 $\times$ 66 mm, Matrix = 512 $\times$ 192 $\times$ 28, zero interpolation in the slice direction, symmetric phase encoding order, Acquisition Time = 2 min 20 s. Intravenous injection of 40 ml paramagnetic contrast bolus at 1.5 ml/s without timing scan.

Interpretation: This case demonstrates that excellent image quality of the thoracic aorta can be achieved with a non-breath-held data acquisition. The intimal flap is well seen (*arrows*) in the ascending aorta on the sagittal oblique (**a**) and axial reformations (**b**). Reformatting the 3D data in multiple planes is most helpful for analysis of dissections.

Diagnosis: Aortic Type A Dissection.
Submitted by Thomas M. Grist, M.D., Madison.

representing entry and re-entry tears. For this purpose, multiplanar reformations are particularly helpful. In a large study assessing 90 patients using conventional angiographic or surgical correlation as a standard of reference, non-breath-hold 3D contrast MRA provided the corrected diagnosis regarding the type of aortic dissection in every case. In addition, patency of the false lumen, as well as entry and re-entry tears, were identified. The only diagnostic errors made in that series involved the evaluation of branch vessels and reflected the non-breath-hold nature of data acquisition. In our experience, breath-held 3D MRA image data sets permit more accurate analysis of the aortic branches. Furthermore, the diagnostic accuracy of identifying entry and re-entry sites can be

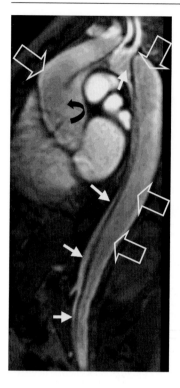

Fig. 4.6. Aortic Dissection: Type I.
Clinical Scenario: Back Pain.
Technique: Sagittal Acquisition, TR/TE/Flip = 7/1.2/45°, Field-of-View = $440 \times 360 \times 90$, Matrix = $256 \times 160 \times 30$. 40 ml Gd injected by hand over 15 seconds and timed with Smartprep.
Interpretation: Dissection flap identified in Ascending Aorta with large entry tear (*curved arrow*) extends into descending thoracic and abdominal aorta. True lumen (*arrow*) is smaller and hugs the inner curve of the arch. False lumen is aneurysmally dilated (*open arrows*).
Diagnosis: Type I Aortic Dissection.
Submitted by Martin Prince, M.D., Ph.D., New York

enhanced by collecting Cine-type images through the areas of suspected tears. Sometimes, these changes are evident only in systole.

Recently, aortic dissections have been further classified according to Svensson LG, Circulation 1999; 99: 1331-1361:

Class 1:   Classical aortic dissection
Class 2:   Intramural hematoma / hemorrhage
Class 3:   Intimal tear without hematoma (limited dissection), eccentric bulge at tear site
Class 4:   Atherosclerotic penetrating ulcer, with surrounding hematoma
Class 5:   Iatrogenic and traumatic dissection

For identifying Class 2 and Class 4 aortic dissections, the aortic wall needs to be assessed. This is best accomplished with spin-echo type sequences. Fat saturation should be used for better delineation of the aortic wall.

Table 4.1. Accuracy of 3D Contrast MRA for Aortic Dissection

Author	Year	Journal	Patients	Sensitivity	Specificity
Prince	1996	AJR	90 (8**)	100 %	100 %
Krinsky	1997	Radiology	108 (98*, 26**)	92–96 %	100 %
Holland	2000	Circulation	Case Report	100 %	
Leiner	2001	Circulation	Case Report	100 %	

*   Correlation available
** Number of Dissections

Aortic Aneurysm

Aneurysms of the thoracic aorta may be classified according to their location (sinus of valsalva, ascending aorta, aortic arch, or descending aorta), their etiology (congenital, atherosclerotic, luetic, mycotic, traumatic, or inflammatory), or their shape (saccular, fusiform, or dissecting). An

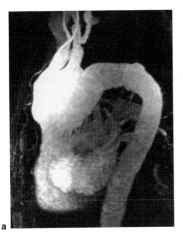
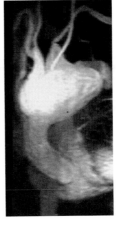

a   b

Fig. 4.7. Aortic Aneurysm.
Clinical Scenario: Elderly man referred to MRA for evaluation of a thoracic aneurysm.
Technique: Body Coil, Sagittal Acquisition, TR/TE/Flip = 10/2.3/60°, Field-of-View = 380 × 280 × 66 mm, Matrix = 512 × 192 × 28, zero interpolation in the slice direction, centric phase encoding order, Acquisition Time = 2 min 10 s. Intravenous injection of 40 ml paramagnetic contrast bolus at 1.5 ml/s without timing scan.
Interpretation: 3D Contrast MRA demonstrates a saccular aneurysm of the thoracic aorta at the aortic arch. The arch vessels are widely patent.
Diagnosis: Aneurysm involving the aortic arch.
Submitted by Thomas M. Grist, M.D., Madison.

aneurysm is diagnosed when the arterial caliber increases to greater than 50 percent of its normal diameter (Figure 4.7). For the thoracic aorta, a diameter exceeding 4 cm is generally considered aneurysmal. When a fusiform aneurysm exceeds 6 cm in diameter, the risk of rupture is increased and surgical repair is recommended for patients who can tolerate major surgery. For those who cannot tolerate surgery, endoluminal stenting may be considered. Saccular aneurysms, mycotic aneurysms, and aneurysms that are rapidly increasing in size at a rate exceeding 1 cm/year are also thought to have an increased risk of rupture.

3D contrast MRA provides a comprehensive overview of the vascular anatomy, particularly the relationship of the aneurysm to branch vessel origins. In the analysis of the 3D MRA data, it is important to consider the fact that the contrast-enhanced images represent a luminogram. As such, 3D MRA can provide topographical information on the aneurysmal lumen as well as its relationship to aortic side branches. True as well as false aneurysms are depicted to equal advantage. A study correlating 3D contrast MRA with conventional angiography and surgery demonstrated a diagnostic accuracy of 100 percent for assessing size and extent

a 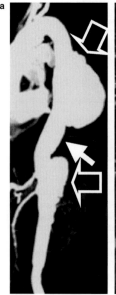 b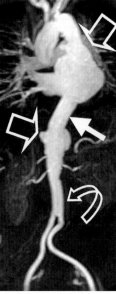

Fig. 4.8. Multiple Aortic Aneurysms. Sagittal Oblique (**a**) and coronal (**b**) MIPs from large Field-of-View 3D contrast MRA. After repairing an aneurysm at the distal descending thoracic aorta, just above the diaphragm with a tube graft (*arrow*) and an infra-renal AAA with aorto-bi-iliac graft (curved arrow), the patient developed recurrent aneurysms (*open arrows*). Submitted by Martin Prince, M.D., Ph.D., New York.

of the aneurysm and its relationship to aortic branches. By evaluating the entire aorta, 3D Contrast MRA shows how many aneurysms are present. (Figure 4.8)

Arterial phase 3D contrast MRA, however, contains little information about the morphology of the aortic wall. It displays the lumen but may fail to show the full extent of an aneurysm that is partially thrombosed. 3D contrast MRA should therefore be complemented by post-contrast

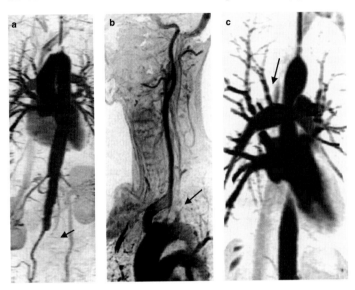

Fig. 4.9. Takayasu's Arteritis.

Clinical Scenario: Middle-aged female with history of numbness in hands and reduced pulses in the upper extremities.

Technique: Sagittal acquisition, TR/TE/FLIP = 6.0/1.4/30°, Field-of-View = 480 × 240 × 96 mm, matrix = 512 × 256 × 36, zero interpolation in phase and slice direction, sequential phase encoding order, acquisition time = 27 sec. Dose-timing scan for timing of contrast, 25 ml Gd infused at 2 ml/s. Separate additional injection of 15 ml for carotid study.

Interpretation: (a) Coronal MIP display demonstrates infrarenal aortic disease with left common iliac occlusion (arrow). (b) Detail view of carotid arteries demonstrates severe stenosis involving the left common carotid with occlusion of the left subclavian artery (arrow). (c) Pulmonary MIP display demonstrates multiple stenoses of the pulmonary arteries.

Diagnosis: Takayasu's arteritis with carotid, subclavian, and iliac stenosis as well as multiple pulmonary stenoses.

Submitted by Thomas M. Grist, M.D., Madison.

images. The remaining contrast within the blood permits easy differentiation between flowing blood and thrombus. The aortic wall can also be assessed. Enhancement of the aortic wall and surrounding soft tissues is indicative of an inflammatory process as found in mycotic aneurysms or aortitis (Figure 4.9). Involvement of the aortic valve should always be considered in the presence of an aneurysm affecting the ascending aorta. Here the acquisition of cine-TrueFISP sequences in a plane along the axis of the aortic outflow tract can determine if aortic stenosis and/or regurgitation is present.

Table 4.2. Accuracy of 3D Contrast MRA for Aneurysm or Pseudoaneurysm

Author	Year	Journal	# of Patients	Sensitivity	Specificity
Prince	1996	AJR	90 (10**)	100 %	100 %
Krinsky	1997	Radiology	108 (98*, 43**)	92-96 %	100 %
Gilkeson	1999	AJR	Case Report ***		
Yamada	2000	30 (5**)	Case Report		
Holland	2000	JMRI	Case Report		
Paiva Magalhaes	2001	Angiology	Case Report		
Lankipalli	2002	Heart	Case Report (2*) ***		

*   Correlation available
**   Number of Dissections
***Pseudoaneurysm

Aortitis

Aortitis may occur as part of a generalized vasculitis for which there are several different etiologies (Figure 4.10). Furthermore, peri-aortic fibrosis associated with atherosclerotic disease may affect the thoracic aorta in a manner similar to the abdominal aorta. If inflammation of the thoracic aorta is suspected, the imaging protocol should be supplemented with additional sequences for analyzing the aortic wall and surrounding tissues. While 3D contrast MRA renders a luminal depiction of the aorta, T2-weighted images (performed with fat saturation) collected pre-Gd and delayed T1-weighted images collected following the administration of paramagnetic contrast material display the periluminal wall and tissues. In active aortitis, the aortic wall will be bright on both T2-weighted as well as on the delayed post Gd T1-weighted images. The degree of contrast enhancement on the delayed post Gd T1-weighted images can be used as a marker reflecting the activity of the disease process.

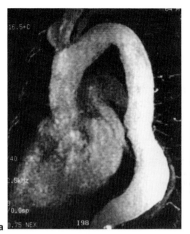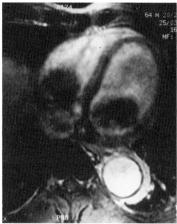

a   b

Fig. 4.10. Peri-Aneurysm Inflammation.
Clinical Scenario: 64-year-old man with evidence of peripheral vascular occlusive disease. Recently, the patient had been complaining of low grade fevers.
Technique: Phased Array Torso Coil, Coronal Acquisition, TR/TE/Flip = 3.8/1.8/40°, 0.5 NEX, Field-of-View = 400 × 400 × 110 mm, Matrix = 256 × 192 × 44, no zero interpolation, sequential phase encoding order, Acquisition Time = 28 s. Test bolus for timing delay. Contrast bolus (0.2 mmol/kg) injected at 2 ml/s with an automated injector. Following 3D MRA, axial ECG-gated 2D SE images were acquired.
Interpretation: Sagittal MIP of the thoracic aorta (**a**) provides evidence of diffuse atherosclerotic disease with vascular wall irregularities, tortuosity, and aneurysmal dilatation. Upon closer inspection, a rim of increased contrast enhancement is visualized along the posterior margin of the descending aorta. On an axial T1-weighted SE image (**b**) acquired following 3D MRA, there is evidence of enhancement of the periaortic tissues.
Diagnosis: Retroperitoneal fibrosis involving lower thoracic aorta.
Submitted by: Jörg F. Debatin, M.D., Essen.

Developmental Abnormalities

MRI can safely assess congenital cardiovascular malformations of the aorta, including arch anomalies (Figure 4.11) and aortic coarctation (Figure 4.12). Coarctation of the descending aorta is present in 5 percent of patients with congenital heart disease and occurs twice as often in males as in females. Coarctation may be described as preductal, juxtaductal, or postductal. The more common juxtaductal or post-ductal types occur as a discrete focal narrowing of the aortic isthmus just distal to the origin of the left subclavian artery and near the aortic end of

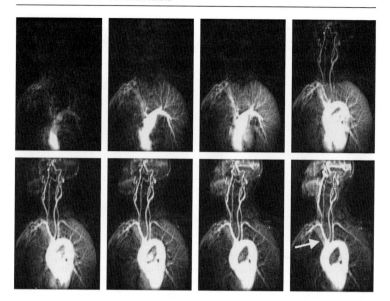

Fig. 4.11. 2D Projection MRA of Bovine Arch. Time-resolved 2D projection MRA obtained in left anterior oblique (LAO) orientation with 7ml Gd injected by hand over 2 seconds shows contrast initially in the right heart. Then over sequential time-resolved images contrast is seen in the pulmonary arteries, left heart, aortic arch and finally in the carotid arteries. Note the common origin of Innominate and left common carotid artery (bovine arch). Submitted by Bernie Redd, M.D., Santa Fe.

the ductus arteriosus (Figure 4.12). The less frequent tubular preductal hypoplasia involves narrowing of a longer segment of the transverse aortic arch and is usually also associated with discrete narrowing at the isthmus. Depending on the severity of the coarctation, an abundance of collateral vessels may be seen. Such collaterals can be particularly extensive near the site of coarctation, bridging the stenosis and merging into the descending aorta (Figure 4.12). It is important to be aware of this collateral anatomy pre-operatively as it facilitates surgical dissection. A bicuspid aortic valve is present in 30 to 85 percent of patients with aortic coarctation. To look for bicuspid aortic valve, obtain a cine (e.g. FIESTA or TRUEFISP) sequence of images in the valve plane perpendicular to the ascending aorta (Figure 4.13).

3D contrast MRA enhances conventional MR imaging protocols by providing an accurate overview of the vascular morphology contained

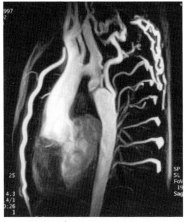

Fig. 4.12. Focal Aortic Coarctation.

Clinical Scenario: 16-year-old patient with clinical suspicion of coarctation of the thoracic aorta. Conventional angiography failed to pass the stenosis. MRA was performed prior to surgery.

Technique: Coronal Acquisition, TR/TE/Flip = 4.3/1.4/25°, Field-of-View = 400 × 400 × 96 mm, Matrix = 256 × 192 × 32, zero interpolation in phase and slice direction, centric phase encoding order, Acquisition Time = 26 s. 3D sequence started 5 s after contrast administration. 0.1 mmol/kg contrast dose injected over 10 s manually was followed by a 20 ml saline flush.

Interpretation: Whole volume MIP of the 3D data set shows high grade coarctation of the descending aorta with extensive collaterals originating from the left subclavian artery and draining into the distal descending thoracic aorta. Enlarged mammarian and intercostal arteries are also seen. The aortic arch is hypoplastic.

Diagnosis: Severe focal coarctation of the thoracic aorta.

Submitted by Jochen Gaa, M.D., Mannheim.

within a large 3D volume. Arch anomalies such as a double aortic arch, aberrant left subclavian artery, right sided aortic arch (Figure 4.14), patent ductus arteriosus, (Figure 3.6) and aortic pseudocoarctation, are easily diagnosed. In the case of aortic coarctation, the 3D MRA images do not merely display the exact location of the aortic stenosis, but also provide information regarding the degree of luminal narrowing without the presence of spin-dephasing artifacts. The 3D acquisitions permit reformatting in any desired plane, allowing exact definition of the size of the aortic lumen. Cine phase contrast acquisitions can provide additional functional information.

Table 4.3. Accuracy of 3D Contrast MRA for Aortic Arch Anomalies and Coarctation‡

Author	Year	Journal	# of Patients	Sensitivity	Specificity
Prince	1996	AJR	90 (8*) ***	100 %	100 %
Carpenter	1997	JVS	28	100 %	
Roche	1999	JCAT	3**	100 %	
O'Connor	1999	Heart	Case report ***	100 %	
Amah	1999	Circulation	Case report ***	100 %	
Grimberge	2000	JMRI	2	100 %	

* Correlation available   ** Surgical correlation available   *** Coarctation

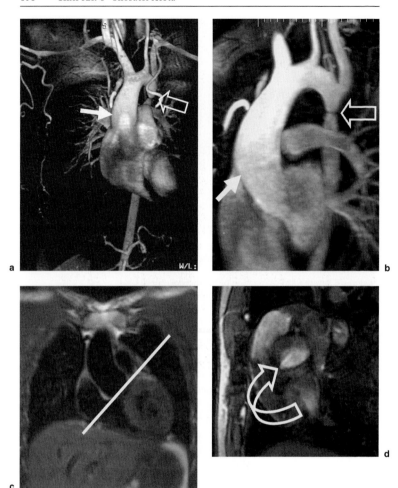

Fig. 4.13. Coarctation with Bicuspid Aortic Valve. Volume rendered coronal view (**a**) and subvolume sagittal oblique MIP (**b**) show aneurysmal ascending aorta (*arrow*) and focal coarctation just beyond left subclavian origin (*open arrow*). To evaluate the aortic valve, a cine (FIESTA) sequence is prescribed off the coronal black blood localizer (**c**) through the aortic valve plane as indicated by the line. A systolic image (**d**) shows the maximally opened bicuspid aortic valve (*curved arrow*) with a fish mouth appearance. Submitted by Martin Prince, M.D., Ph.D., New York.

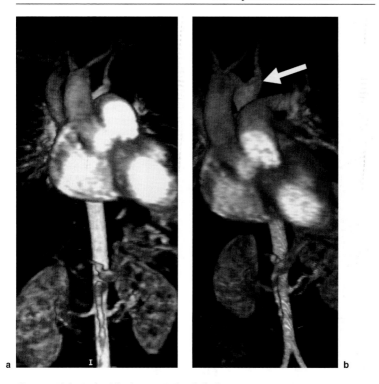

Fig. 4.14. Right Arch with Aberrant Left Subclavian Artery.
Clinical Scenario: 6-year-old female: "food sticks".
Technique: Coronal acquisition using 20ml Gd timed with Smartprep.
Interpretation/Diagnosis: Coronal volume rendered view (**a**) shows right sided aortic arch and aberrant left subclavian artery. Oblique view (**b**) shows the left subclavian origin is dilated – diverticulum of Kommerell (*arrow*).
Submitted by John van Tassel, M.D. and Joan Minn, M.D., New York.

Post-surgical Evaluation of the Thoracic Aorta

Various aortic grafts are used in the surgical treatment of thoracic aortic pathology. All of these grafts are now MR compatible. As a result, MRI can be used for the non-invasive postoperative follow-up of these patients. 3D contrast MRA is most helpful in depicting the postoperative vascular luminal morphology, (Figure 4.15), including aneurysms and stenoses arising at graft anastomoses. The incorporation of an artificial

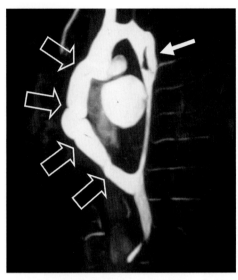

Fig. 4.15. Extra-anatomic Coarctation Repair.

Clinical Scenario: Follow-up Coarctation Repair × 2.

Technique: Oblique sagittal acquisition, TR/TE/Flip = 5/2/50°, Field-of-View = $320 \times 240 \times 90$ mm, Matrix = $256 \times 160 \times 32$. Sequential ordering of k-space following injection of 20 ml Magnevist at 2ml/s via power injector following a test dose using the timing equation Td=Tc=Ti/2-Ta/2 for linear sequential k-space order.

Interpretation: An initial left subclavian artery to descending aorta bypass (*solid arrow*) is widely patent but unsu<Keines> essful due to the long segment of descending thoracic coarctation. A subsequent, extra-anatomic bypass (*open arrows*) from ascending aorta to lower descending thoracic aorta is widely patent and completely bypass the entire segment of coarctation.

Diagnosis: Widely patent extra-anatomic bypass with intact anastomoses and no complications.

Submitted by Neil Rofsky, M.D., and Glenn Krinsky, M.D., New York.

aortic valve in a composite aortic graft of the ascending aorta may cause artifactual signal voids in the very proximal aortic outflow tract. Beyond this limitation, the vascular morphology is well depicted. The technique is particularly helpful in the evaluation of complex cases in which multiple grafts coexist.

While MIPs provide an overview of the aortic morphology, and while multiplanar reformations permit detailed analysis of branch vessel and luminal irregularities, volume rendered displays provide a more three-dimensional appreciation of the vascular morphology. These displays can be helpful in evaluating complex post-surgical morphology.

In order to assess for graft infection, it is crucial to include a 2D T1-weighted ECG gated SE or GRE sequence with flow compensation following the administration of paramagnetic contrast. Because many grafts involve the ascending aorta beginning at the aortic valve, ECG gating is essential to resolve cardiac motion. Nonperfused fluid collections surrounding the aortic graft can then be visualized. In the early postoperative period, it is important to differentiate organizing hematomas from graft infection. This may require correlation with clinical parameters. Also, note that some surgeons wrap the native aorta around the surgical graft, which creates a potential space that can give an impression of leaking aorta. In some instances, this space may be deliberately drained into the right atrium. Thus, it may be necessary to consult the thoracic surgeon when analyzing postoperative cases.

Table 4.4. Accuracy of 3D Contrast MRA for Thoracic Aorta Branches

Author	Year	Journal	# of Patients	Sensitivity	Specificity
Prince	1996	AJR	90 (19*)	90 %	96 %
Carpenter	1997	JVS		73 %	89–98 %
Krinsky	1997	Radiology	108 (98*,7**)	92–96 %	100 %
Krinsky	1998	JCAT	160 (27*)	38 %	95 %
Stone	2000	JCAT	16	100 %	89 %
Cosottini	2000	ER	50	90–100 %	95–100 %
Yamada	2000	JMRI	30 (72**)	100 %	100 %
Fellner	2000	JMRI	16 (12*,10**)	100 %	
Wintersperger	2000	Radiologe	14	100 %	96 %

* Correlation available   ** Number of lesions

Aortic Branch Vessels

Accuracy for 3D contrast MRA in assessing the great vessel origins is given in Table 4.4. Application to coronary arteries is promising (Figure 4.16), but still under development. Coronary bypass grafts, however, can be reliably assessed (Table 4.5). Another emergency applicaton is the evaluation of intercostal and spinal arteries. 3D Contrast MRA is particularly useful for demonstrating spinal arterio-venous malformations (Figure 4.17).

Table 4.5. Accuracy of 3D Contrast MRA for Coronary Bypass Graft

Author	Year	Journal	# of Patients	Sensitivity	Specificity
Wintersperger	1997	RFGRNBV	19 (53**)	94.8 %	85.7 %
von Smekal	1997	RFGRNBV	21 (26**)	67 %	
Wintersperger	1998	Radiology	27 (76**)	96 %	67 %
Boehm	1999	HSF	20	92–100 %	
Brenner	1999	EJCS	85 (247**)	89.9 %	93.8 %
Engelmann	2000	IJC	40 (133**)	76–100 %	
Molinari	2000	IJCI	18 (51**)	91 %	97 %
Vetter	2001	ATS	30	95.5 %	66.7 %

** Number of lesions

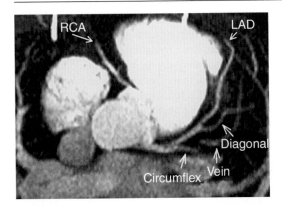

Fig. 4.16. Coronary 3D Contrast MRA. Coronary arteries in a normal volunteer imaged with a magnetization prepared, contrast-enhanced volume targeted 3D acquisition. EKG gating and breath-holding eliminate physiologic motion and an inversion pulse with 300 ms inversion time nulls myocardial signal. 40ml Gd are injected at 2 ml/s and timed empirically using centric ordering of k-space.

Submitted by Debiao Li, Ph.D., Chicago and reprinted from Radiology. 2001;219:270-277.

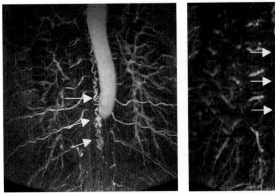
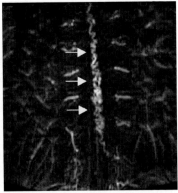

a   b

4.17. Spinal AVM. Coronal MIP (a) includes a portion of descending aorta (a), multiple intercostal arteries and a spinal arteriovenous malformation (*arrows*). A thinner MIP centered on the spinal cord (b) shows more detail of the vascular malformation (*arrows*). Submitted by James F.M. Meaney, M.D. Dublin.

Table 4.6. Accuracy of 3D Contrast MRA for Intercostal and Adamkiewicz Arteries

Author	Year	Journal	# of Patients	Sensitivity
Yamada	2000	JCAT	26 (3*)	69 %
Ingu	2001	ATS	Case Report	100 %
Myerson	2000	JCMR	1 **	100 %

* Correlation available   ** Pseudoaneurysm

Pitfalls

Incomplete Coverage of the Anatomy

The tortuosity inherent to the thoracic aorta and its branches may result in the inadvertent exclusion of important portions of the arterial anatomy from the 3D imaging volume. To prevent this, the localizing process should be carefully conducted using breath-held technique if the 3D contrast MRA sequence is also collected during breath-holding. Furthermore, a 3D data set can be collected initially without paramagnetic contrast to assure that the relevant anatomy is encompassed within the imaging volume before injecting the contrast agent. It may also be necessary to use sections as thick as 3 or 4 mm for complete coverage of tortuous, unfolded aortas, particularly on slower scanners. Preferably, those 3–4 mm thick slices should then be zero interpolated down to 1.5–2 mm.

Blurring of Arch Vessel Origins

Usually caused by respiratory motion, this artifact can be avoided by collecting the data in apnea.

Ringing (Stripe) Artifact in the Aortic Lumen

This represents the most common and potentially harmful artifact. One or more dark longitudinal stripes are seen within the aortic lumen, simulating the presence of a dissection (Figure 1.5). They reflect a change in the T1 of arterial blood during the acquisition of the central portion of k-space. This phenomenon points to faulty timing of the contrast bolus. Usually the bolus arrives too late, so that the plateau phase has not been reached by the time the center of k-space is collected.

Periaortic Enhancement

A thin rim of atelectatic lung adjacent to and compressed by an enlarged aorta may enhance brightly. This may give the false impression of an enhancing or inflammatory aneurysm.

CHAPTER 5

Abdominal Aorta

Background

Advantages of cross-sectional imaging over conventional catheter angiography are well established for the assessment of the abdominal aorta. Although ECG-gating is not required, clinical acceptance of non-contrast black-blood spin echo (SE) and bright-blood gradient recalled echo (GRE) scans has been limited. CT angiography has been the preferred modality for cross-sectional imaging of the abdominal aorta. Three-dimensional contrast MRA, however, has overcome limitations inherent to conventional MR techniques including long imaging times and reduced vessel-to-background contrast in regions of slow flow. It is now beginning to surpass CT angiography as the modality of choice for imaging the abdominal aorta.

Technique

Patients are imaged in the supine position. The arms should be placed either above the head or, for more comfort, folded across the chest. Special care with the latter position is needed because folding the arms may kink IV lines placed in the antecubital fossa, making intravenous contrast injection less controllable. If available, body or torso phased array coils may be used for better signal-to-noise, compared to most body coil designs. In tall patients, it may be necessary to use the standard body coil to ensure coverage of the entire aorto-iliac system, from diaphragm to common femoral arteries.

The coronal plane is used to display abdominal aortic anatomy with the fewest number of sections. In rare instances, if concomitant assessment of the superior mesenteric artery is desired, data can be acquired in the sagittal plane. A set of axial localizer images through the kidneys are generally used to prescribe the coronal or sagittal 3D contrast MRA acquisition. If an automatically triggered pulse sequence is used, a localizer image in the sagittal plane may be preferable for selecting both the trigger voxel and the coronal 3D contrast MRA volume. Localizing sequences should be collected with the same degree of inspiration as the planned 3D MRA volume acquisition.

Generally, the coronal 3D imaging volume should encompass the kidneys, aorta, and iliac arteries. The top of the imaging volume should be positioned above the origin of the celiac trunk. If the aorta is extremely tortuous, it may be necessary to exclude part of its course in a coronal acquisition. In extreme cases, a sagittal acquisition may be more suitable. It is useful to examine the localizer sequence carefully to identify the location of tortuous iliac arteries so that they are not inadvertently excluded.

To assure coverage of the desired anatomy and the absence of aliasing artifacts, it is useful to acquire a 3D data set prior to administration of the contrast bolus. These images can later be used as a baseline for image subtractions. Individualized timing of the contrast bolus is crucial for optimal image quality. In determining the timing protocol, keep in mind that large abdominal aortic aneurysms and the false lumen of an aortic dissection may fill slowly. Two 3D MRA data sets can be collected immediately following one another to reduce the chance of a bolus timing error. The first is timed for optimal aortic contrast opacification; a second set is acquired following a short 5–10 second breathing interval. Bolus timing is completely eliminated if time-resolved scanning is available. Time-resolved aortic imaging has been proposed at 5–10 seconds/data set to strike a balance between maximizing both temporal and spatial resolution. Alternatively, sub-second time-resolved MRA of the aorta with a small test bolus of 5–6 ml Gd (injected at 6 ml/s) has been proposed as a test bolus technique. Timing information from this initial low-dose time-resolved acquisition is then used to plan a high spatial resolution 3D MRA at a single time point with a higher contrast dose.

The abdominal aorta is generally well displayed with a contrast dose of 0.2 mmol/kg. Several investigators have demonstrated excellent results with smaller doses of 0.1 mmol/kg. It is likely that smaller doses will prevail as MR imaging gradient performance continues to advance and faster scanning becomes more common place.

3D contrast MRA image sets of the abdominal aorta are best interpreted on an independent workstation with 3D reconstruction capabilities. While MIPs should be used for purposes of documentation and demonstration, diagnostic analysis must always include multiplanar 3D reformations traced through the origin of each major aortic branch vessel.

Complimentary Sequences

To permit analysis of the abdominal aortic wall and facilitate delineation of thrombosed regions within the abdominal aorta, a T1-weighted sequence post-contrast should be acquired (Figure 5.1). Alternatively, the 3D MRA scan can be repeated for this purpose. On delayed post-contrast 3D imaging a lower flip (about 20°–30°) may improve visualization of background tissues. Alternatively, axial SE or GRE images with first order gradient moment nulling and respiratory compensation can be collected. They emulate the appearance of contrast-enhanced CT. A thick rind of enhancement involving the aortic wall and periaortic tissues is indicative of inflammation.

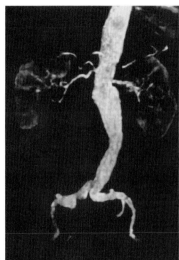

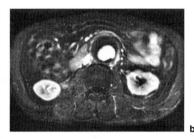

b

Fig. 5.1. Abdominal Aortic Aneurysm (AAA).

Clinical Scenario: 62-year-old male referred for pre-operative AAA evaluation.

Technique: Phased Array Torso Coil, Coronal Acquisition, TR/TE/Flip = 4.2/2.0/40°, 0.5 NEX, Field-of-View = 380 × 380 × 110 mm, Matrix = 256 × 192 × 44, no zero interpolation, sequential phase encoding order, Acquisition Time = 28 s. Test bolus for timing delay. Contrast bolus (0.2 mmol/kg) injected at 2 ml/s with an automated injector. Following 3D contrast MRA, axial 2D SE images were acquired.

a

Interpretation: 3D contrast MRA MIP projection (**a**) demonstrates aneurysmal dilatation of the infrarenal aorta extending into both iliac arteries. An axial T1-weighted spin echo image acquired after the 3D contrast MRA sequence (**b**) shows the aortic lumen as well as a surrounding area of thrombosis, which is part of the aneurysm. Acquisition of post-contrast T1-weighted spin echo or gradient echo images is crucial for assessment of aortic aneurysms as they permit delineation of thrombosed regions and depict the aortic wall.

Diagnosis: Partially thrombosed infrarenal AAA extending into both iliac arteries.

Submitted by Jörg F. Debatin, M.D., Essen.

Clinical Applications

In many centers, 3D contrast MRA is emerging as the technique of choice for assessing abdominal aorta morphology and pathology. Recent scanner designs are fast enough to permit data collection within the confines of a single breath-hold lasting far less than 30 seconds. These detailed 3D data sets provide a comprehensive depiction of the abdominal aorta and its major branches, thus, offering high diagnostic accuracy (Table 5.1).

Abdominal Aortic Aneurysm

Most abdominal aortic aneurysms (Figure 5.2) are atherosclerotic in etiology and almost always involve the aorta distal to the origin of the renal arteries. They are characteristically fusiform in configuration, although occasionally a saccular aneurysm may be seen. Saccular aneurysms, however, may be mycotic pseudo-aneurysms or related to prior trauma. Analysis of an aneurysmal aorta should always be based on both the arterial phase 3D contrast MRA displaying the aortic lumen in combination with delayed, post-contrast scans, depicting the thrombosed portion of the lumen. These delayed scans also evaluate enhancement of the aortic wall and surrounding tissues in inflammatory or mycotic aneurysms.

Evaluation of patients with abdominal aortic aneurysm should include a systematic description of the following morphologic details: maximum aneurysm diameter, proximal extent of the aneurysm, relationship to renal arteries, distal extent of the aneurysm, relationship to iliac arteries, concomitant occlusive disease involving renal, mesenteric, and iliac arteries, any renal anomalies, including circumaortic renal veins and ectopias, as well as inflammatory changes seen around the aneurysm. With 3D contrast MRA, these details of aneurysmal morphology are well depicted. The large coronal field-of-view reveals extension of the aneurysm into the iliac arteries. Multiplanar reformations help unfold even highly tortuous vascular morphology. Based on subvolume MIPs, as well as multiplanar reformations, exact dimensions of the aneurysm can be determined prior to any surgical or percutaneous intervention. 3D contrast MRA is also effective in demonstrating the status of renal arterial origins and their relationship to the aortic aneurysm. High diagnostic accuracy of 3D contrast MRA regarding morphological analysis of aortic aneurysms has been confirmed by several clinical series (Table 5.1).

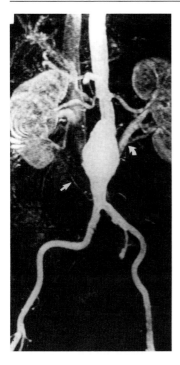

Fig. 5.2. Abdominal Aortic Aneurysm (AAA).

Clinical Scenario: 66-year-old asymptomatic male referred for pre-operative AAA evaluation.

Technique: Body Coil, Coronal Acquisition, TR/TE/Flip = 10/3.2/60°, 0.5 NEX, Field-of-View = 450 × 340 × 90 mm, Matrix = 512 × 160 × 30, no zero filling, sequential phase encoding order, Acquisition Time = 36 s. Injection of 40 ml contrast agent at 2 ml/s by hand followed by saline flush. Data acquisition started at end of contrast injection.

Interpretation: 4.5 cm infrarenal AAA arising 2.5 cm below the origin of the left renal artery and 2 cm below the origin of the right renal artery, extending to within 2 cm of the aortic bifurcation. The MIP image also demonstrates a retro-aortic left renal vein (*curved arrow*) and an accessory right renal artery arising from the aorta below the AAA (*straight arrow*). A tube graft repair was performed and the accessory right renal artery was re-implanted above the level of the graft.

Diagnosis: Infrarenal AAA with accessory renal artery and retro-aortic left renal vein.

Submitted by Helen M. Fenlon, M.D., and E. Kent Yucel, M.D., Boston.

Table 5.1. Diagnostic Performance of 3D Contrast MRA for Abdominal Aortic Aneurysms

Author	Year	Journal	# of Patients	Sensitivity	Specificity
Petersen	1995	J Vasc Surg	38	Accuracy = 95 %	
Laissy	1995	Eur J Radiol	20	93-96 %	100 %
Prince	1995	J Vasc Surg	43	94 %	98 %
Arlart	1997	RFGRNBV	24	100 %	100 %
Hany	1997	Radiology	39 (6**)	100 %	
Maspes	1999	Radiol Med	47 (11**)	100 %	100 %
Kelekis	1999	MRI	32 (12**)	Accuracy = 97 %	
Di Cesare	2000	Radiol Med	24 (15*)	Accuracy = 100 %	
Aortocaval Fistula					
Gaa	1999	Eur Radiol	case report	100 %	
Walter	2000	JCMR	case report	100 %	
Mycotic Aneurysm					
Torigian	2002	JMRI	case report	100 %	

*   Correlation available
** Number of lesions

Inflammatory Aneurysm

While a variety of etiologies have been described for retroperitoneal fibrosis, there is a definite association of this condition with aortic aneurysms. Retroperitoneal fibrosis is characterized by a mass of grey-white tissue with discrete margins covering the aorta and the vena cava. It is usually centered on the lower lumbar spine and extends from the renal pedicles to the pelvic brim, where it often bifurcates to follow along the pelvic vasculature. Although usually midline, the disease may involve one side more than the other. If fibrosis extends to involve the ureters, renal obstruction with hydronephrosis may result. A combination of 3D contrast MRA and delayed post-contrast imaging is well suited for a comprehensive analysis of retroperitoneal fibrosis (Figure 5.3). Based on the degree of enhancement of the aortic wall, MRI can be used for follow-up and assessment of therapeutic effectiveness in these patients. Aneurysms, as well as regions of stenosis, are well depicted. Delayed 3D acquisitions are useful as they may display contrast within dilated ureters and intrarenal collecting systems, as well as infectious complications of aortic graft repair (Figure 5.4).

Aortic Stenting

Based upon encouraging initial data, percutaneous stent grafting is increasingly employed as a less invasive alternative for the treatment of infrarenal abdominal aortic aneurysms. The covered stent is placed

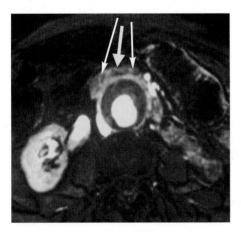

Fig. 5.3. Retroperitoneal Fibrosis. Axial 2D TOF obtained post 3D Gd MRA shows enhancing soft tissue anterior to the abdominal aortic aneurysm (*arrow*) confirmed at surgery to be retroperitoneal fibrosis. Submitted by Martin Prince, M.D., Ph.D., New York.

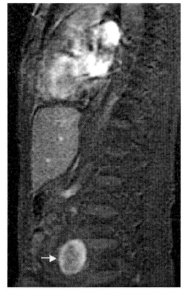

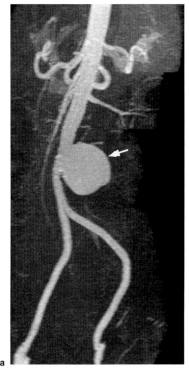

Fig. 5.4. Infection Following Aorto-Bifemoral Graft.

Clinical Scenario: 60-year-old male with fever 8 weeks following aorto-bifemoral graft.

Technique: Body Coil, Coronal Acquisition, TR/TE/Flip = 8/2.1/60°, Field-of-View = 360 × 270 × 88 mm, Matrix = 512 × 192 × 44, 1 NEX, zero filing interpolation of slices, sequential phase encoding order, Acquisition Time = 28 s. Test bolus for timing scan. 40 ml Gd injected at 1.4 ml/s.

Interpretation: The arterial phase image (**a**) demonstrates a saccular aneurysm at the proximal graft anastomosis suspicious for an inflammatory pseudo-aneurysm. Delayed images (**b**) show aneurysmal wall enhancement.

Diagnosis: Mycotic pseudo-aneurysm at graft anastomosis confirmed at surgery.

Submitted by Thomas M. Grist, M.D., Madison.

within the aorta, positioned to exclude the aneurysm. Long-term success of this endoluminal procedure is predicated upon the availability of accurate imaging data before, as well as following, the procedure.

3D contrast MRA has been shown to be well suited for the characterization of abdominal aortic aneurysms. To assure uncomplicated delivery, pelvic arteries should be included in the coronal acquisition volume. In contrast to surgery, aneurysmal stenting requires long-term imaging follow-up to document the structural integrity of the device as well as shrinkage of the aneurysm. Expectation of severe stent-induced artifacts and safety concerns have prevented 3D contrast MRA from being used for follow-up after stenting. Recent in-vitro and in-vivo analysis of one of the more commonly used stenting devices, the Vanguard bifurcated stent graft (Boston Scientific, Oakland, NJ.), have shown these concerns to be unfounded. The nitinol from which the stent is constructed is non-magnetic; there is no torque on the stent from the magnetic field. The very short echo time of less than 2 ms, inherent to fast 3D MRA acquisitions, limits stent-related magnetic susceptibility artifacts, which have been associated with other sequences. Nitinol frame filaments of the stent graft are identifiable on individual sections and reformations as distinct areas of signal void, allowing for a detailed assessment of stent structure. Stent graft deformities are thus easily excluded. Furthermore, the stent lumen can be fully assessed with the exception of one critical area: overlapping platinum markers at the junction between two stent components in one of the iliac legs may simulate the presence of a stenosis (Figure 5.5). Tissues surrounding the stent are also well visualized. Both graft and perigraft leaks are easily recognized on 3D contrast MRA. In fact, a recent study has shown MRA to be more sensitive than CTA in detecting endoleaks. Delayed data sets need to be collected for this purpose.

Clearly, imaging characteristics directly reflect the underlying material used for stent construction. It is therefore important to point out that favorable imaging experience remains limited to selected nitinol or platinum based stents. Nevertheless, these data suggest that 3D contrast MRA may evolve into the imaging modality of choice for post-stenting follow-up.

Dissection of the Abdominal Aorta

Dissection of the aorta occurs when the intima is interrupted and peels away from the media, allowing blood to enter the aortic wall and separate layers of media. It usually occurs between the middle and outer third of the media. Dissection is the most frequent and most important acute disease involving the abdominal aorta. Without treatment, it can be fatal. With prompt diagnosis and appropriate therapy, however, the majority of patients survive.

In a type B (Stanford classification) dissection, separation of the intima and adventitia affects only the descending or abdominal aorta. While there is only one true lumen, several false lumen may exist.

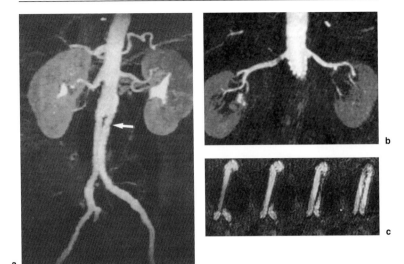

Fig. 5.5. Abdominal Aortic Aneurysm (AAA) Stent.

Clinical Scenario: 51-year-old male 3 months following percutaneous stent grafting of an infrarenal AAA. MRA is performed to document stent graft patency and rule out stent-related complications (stent dislocation or distortion, perigraft leaks).

Technique: Phased Array Torso Coil, Coronal Acquisition, TR/TE/Flip = 4.0/1.9/ 40°, 0.5 NEX, Field-of-View = 400 × 300 × 110 mm, Matrix = 256 × 192 × 44, no zero interpolation, sequential phase encoding order, Acquisition Time = 28 s. Test bolus for timing delay. Contrast bolus (0.2 mmol/kg) injected at 2 ml/s with an automated injector.

Interpretation: MIP projection permits full assessment of the contrast-enhanced aortic lumen within the stent, thereby documenting stent graft patency (**a**). A wider area of signal loss is seen at the insertion of the iliac stent leg into the aortic stent portion (*arrow*). This reflects the overlap of two radio-opaque platinum markers and should not be mistaken for a stenosis. The low level of artifact on the 3D GRE images permit delineation of stent contours in both the aortic (**b**) and iliac segments (**c**), as seen on coronal source images.

Diagnosis: Normal MRA 3 months following endovascular stenting of an infrarenal AAA. Submitted by Jörg F. Debatin, M.D., Essen.

Type B dissections usually originate in the thoracic aorta just distal to the left subclavian artery and extend a variable distance, sometimes even into the iliac arteries. They may be post-traumatic in origin. Hypertension and long-standing atherosclerosis weaken the aortic wall and predispose to dissection. Hypertension and severe atherosclerosis are the most common risk factors for dissection of the abdominal aorta. Dissection frequently coexists with aneurysmal disease (Figure 5.6).

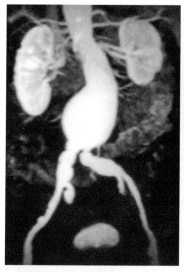
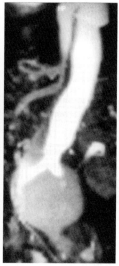

a

b

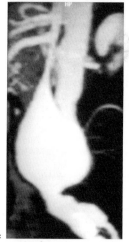

c

Fig. 5.6. Dissecting Abdominal Aortic Aneurysm (AAA).

Clinical Scenario: 76-year-old patient with abdominal pain persisting over a few weeks.

Technique: Phased Array Torso Coil, Coronal Acquisition, 40 contiguous 1.75 mm sections were acquired during a single 26 s breath-hold. Contrast (0.15 mmol/kg) was administered intravenously with a power injector at a rate of 2 ml/s beginning 22 seconds before the start of data acquisition. The time delay was determined with a test bolus.

Interpretation: MIP projection displays a large infrarenal abdominal aneurysm with extension into both common iliac arteries (**a**). Additionally, a dissecting membrane is visualized in the abdominal aorta. The false lumen (larger diameter) is perfused earlier than the true lumen (smaller diameter) of the dissected abdominal aorta. Note a contrast material jet from the false lumen into the aortic aneurysm (**b**). The delayed scan demonstrates both lumen filled with contrast material (**c**).

Diagnosis: Simultaneous appearance of an infrarenal aneurysm and a dissection of the abdominal aorta.

Submitted by Lars Kopka, M.D. and Jens Rodenwaldt, M.D., Göttingen.

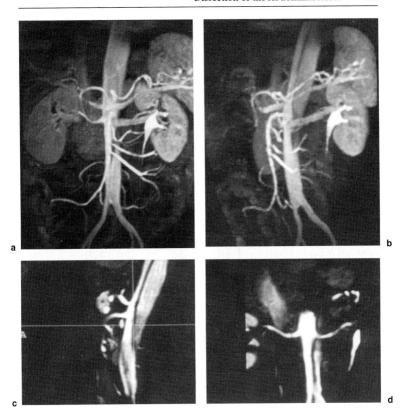

Fig. 5.7. Aortic Dissection.

Clinical Scenario: 72-year-old man with a chronic type B dissection. The patient was referred for 3D MRA to evaluate branch vessel involvement.

Technique: Phased Array Torso Coil, Coronal Acquisition, TR/TE/Flip = 4.0/1.9/ 40°, 0.5 NEX, Field-of-View = 380 × 380 × 110 mm, Matrix = 256 × 192 × 44, no zero interpolation, sequential phase encoding order, Acquisition Time = 28 s. Test bolus for timing delay. Contrast bolus (0.2 mmol/kg) injected at 2 ml/s with an automated injector.

Interpretation: Frontal MIP image (**a**) obscures the dissecting membrane. It is seen to better advantage on the oblique MIP projection (**b**). From MIP images, it is not possible to determine which vessels arise from the true or false lumen. For this determination, individual multiplanar reformations are mandatory. The sagittal reformation (**c**) demonstrates that both the superior mesenteric artery and the celiac trunk arise from the true lumen. Similarly, the coronal reformation (**d**) shows both renal arteries arise from the anteriorly located true lumen.

Diagnosis: Chronic dissection without impairment of flow to parenchymal organs.

Submitted by Jörg F. Debatin, M.D., Essen.

Three-dimensional contrast MRA can provide answers to most questions pertaining to the assessment of a dissection in the abdominal aorta (Figure 5.7). Intimal flaps are easily identified on individual source images as well as multiplanar reformations. Relying exclusively on MIP images can result in diagnostic errors because the intimal membrane may be obscured, resulting in a failure to recognize the dissection (Figure 5.7). In the abdomen, the true lumen is frequently compressed and located around the left posterior aspect of the aorta. The 3D nature of the data set facilitates viewing of branch vessel origins and determines whether the vessels originate from the true or false lumen. Extension of the dissecting flap into a branch vessel should be looked for as this can lead to ischemia of tissues supplied by that branch vessel. The degree of parenchymal enhancement, particularly in the kidneys, can be used as an indicator of whether relative ischemia is present.

Non-invasiveness and high diagnostic accuracy (Table 5.1) allow 3D contrast MRA to emerge as the modality of choice for assessment of aortic dissections. The exam can be repeated with ease, which is important in patients with chronic dissections as they are prone to extension of the dissection, redissection, aneurysm formation, and even aortic rupture.

Aortic Stenosis/Occlusion

Atherosclerotic occlusive disease commonly affects the infrarenal portion of the abdominal aorta and typically extends for a variable distance into iliac and femoral arteries. Atherosclerotic occlusive disease of the aorta may occur if plaques become large or are complicated by hemorrhage. Frequently, the disease progresses to ulceration and/or calcification, which can complicate arterial catheterization and surgical intervention. Diabetes and cigarette smoking dramatically increase the severity of atherosclerotic occlusive disease. Once the aorta reaches a critical degree of atherosclerotic narrowing, it may go on to complete thrombosis. Other causes of aortic stenosis or occlusion include congenital abdominal coarctation and periaortic fibrotic processes, which may rarely be seen following radiation therapy.

Le Riche syndrome (Figure 5.8) is caused by complete aortic occlusion, which usually occurs inferior to the origin of the renal arteries. Patients with this vascular disorder have a classic clinical presentation with gluteal claudication, impotence, and lower extremity wasting. Three-dimensional contrast MRA is preferred over conventional angiog-

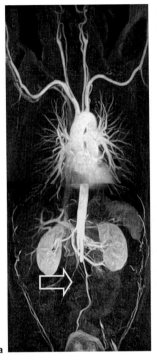

a

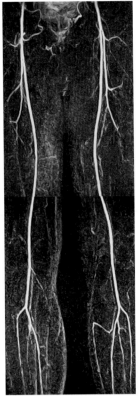

b

Fig. 5.8. LeRiche Syndrome.

Clinical Scenario: Suspected aorto-iliac disease.

Technique: Whole body MRA with Angiosurf.

Interpretation: Occlusion of infrarenal aorta (*open arrow*) as well as common, internal and external iliac arteries. Common femoral arteries are reconstituted via inferior epigastric arteries and via pelvic collaterals including a prominent inferior mesenteric/hemorrhoidal artery. Runoff arteries are normal. Whole body MRA is the preferred technique for evaluating suspected aortic occlusion because it shows the aorto-iliac pathology, collaterals and runoff vessels.

Diagnosis: LeRiche Syndrome.

Submitted by Jörg F. Debatin, M.D., Essen.

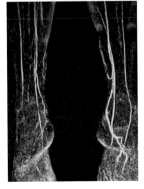

c

raphy for evaluating patients with symptoms of aortic occlusive disease. Conventional catheter angiography in these patients mandates accessing the arterial system via the bracheal approach, which increased the risk for catheter-induced complications. Intravenous injection of paramagnetic contrast is sufficient to display the arterial anatomy proximal, as well as distal, to the occlusion. In addition to depicting the aorta with its stenosis and wall irregularities, 3D contrast MRA is also capable of displaying collateral vessels and distal vascular runoff. These images are adequate for presurgical planning and thereby obviate the need for further invasive imaging.

Pitfalls

Incomplete Coverage of the Anatomy

The tortuosity inherent to the abdominal aorta and its branches may result in inadvertant exclusion of relevant arterial territories from the 3D imaging volume. Therefore, the localizing process should be carefully conducted to ensure coverage of the entire abdominal aorta and all its branches. A first 3D data set can also be collected without paramagnetic contrast as a trial run.

Blurring of Branch Vessel Origins

This artifact is usually caused by respiratory motion. It can be avoided by collecting data in apnea.

Ringing-Artifact in the Aortic Lumen

This represents the most common and potentially harmful artifact. One or more dark lines are seen within the aortic lumen simulating the presence of a dissection. They reflect a change in the T1 of arterial blood during acquisition of the central portion of k-space. The artifacts point to faulty timing of the contrast bolus. Usually the bolus arrives too late so that the plateau phase has not been reached by the time the center of k-space is collected. This occurs less frequently if a centric phase encoded 3D sequence is employed and is entirely eliminated on fast multiphase, time-resolved MRA.

CHAPTER 6

Renal Arteries

Background

Renal artery stenosis has long been recognized as a cause of hypertension and end-stage renal disease. Renovascular disease is implicated as the underlying cause in 1–5% of patients with hypertension and 5–15% of patients with end-stage renal disease entering dialysis each year. A large autopsy study has shown a renal artery stenosis incidence of 10% in patients with diabetes mellitus in combination with hypertension, 22% in patients with abdominal aortic aneurysms (AAA), and 45% in patients with peripheral vascular disease. Availability of cost-effective treatment options, including percutaneous transluminal angioplasty, stents, and surgical revascularization, has motivated an extensive search for a non-invasive, cost-effective alternative to DSA, the traditional standard of reference.

Ultrasound is limited in its resolution, consistency (large inter-operator variability) and accuracy. Furthermore, ultrasound does not provide images that can be used to plan therapy. CT-angiography exposes the patient to ionizing radiation and the risk of contrast-induced nephrotoxicity. Particularly, in patients with renal disease this should be avoided. Magnetic resonance imaging has been considered promising due to its higher resolution, higher accuracy, reproducibility and non-invasiveness. In addition, as previously indicated, paramagnetic contrast agents are free of nephrotoxicity.

Multiple imaging strategies, including 2D and 3D TOF and phase contrast sequences, have been evaluated for renal artery MRA. Most studies reported some success in the assessment of proximal renovascular disease with these flow-based techniques. However, the widespread clinical application of MRA, prior to the introduction of intravenous administration of paramagnetic contrast agents, had been hampered by in-plane flow saturation, respiratory motion, and limited spatial resolution. 3D contrast MRA overcomes these limitations (Figure 6.1). Renal arteries are assessed in their entirety, including major segmental branch vessels and small accessory renal arteries. In addition, speed, operator independence, high spatial and contrast resolution, and lack of side effects have contributed to making 3D contrast MRA the technique of choice for detecting renovascular disease.

Technique

Diagnostic image quality mandates high-resolution (512 matrix) data acquisition in apnea. This, in turn, requires short acquisition times, and thus high performance gradient systems. Non-breath-hold 3D contrast MRA of the renal arteries should not be performed as significant lesions are easily overlooked and normal arteries may falsely appear stenotic due to image corruption by respiratory motion artifacts. Informing the patient about the importance of breath-holding prior to the exam increases patient cooperation. The depth of inspiration can be practiced so that a mask acquisition can be obtained pre-contrast for subtraction. Patients should also be told when to expect breath-holding to begin. Some may benefit from oxygen and hyperventilation immediately prior to the breath-hold so they can more easily suspend breathing for the entire scan.

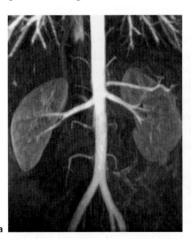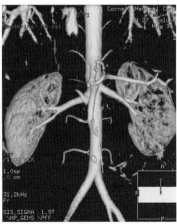

Fig. 6.1. Normal Renal MRA. (**a**) MIP, (**b**) volume rendering with shaded surface.

Patients should be imaged in the supine position using a torso phased array coil for more signal-to-noise. The torso surface coil should permit at least 36 cm in craniocaudal coverage. This is important to avoid missing collateral arteries which may originate from as low as the common iliac arteries. A multiplanar localizer should be acquired to properly plan the prescription of the 3D MRA volume acquisition. The same localizing sequence may also be used to prescribe the timing bolus scan. Ideally, this localizer is collected with the same degree of inspiration as the following 3D contrast MRA acquisition so that the position of the organs does not change.

The repetition time of the 3D acquisition needs to be sufficiently short to permit collection of a large enough 3D volume to encompass the renal arteries with at least 160 phase encoded steps (ky). Twenty-eight contiguous sections, each 2.5 mm–3 mm thick, represent the minimum volume; 2-fold zero-padding in the slice direction is mandatory and the frequency encoding should be 512. Acquisition of more sections with higher resolution is preferable as it allows for thinner sections and more extensive anterior and posterior coverage. This results in a higher through-plane resolution and a greater margin for positioning error.

Since the data acquisition time is short, properly timing the intravenous infusion of paramagnetic contrast is especially important. The exact timing protocol needs to be individualized for each patient using either a timing bolus scan or an automated triggering algorithm. Guessing the contrast travel time will rarely be as good as a precisely timed scan, and about 20% of renal 3D MRA exams may be uninterpretable. If automated triggering is not available, a timing sequence should be employed following administration of a small 1–2 ml contrast test bolus. With automatic triggering (SmartPrep) or Fluoroscopic triggering, it is useful to recess the absolute center of k-space 3–4 seconds in from the beginning of 3D data acquisition to avoid ringing artifact from premature triggering (Figure 6.2).

Different doses of paramagnetic contrast ranging between 0.1 mmol/kg and 0.3 mmol/kg have been advocated for 3D contrast MRA of the renal arteries. A dose beyond 0.2 mmol/kg probably does not improve diagnostic accuracy. Currently most centers use a dose of 0.1 mmol/kg–0.2 mmol/kg or a fixed volume of 20–30 ml independent of weight.

The 3D contrast MRA volume acquisition should be prescribed in the coronal plane. Most new scanners may allow obliquing the orientation of the coronal volume to align with the aorta for the most efficient coverage of the anatomy with the smallest number of sections. The top of

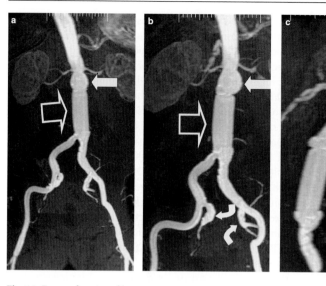

Fig. 6.2. Recessed center of k-space.

Clinical Scenario: A 69-year-old male post aneurysm repair.

Technique: Coronal Acquisition, TR/TE/Flip = 6.2/1.2/30°, Field-of-View = 380 × 380 × 96, Matrix = 512 × 160 × 30 with 2-fold zero-filling in the slice direction. 30 ml Gd was hand injected over 15 seconds and timed with SmartPrep using centric view ordering with the absolute center of k-space recessed 4 seconds from the beginning of the scan.

Interpretation: Coronal MIP (**a**), Oblique MIP (**b**) and sub-volume sagittal MIP (**c**) show tube graft repair of infra-renal abdominal aortic aneurysm (*open arrow*). A recurrent aneurysm is developing above the proximal anastomosis (*arrow*). Also note fusiform aneurysms of the internal iliac arteries (*curved arrows*). Note that aorta, renal arteries and iliac arteries are all uniformly enhanced with no venous contamination. This is facilitated by recessing the absolute center of k-space in from the beginning of the scan so that it is obtained during peak contrast enhancement; venous contamination is avoided by using the leading edge of Gd bolus arrival to acquire data prior to the absolute center.

Diagnosis: Recurrent aneurysm above proximal anastomosis of AAA tube graft repair. Submitted by Richard Watts, Ph.D., Bernard Ho and Minh T. Chao, New York.

the coronal volume should be above the origin of the celiac trunk and preferably below the heart to avoid cardiac motion artifacts. The volume should extend anteriorly to encompass the entire aorta and posteriorly at least to the mid-kidney on both sides. Including all renal parenchyma is preferable as this allows contrast-enhanced imaging of any unsuspected renal masses or anomalies (Figure 6.3). The inferior extent should include the common iliac arteries as accessory renal arteries may arise

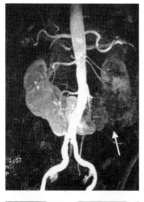

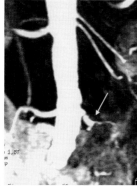

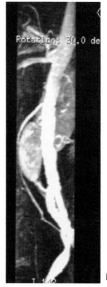

Fig. 6.3. Horseshoe Kidney.
Clinical Scenario: 55-year-old male with hypertension and hematuria.
Technique: Coronal acquisition, TR/TE/FLIP = 8.7/1.4/45°, Field-of-View = 360 × 270 × 80 mm, matrix = 512 × 192 × 24, zero interpolation in phase and slice direction, sequential acquisition order, acquisition time = 30 s. Dose-timing scan used for contrast administration. 38 ml Gd contrast agent.
Interpretation: (**a**) Coronal view demonstrates large horseshoe kidney with multiple renal arteries. An area of hypoperfusion is seen in the left inferior renal parenchyma (arrow). (**b**) Lateral view demonstrates renal parenchymal tissue anterior to aorta, with superior mesenteric artery draped over renal parenchyma. (**c**) Magnified view demonstrates multiple renal arteries with encasement of inferior left renal artery by renal mass.
Diagnosis: Horseshoe kidney with renal cell adenocarcinoma.
Submitted by Thomas M. Grist, M.D., Madison.

this low. A field-of-view of about 34–40 cm is generally sufficient to cover this anatomy without excessive aliasing. To assure optimal coverage of the desired anatomy, it is useful to acquire a 3D data set prior to contrast administration. These pre-contrast images can later also be used as a baseline for image subtractions.

Complementary Sequences

Renal MRA protocols should include a sequence for asssessing the renal parenchyma. A delayed 3D sequence collected about 60 seconds post-contrast administration is well suited for that purpose. Alternatively, a 2D multiplanar spoiled GRE image set may be acquired. Renal masses, cysts, and other pathologies, such as infarcts, are well visualized on these images (Figure 6.4). In addition, particularly in patients with arterial hypertension, the adrenal glands should be assessed for possible presence of a mass. Finally a delayed coronal 3D gradient echo sequence is useful to assess excretion of Gd, another indicator of renal function (Figure 6.5). Use of a wide bandwidth to get the shortest possible echo time to avoid T2* effects of highly concentrated Gd in the collecting system is recommended. A higher flip angle may also be useful. Typically, a delay of about 10 minutes after Gd injection is optimal. If there is too little Gd excretion to get an adequate assessment, 10 mg–20 mg lasix IV may be useful.

MR also offers a functional approach to the assessment of vascular disease. It is possible to measure renal arterial flow with gated, breath-held, cine phase contrast (Figure 6.6). This sequence should be performed following coronal 3D contrast MRA to take advantage of the increased signal-to-noise ratio provided by the paramagnetic agent. For measuring flow, renal arteries need to be imaged in a plane perpendicular to their course, transecting them proximal to the first bifurcation. Typically, a sagittal or sagittal-oblique imaging plane is utilized and the scan is made short enough to complete in a breath-hold. Flow volumes per unit time can be derived from these images (Figure 6.6). These data have been shown to correlate well with para amino hippurate (PAH) clearance-based renal flow volume determinations. Based on these data, a renal index relating flow volume to renal mass can be determined. Furthermore, flow profiles may be determined based on flow velocities over time. These functional data may help select patients for revascularization and aid quantifying the therapeutic effectiveness of these procedures. In clinical practice, however, these techniques do not play a central role.

In several centers, 3D contrast MRA is complimented by 3D phase contrast acquisitions (Figure 6.7). Areas of hemodynamically significant stenosis are detected by their associated turbulence, seen as a signal void on 3D phase contrast images. The presence of a signal void at, or immediately downstream from, a stenosis indicates that there is a pressure drop across the stenosis (Figure 6.7). For the 3D phase contrast to be optimally sensitive

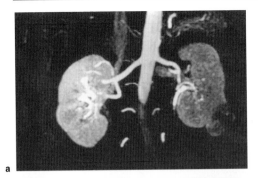

a

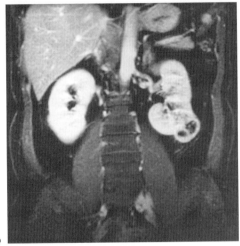

b

Fig. 6.4. Other Cause for Arterial Hypertension.

Clinical Scenario: 53-year-old female with progressively uncontrollable arterial hypertension referred for MRA of the renal arteries to exclude renal artery stenosis.

Technique: Phased Array Torso Coil, Coronal Acquisition, TR/TE/Flip = 4.0/1.8/40°, 0.5 NEX, Field-of-View = 380 × 380 × 88 mm, Matrix = 256 × 192 × 44, no zero interpolation, Sequential Phase Encoding Order, Acquisition Time = 26 s. Test bolus for timing delay. Contrast bolus (0.2 mmol/kg) injected at 2 ml/s. Subsequently, 2D multiplanar GRE (MPSPGR) TR/TE/Flip = 150/1.8/60°, Fat Saturation.

Interpretation: MIP projection of a 3D Contrast MRA (**a**) revealed normal renal arteries without evidence of stenosis. Upon closer inspection, a heterogeneous mass is seen arising from the lower pole of the left kidney. The presence of a mass is confirmed on the 2D MPSPGR image (**b**), collected following the 3D contrast MRA data set.

Diagnosis: Renal cell carcinoma arising from left lower pole.

Submitted by Jörg F. Debatin, M.D., Essen.

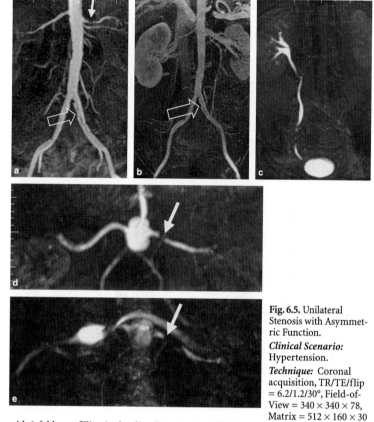

Fig. 6.5. Unilateral Stenosis with Asymmetric Function.

Clinical Scenario: Hypertension.

Technique: Coronal acquisition, TR/TE/flip = 6.2/1.2/30°, Field-of-View = 340 × 340 × 78, Matrix = 512 × 160 × 30 with 2-fold zero filling in the slice direction. 30 ml Gd injected by hand as fast as possible and timed with (**a**) followed by a venous phase (**b**) and a 10 minute delayed phase (**c**). Post-Gd axial phase contrast (**e**) was obtained with a VENC = 40 cm/s.

Interpretation: Coronal MIP (**a**) shows a severe left renal artey stenosis (*arrow*). Venous phase (**b**) shows the left kidney is smaller than the right and there is loss of the normal cortico-medullary differentiation in the ischemic left kidney. Delayed phase (**c**) shows asymmetry in Gd excretion indicating decreased left renal function. Axial sub-volume MIP (**d**) shows the left renal artery stenosis (*arrow*) is near occlusive. On post Gd 3D phase contrast MRA (**e**) there is a jet of dephasing causing over-estimation of the severity of the stenosis making it appear like a several cm occlusion. These factors all point to a hemodynamically significant stenosis which was confirmed at stent placement to have a 60 mm pressure gradient. Also note focal iliac artery dissection (*open arrow* in **a** & **b**)

Diagnosis: Hemodynamically significant left renal artery stenosis.

Submitted by Martin Prince, M.D., Ph.D., New York.

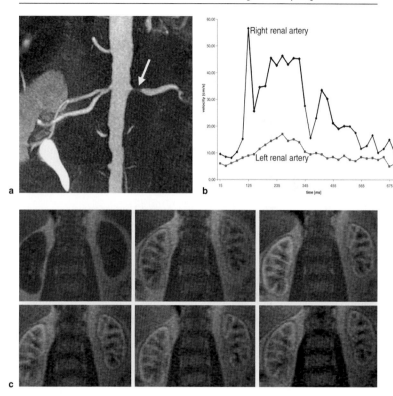

Fig. 6.6. Renal Artery Flow and Perfusion.

Clinical Scenario: Hypertension.

Technique: 3D MRA with parallel imaging (iPAT, acceleration factor 2): Coronal acquisition, TR/TE = 3.8/1.5, Field-of-View = 380 × 320 (87% FoV), Matrix = 512 × 512 × 80 (80% phase resolution) = Spatial resolution (mm) 1 × 1 × 0.8, Acquisition time = 26s, injection of 15 ml gadobutrol at 2ml/s, timed using a test bolus. Perfusion imaging with saturation recovery: Coronal acquisition, TR/TE = 250/1.0, Field-of-View = 400 × 348 (87%FoV), 4 slices, Matrix = 256 × 128 (50% phase resolution), Acquisition time / phase = 1.0 s, Total acquisition time = 60s, injection of 0.05mmol/kg gadobutrol at 2ml/s.

Interpretation: Coronal MIP (**a**) shows high-grade left renal artery stenosis exceeding 90% (*arrow*) and a mild right renal artery stenosis. Flow curves (**b**) show loss of early systolic velocity peak in the left renal artery while the right renal artery has a normal flow profile. The dynamic perfusion images (**c**) reveal delayed and decreased left renal perfusion.

Diagnosis: Hemodynamically and functionally significant left renal artery stenosis.

Submitted by Stefan Schoenberg, M.D., Munich, Lars Johanson, M.S., Uppsala.

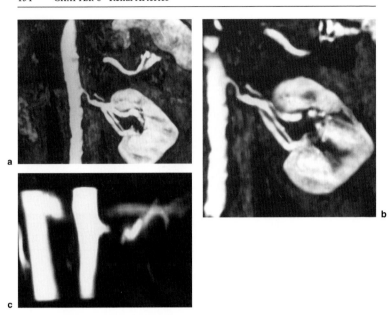

Fig. 6.7. Utility of combining 3D Contrast MRA and 3D Phase Contrast MRA to evaluate Renal Arteries.

Clinical Scenario: 43-year-old male post right nephrectomy with rising serum creatinine and increasingly difficult-to-control hypertension.

Technique: Phased Array Torso Coil, Coronal Acquisition, TR/TE/Flip = 14/2.6/45°, Field-of-View = 320 × 320 × 42 mm, Matrix = 256 × 128 × 12, Sequential Ordering of k-space, Acquisition Time = 29 s, with bolus injection of 40 ml paramagnetic contrast at 2 ml/s timed empirically. Subsequently, axial 3D phase contrast MRA (TR/TE/Flip = 20/8/35°; Field-of-View = 320 × 320 × 70 mm; VENC = 30 cm/s, speed images reconstructed with phase difference method.

Interpretation: Thick (**a**) and thin (**b**) subvolume coronal oblique MIPs show an atherosclerotic abdominal aorta and a proximal left renal artery stenosis. Coronal oblique MIP from the 3D phase contrast MRA data (**c**) shows a short region of complete signal drop-out (severe dephasing) at, and just distal to, the stenosis. This dephasing is a marker of swirling, turbulent flow and indicates the presence of a pressure gradient across the stenosis.

Diagnosis: Hemodynamically significant left renal artery stenosis.

Submitted by Martin R. Prince, M.D., Ph.D., New York. Reprinted with permission from Radiology 1997;205:128-136.

to turbulent flow, the echo time should be 8 ms and the velocity encoded value (VENC) should be 25 cm/s – 50 cm/s. For patients under 65 years of age with normal cardiac function, a slightly higher VENC of 40 cm/s - 60 cm/s is recommended. For older patients exceeding 70 years of age, as well as for patients with congestive heart failure, elevated serum creatinine, or aortic aneurysmal disease, a VENC of 30 cm/s is more appropriate.

Clinical Applications

There are several reasons for the clinical acceptance of 3D contrast MRA:
1. Image data are acquired rapidly during a breath-hold, which eliminates respiratory motion artifacts and shows the differential contrast enhancement between normal and ischemic kidneys;
2. The 3D acquisition provides high spatial resolution with near isotropic voxels, permitting assessment of both renal arteries in their entirety, major branch vessels, and even small accessory renal arteries in any obliquity;
3. The data can be acquired in the coronal plane using a large field-of-view, thereby permitting a full display of the aorto-renal-iliac arterial morphology.

These attributes have resulted in a high diagnostic accuracy, as documented in numerous studies (Table 6.1) and a meta-analysis study.

Table 6.1. Diagnostic performance of 3D contrast MRA for Renal Arteries

Author	Year	Technique	# of Patients	Sensitivity	Specificity
Prince	1995	3D-Gd	19	100 %	93 %
Grist	1996	3D-Gd	35	89 %	95 %
Snidow	1996	3D-Gd	47	100 %	89 %
Holland	1996	3D-Gd	63	100 %	100 %
Steffens	1997	3D-Gd	50	96 %	95 %
Rieumont	1997	3D-Gd	30	100 %	71 %
De Cobilii	1997	3D-Gd	55	100 %	97 %
Arlart	1997	3D-Gd	24	66.6 %	100 %
Bakker	1998	3D-Gd	50	97 %	92 %
Hany	1998	3D-Gd	103	93 %	90 %
Thornton	1999	3D-Gd	62	88 %	98 %
Schoenberg	1999	3D-Gd	26	94–100 %	96–100 %
Thornton	1999	3D-Gd	42	100 %	98 %
Cambria	1999	3D-Gd + PC	25	97 %	100 %
Thornton	1999	3D-Gd	42	100 %	98 %
Steinborn	1999	3D-Gd	27	75-98 %	98-100 %

$\rightarrow$

Table 6.1. Continued

Author	Year	Technique	# of Patients	Sensitivity	Specificity
Ghantous	1999	3D-Gd	12	–	100 %
Gilfeather	1999	3D-Gd	54	*	*
Marchand	2000	3D-Gd		88-100 %	71-100 %
Shetty	2000	3D-Gd	51	96 %	92 %
Winterer	2000	3D-Gd	23	100 %	98 %
Bongers	2000	3D-Gd	43	100 %	94 %
		Captopril Renogram		85 %	71 %
Volk	2000	Time resolved 3D-Gd	40	93 %	83 %
Oberholzer	2000	3D-Gd at T1	23	96 %	97 %
Korst	2000	3D-Gd	38	100 %	85 %
De Corbilii	2000	3D-Gd	45	94 %	93 %
		Doppler US		71 %	93 %
Mittal	2001	3D-Gd	26	96 %	93 %
Voiculescu	2001	3D-Gd	36	96 %	86 %
Quanadli	2001	3D-Gd	41	97 %	64 %
		Doppler + Captopril		69 %	82 %
		Captopril Scintigraphy		41 %	82 %
Masunaga	2001	3D-Gd	39	100 %	100 %
Voiculescu	2001		36	96 %	86 %
Hood	2002	3D-Gd	21	100 %	74 %
		3D-Gd+PC		100 %	100 %
Jha	2002	3D-Gd	64	89.4 %	94.1 %
Schoenberg	2002	3D-Gd+flow	43	Kappa = 0.75	

*Accuracy assessed by inter-observer agreement, standard deviation of MRA = 6.9 %, Angio = 2.5 %

Renal Artery Stenosis

Most renal artery stenoses are due to atherosclerosis (Figure 6.8). In the typical diffuse form, atherosclerotic disease in the aorta overflows into the renal artery origins, thereby compromising blood flow. These atherosclerotic stenoses are often progressive, tend to involve the ostium or proximal third of the renal artery, and are frequently eccentric. The other significant cause of renal artery stenosis is fibromuscular dysplasia (FMD). FMD has several presentations depending upon the layer of blood vessel wall that is affected. In the most common type, medial hyperplasia, the artery develops a characteristic pattern of webs and small aneurysms called, "string of beads" (Figure 6.9). Medial hyperplasia affects younger patients and women more frequently than men. In contrast to atherosclerotic stenoses, FMD tends to affect the mid- and

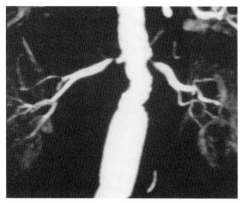

Fig. 6.8. Bilateral Renal Artery Stenoses.

Clinical Scenario: 65-year-old male with renal insufficiency, congestive heart failure, and hypertension. The patient had a heart transplant for ischemic cardiomyopathy.

Technique: Body Coil, Coronal Acquisition, TR/TE/Flip = 8/2.1/60°, Field-of-View = 360 × 270 × 88 mm, Matrix = 512 × 192 × 44, 1 NEX, zero filling interpolation of slices, Sequential Phase Encoding Order, Acquisition Time = 28 s, test bolus for timing scan, 40 ml paramagnetic contrast injected at 1.4 ml/s.

Interpretation: The MIP image demonstrates severe bilateral ostial and proximal renal artery stenosis with significant aortic atherosclerotic plaque.

Diagnosis: Bilateral renal artery stenosis causing renal insufficiency. A bilateral renal endarterectomy was performed, based on the MRA, resulting in improved renal function and resolution of the congestive heart failure.

Submitted by Thomas M. Grist, M.D., Madison.

distal renal artery. Another form that is more rare, intimal hyperplasia, tends to present in male children with long tubular narrowing of the renal arterial mid-section (Figure 6.10).

Diagnostic performance of 3D contrast MRA in the detection of renal arterial disease has been extensively evaluated. Most of these studies employed conventional angiography or digital subtraction angiography (DSA) as the gold standard. The sensitivity of 3D contrast MRA has been reported to vary between 88%–100%, specificity between 71%-100% (Table 6.1). A large meta-analysis in Annals of Internal Medicine, 2001; 135:401-411 found 3D Gd MRA equivalent to CTA in diagnosing renal artery stenosis and superior to ultrasound, Captopril renography and MRA with TOF instead of Gd.

Analysis of some of the discrepant results between conventional catheter angiography and 3D contrast MRA calls into question the validity of using DSA as the gold standard. The limitations inherent to conventional angiographic projection techniques are well known. Even with selective DSA and multiple projections, eccentric and orificial stenoses can be overlooked. The 3D nature of the MRA image set overcomes this

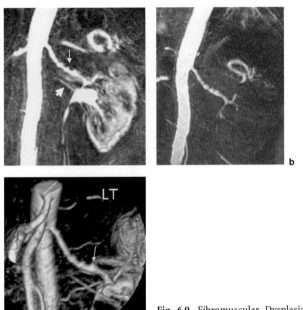

Fig. 6.9. Fibromuscular Dysplasia: Impact of Acquisition Parameters.

Clinical Scenario: 35-year-old woman with hypertension. MRA ordered initially as diagnostic tool (a), then one year later for follow-up of potential complications (b).

Technique: Images demonstrate the impact of acquisition parameters on spatial resolution and image quality. (a) Initial diagnostic MRA exam performed with sequential acquisition, larger field-of-view. Image parameters included TR/TE/flip = 6.0/1.4/45°, Field-of-View = 360 × 270 × 80 mm, Matrix = 512 × 192 x 20, zero interpolation end phase in slice direction, sequential or acquisition order. (b) Performed with high-resolution, near isotropic imaging including TR/TE/FLIP = 4.7/1.0/30°, field-of-view = 280 × 280 × 72 mm, matrix = 320 × 192 × 32, zero interpolation end phase in slice direction, elliptical-centric phase encoding order. Dose-timing was used in both cases, 40 ml Gd-contrast agent.

Interpretation: (a) The initial diagnostic MRA demonstrates irregular stenoses mixed with aneurysmal enlargement of left renal artery consistent with medial fibroplastic type of fibromuscular dysplasia. In addition, however, contrast agent in collecting system from dose-timing scan obscures segmental renal artery. (b) Elliptical-centric scan demonstrates higher spatial resolution due to a combination of smaller field-of-view, thinner slices, and higher matrix size. Note the absence of renal venous enhancement seen with elliptical centric ordering. (c) Volume-rendered image of follow-up MRA demonstrates left renal artery aneurysm (arrow).

Diagnosis: Fibromuscular dysplasia.

Submitted by Sean Fain, Ph.D., and Thomas M. Grist, M.D., Madison.

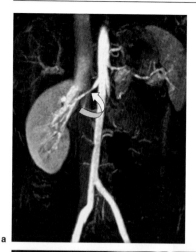

a

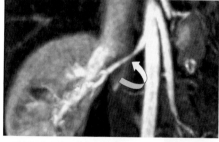

b

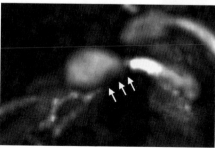

c

Fig. 6.10. Intimal Hyperplasia.

Clinical Scenario: 14-year-old male with history of left nephrectomy for FMD and now has recurrent hypertension.

Technique: Coronal Acquisition, TR/TE/Flip = 6.2/1.2/45°, Field-of-View = 360×360×84, Matrix = 256 × 160 × 32. 20 ml Gd injected by hand and timed with SmartPrep. Post Gd 3D phase contrast MRA (c) obtained with VENC = 50 cm/s.

Interpretation: Coronal MIP (**a**) and subvolume MIP (**b**) show mid right renal artery moderate-to-severe stenosis (*curved arrow*). Axial 3D phase contrast MRA shows dephasing of signal (*arrows*) in the region of the stenosis causing the appearance of total occlusion. This dephasing indicates the stenosis is hemodynamically significant. At surgery, multiple thin webs were identified in the mid-renal artery and histo-pathology revealed intimal hyperplasia which is known to typically cause long tubular mid-renal artery narrowing in young males.

Diagnosis: Intimal Hyperplasia with hemodynamically significant stenosis.

Submitted by Martin Prince, M.D., Ph.D., New York.

limitation by permitting interactive reformatting to find the optimal obliquity for demonstrating these lesions.

Three-dimensional contrast MRA permits visualization of renal artery pathology affecting both the proximal as well as distal renal arteries. Changes associated with fibromuscular dysplasia are seen on reformations but may be partially obscured on MIPs (Figure 6.9) if the resolution is insufficient.

Once a stenosis is identified, the information on symmetry of kidney size, parenchymal thickness Gd excretion as well as the presence of turbulent dephasing and post-stenotic dilatation should be used to assess the hemodynamic significance of the stenosis. Also be aware of other causes of hypertension such as adrenal tumors, juxtaglomerular cell tumor, page kidney (Figure 6.11), etc.

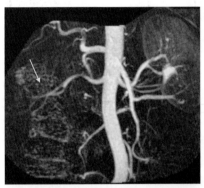

a

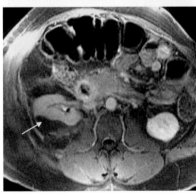

b

Fig. 6.11. Hypertension, other causes.

Clinical Scenario: 42-year-old male with marked hypertension. Recent history of motor vehicle accident.

Technique: (a) Coronal acquisition, TR/TE/flip = 4.7/1.0/30°, Field-of-View = 280 × 280 × 96 mm, Matrix = 320 × 192 × 32, zero interpolation end phase in slice direction, elliptical-centric phase encoding order. Dose timing used for contrast timing, 30 cc Gd. (b) Fat-suppressed T1 weighted gradient echo scan in axial plane following contrast administration.

Interpretation: (a) The MRA image demonstrates poor perfusion of the right kidney relative to the left, with little excretion of Gd contrast agent following dose-timing scan (arrow). (b) Axial gradient echo image demonstrates subcapsular hematoma (arrow) with compression of the right renal parenchyma, consistent with hypertension associated with "Page" kidney.

Diagnosis: Subcapsular hematoma with hypertension and poor perfusion of right kidney.

Submitted by Thomas M. Grist, M.D., Madison.

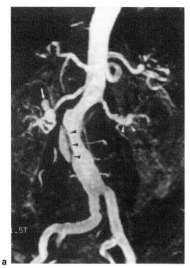

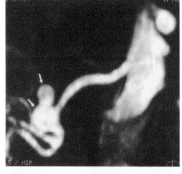

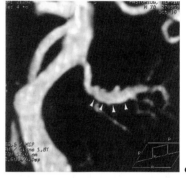

Fig. 6.12. Renal Artery Aneurysms.

Clinical Scenario: 70-year-old male presenting emergently with hypertension and back pain.

Technique: Coronal Acquisition, TR/TE/Flip = 5.2/1.2/45°, 0.5 NEX, Field-of-View = 360 ×360×94 mm, Matrix = 256×128×36, Centric Ordering of k-space, Acquisition Time = 27 s, 40 ml paramagnetic contrast infused at 2 ml/s and timed with SmartPrep.

Interpretation: Coronal (**a**) and oblique subvolume MIPs (**b, c**) show bilateral distal renal artery aneurysms. On the distal right renal artery there are two saccular aneurysms (*arrow*). The left renal artery has fusiform aneurysmal dilatation distally (*white arrowheads*). Note the aneurysmal dilatation of the infra-renal abdominal aorta with a focal dissection (*black arrowheads*). The dissection likely accounts for the patient's emergent presentation with back pain.

Diagnosis: Bilateral renal artery aneurysms and infrarenal aortic dissection.

Submitted by Martin R. Prince, M.D., Ph.D., New York.

Renal Arterial Aneurysm

Aneurysms of the renal arteries can occur as a manifestation of atherosclerotic disease (Figure 6.12). They are also seen in the presence of FMD, neurofibromatosis, and polyarteritis nodosa. Although no systematic series has been reported, in our experience, aneurysms involving the main renal arteries are seen well on 3D contrast MRA but the smaller, intraparenchymal aneurysms of polyarteritis nodosa may not be as reliably detected. The three-dimensional nature of the data set is most helpful in evaluating the neck of the aneurysm. Again, interactive viewing of reformations is crucial for determining whether the aneurysm is saccular or fusiform in nature. The latter differentiation may have therapeutic implications as it helps triage patients to percutaneous coiling techniques, open surgery or medical management with frequent follow-up imaging.

Renal Transplant Donors

Defining renal vascular anatomy is an integral component in the evaluation of potential living-related kidney donors. Prior to harvesting a kidney, it is important to make sure that the donor will be left with a normal kidney. Failure to identify accessory renal arteries before surgery can complicate the transplantation procedure and may compromise the outcome. Accurate determination of number, length, and location of renal arteries is essential for proper surgical planning, especially with the minimally invasive harvesting techniques. Similarly, it is important to identify anatomic variation in the renal venous anatomy.

Three-dimensional contrast MRA is well suited for this task. The large coronal acquisition plane assures visualization of accessory renal arteries originating from the lower aspect of the abdominal aorta or common iliac arteries (Figure 6.3). The lack of in-plane saturation enables visualization of even very small vessels. To fully exploit the potential of contrast-enhanced 3D MRA for the detection of accessory renal arteries, it is necessary to analyze image data in the reformation mode. The data must be viewed in both the coronal and axial planes. Axial reformation allows easy differentiation between lumbar arteries, accessory renal arteries, and overlying mesenteric arterial branches.

Renal Transplants

Arterial inflow stenosis is an important correctable cause of renal allograft failure. Early diagnosis allows salvaging the allograft by either angioplasty or surgical revascularization. For a long time, the standard of reference for detecting transplant arterial stenosis has been conventional catheter angiography. Three-dimensional contrast MRA now represents a safer, less invasive alternative (Figure 6.13). It is relatively operator-inde-

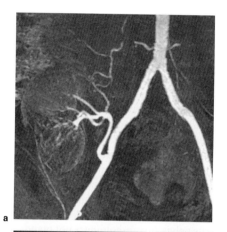

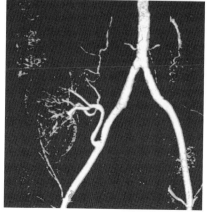

Fig. 6.13. Normal Transplant Renal Artery. Coronal MIP (**a**) and Volume Rendered image (**b**) show a widely patent transplant renal artery with a widely patent anastomosis to the external iliac artery. The MIP is better for identifying stenoses and the volume rendered image is better for displaying the three-dimensional relationship of the arteries. Submitted by Thomas M. Grist, M.D., Madison

pendent and provides high-resolution angiographic images that depict pelvic transplant arterial venous and parenchymal anatomy in a manner analogous to conventional contrast arteriography.

Prior to imaging a renal transplant patient, conventional pelvic films, if available, should be reviewed to identify any metal clips that may create artifacts on MR images. If many clips are present, a wide bandwidth with the shortest possible echo time should be used or alternative studies could be considered. The transplant renal artery examination is performed in a manner similar to native renal artery imaging but shifted lower into the pelvis to cover the transplant kidney. Before injecting contrast, an axial T2-weighted sequence with fat saturation is useful to assess for perinephric fluid collections (urinomas, lymphoceles, and hematomas) and hydronephrosis. Three-dimensional contrast MRA is performed in the coronal plane encompassing the lower abdominal aorta and extending down to just below the femoral heads. Generally, about 30–40 sections (interpolated to 80 sections with zero padding), each 2.5 mm or less, are sufficient to include the aorta and the entire transplant kidney. Care must be taken to extend the posterior coverage sufficiently to include tortuous common and internal iliac arteries. Also be sure to include the entire external iliac artery because it can be injured at the time of surgery by the surgical clamp (Figure 6.14). Since a transplant kidney may have more than one artery, always look for signs of focal infarction that may suggest occlusion of an accessory artery (Figure 6.15). Since transplant kidneys are located in the pelvis, breath-holding is not mandatory. Post-contrast T1-weighted images should be obtained to assess renal excretion of contrast, which normally is seen within 5 minutes of the intravenous contrast injection.

Proper data analysis requires interactive reformatting to unfold the transplant artery (Figure 6.16). It is especially important to visualize the anastomosis in two perpendicular views because this is where most transplant stenoses are located. Interpretation of source images should also be performed to insure that any apparent signal dropout on MIP images is not due to susceptibility artifacts associated with a metal clip near the transplant anastomosis. The susceptibility artifact has a characteristic feature of complete signal loss in the soft tissues outside the lumen that may extend into the lumen. The focus of signal loss is often associated with a build-up of signal on one margin of the artifact. The transplant renal vein should also be analyzed in a similar fashion on the equilibrium phase images. Since renal transplants in diabetic patients may include a pancreas transplant, this should also be assessed (Figure 6.17).

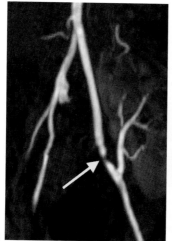

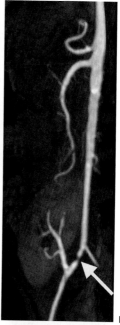

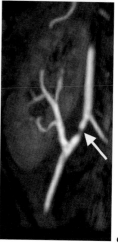

Fig. 6.14. Transplant Artery Inflow Stenosis.

Clinical Scenario: Hypertension post renal transplantation.

Technique: Coronal Acquisition, TR/TE/Flip = 6.2/1.2/45°, Field-of-View = 340 × 340 × 84, Matrix = 256 × 160 × 32. 30 ml Gd injected by hand and timed with SmartPrep.

Interpretation: Subvolume coronal (**a**), sagittal (**b**) and magnified sagittal (**c**) MIPs show a transplant kidney in the left pelvis which enhances with Gd and has a widely patent transplant renal artery. However, there is severe stenosis of the external iliac artery (*arrow*) just proximal to the transplant anastomosis which impedes flow to the kidney. This is known as "clamp injury" because the artery is stenotic at the site of vascular clamp placement during transplantation surgery.

Diagnosis: Iliac artery stenosis proximal to transplant renal artery anastomosis.

Submitted by Martin Prince, M.D., Ph.D., New York.

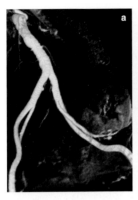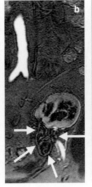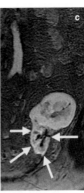

Fig. 6.15. Transplant Kidney with Atrophic Lower Pole.

Clinical Scenario: Hypertensive post-transplantation.

Technique: Coronal acquisition, TR/TE/Flip = 6.2/1.2/30°, Field-of-View = 340 × 340 × 78, Matrix = 512 × 160 × 30 with 2-fold zero filling in the slice direction. 30 ml Gd injected by hand as fast as possible and timed with SmartPrep (**a** and **b**) followed by a venous phase (**c**).

Interpretation: Volume rendered image of arterial phase data (**a**) shows a single widely patent transplant renal artery with end-to-end anastomosis to the left internal iliac artery. Coronal source image of arterial phase (**b**) and venous phase (**c**) show a severely atrophic lower pole (*arrows*) with delayed enhancement. This indicates there likely was a second renal artery supplying the lower pole which was not connected at the time of transplantation.

Diagnosis: Occluded accessory transplant renal artery.

Submitted by Martin Prince, M.D., Ph.D., New York.

Table 6.2. Accuracy of 3D contrast MRA for Renal Transplants

Author	Year	Journal	# of Patients	Sensitivity	Specificity
Johnson	1997	3D Gd	11	67 %	88 %
		3D PC		60 %	76 %
		2D TOF		47 %	81 %
		3D Gd+PC		100 %	100 %
Luk	1999	3D Gd	9	-	100 %
Ferrieros	1999	3D Gd	24	100 %	98 %
Chan	2001	3D Gd	17	100 %	75 %
Huber	2001	3D Gd	41	100 %	93-97 %

Post-Revascularization Renal MRA:

After renal artery stenting, there is artifactual signal dropout at the site of the stent. To avoid misinterpreting stent artifact as occlusion, look for the characteristic spot of bright signal adjacent to the stent signal void

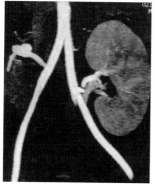

Fig. 6.16. Renal Transplant Patient with Hypertension.

Clinical Scenario: 45-year-old male with hypertension and renal insufficiency following renal transplantation.

Technique: Body Coil, Coronal Acquisition, TR/TE/Flip = 8/2.1/60°, Field-of-View = 360 × 270 × 90 mm, Matrix = 512 × 160 × 60, 1 NEX, zero filling interpolation of slices, Sequential Phase Encoding Order, Acquisition Time = 32 s. Test bolus for timing scan. 40 ml paramagnetic contrast injected at 1.4ml/s.

Interpretation: The MIP image demonstrates a severe stenosis involving the transplant artery.

Diagnosis: Severe renal transplant artery stenosis.

Submitted by Thomas M. Grist, M.D., Madison.

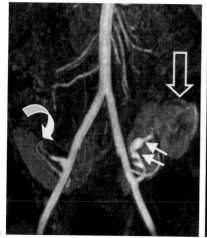
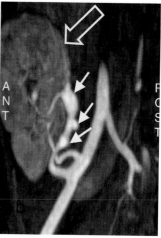

a   b

Fig. 6.17. Transplant Renal Artery Aneurysms.

Clinical Scenario: Post renal-pancreas transplant with multiple episodes of pancreatitis.

Technique: Coronal Acquisition, TR/TE/Flip = 9.2/1.2/45°, Field-of-View = 360 × 360 × 84, Matrix = 256 × 160 × 32. 40 ml Gd injected by hand and timed with SmartPrep.

Interpretation: Coronal MIP (**a**) and subvolume sagittal MIP (**b**) show transplant pancreas (*curved arrow*), transplant kidney (*open arrow*) and multiple transplant renal artery aneurysms (*arrows*) caused by repeated episodes of transplant pancreatitis. Note that all three transplant arteries are widely patent.

Diagnosis: Transplant Pancreatitis with transplant renal artery aneurysms.

Submitted by Martin Prince, M.D., Ph.D., New York.

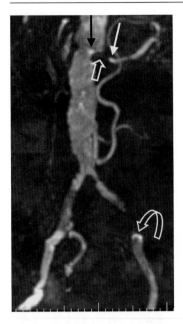

Fig. 6.18. Renal Artery Stent Artifact. Apparent renal artery occlusion (*open arrow*) is actually a stent artifact with the characteristic foci of bright signal (*solid black and solid white arrows*) at the edges of the apparent occlusion. Similar artifact is present at the edge of artifact from a left common iliac stent (*curved open arrow*). Submitted by Martin Prince, M.D., Ph.D., New York.

(Figure 6.18). You can confirm that there is a stent by analyzing the source images for signal drop-out in the tubular stent shape. For stents made of nitinol or platinum, there is minimal metal susceptibility artifact but it may still be difficult to image inside the stent due to RF attenuation by the Faraday Cage effect of the stent mesh. This can sometimes be overcome by using a higher flip angle (Figure 6.19), typically 60°–120°. For patients who have undergone revascularization, it is important to be aware of the new vascular anatomy. Renal endarterectomy patients are the easiest to image. Patients with aorto-renal (Figure 6.20), spleno-renal (Figure 7.9) or hepato-renal (Figure 6.21) grafts may be more difficult since the image volume must be expanded to include the entire course of the renal bypass.

Pitfalls

Incomplete Coverage of the Anatomy

The coronal acquisition needs to be adapted to the patient's anatomy.

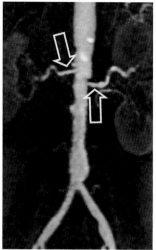

Fig. 6.19. High Flip Angle Imaging of Platinum Stents.

Clinical Scenario: Hypertension post platinum renal artery stents

Technique: Coronal Acquisition, TR/TE/flip = 6.5/1.2/70, Field-of-View = 360 × 360 × 60, Matrix = 256 × 160 × 30, 40 ml Gd injected at 2ml/s by hand and timed with SmartPrep utilizing elliptical centric ordering of k-space

Interpretation: Volume rendered image of bilateral renal artery platinum stents (*open arrows*). Platinum is non-magnetic but the wire produces a Faraday cage effect that attenuates the RF signal. This RF attenuation is overcome by increasing the flip angle. Note the stents are widely patent. Fine wire is visualized projecting in to the aorta lumen.

Diagnosis: Widely patent renal artery stents and 3cm infrarenal abdominal aortic aneurysm.

Submitted by David Trost, M.D., Tom Sos, M.D., and Martin Prince, M.D., Ph.D. New York.

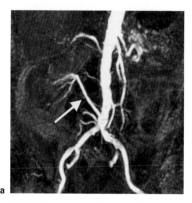
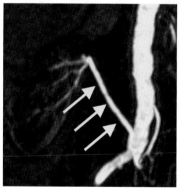

a   b

Fig. 6.20. Aorto-renal Bypass Graft.

Clinical Scenario: Hypertension post renal revascularization.

Technique: Coronal Acquisition, TR/TE/Flip = 6.2/1.2/45°, Field-of-View = 340 × 340 × 84, Matrix = 256 × 160 × 32. 30 ml Gd injected by hand and timed with SmartPrep.

Interpretation: Coronal MIP (**a**) and subvolume MIP (**b**) show an atherosclerotic aorta with revascularization of the right kidney with a bypass graft (*arrows*) from distal aorta to distal native renal artery. Better detail of subvolume MIP reveals the graft to be widely patent with widely patent proximal and distal anastomoses.

Diagnosis: Widely patent aorto-renal bypass graft.

Submitted by Martin Prince, M.D., Ph.D., New York.

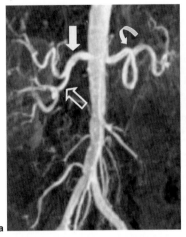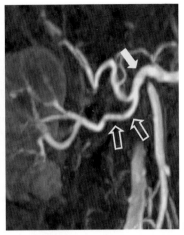

a   b

Fig. 6.21. Hepato-renal Bypass Graft.

Technique: Coronal Acquisition, TR/TE/Flip = 9.2/1.2/45°, Field-of-View = 360 × 360 × 84, Matrix = 256 × 160 × 32. 40 ml Gd injected by hand and timed with SmartPrep.

Interpretation: Coronal MIP (**a**) and subvolume MIP (**b**) show splenic artery (*curved arrow*), common hepatic artery (*solid arrow*) and a widely patent right renal artery anastomosed end-to-end to the gastroduodenal artery (*open arrow*). There are no renal arteries arising from the aorta.

Diagnosis: Widely patent hepato-renal bypass.

Submitted by Qian Dong, M.D., Ann Arbor.

Sometimes, the kidneys are positioned substantially posterior to the aorta. Particularly, if limited to the acquisition of 28 sections, portions of the renal arteries may be cut off. A 3D data set can be collected without paramagnetic contrast first, as a test run, to ensure that all the vascular anatomy of interest is covered before injecting contrast for the arterial phase run.

Blurring of Vessel Origins

This artifact is caused by respiratory motion. It can be avoided by collecting the data in apnea. Practicing breath-holding improves patient compliance.

Ringing-Artifact in the Aortic Lumen

This represents a potentially harmful artifact. One or more dark lines are seen within the arterial lumen, thereby considerably complicating image interpretation. These artifacts point to faulty timing of the contrast bolus. Usually the bolus arrives too late so that the plateau phase has not been reached by the time the center of k-space is collected.

Venous Overlap

This represents the most common artifact. Again, it points to faulty timing of the contrast bolus. The contrast agent has arrived too early. Paramagnetic contrast is present within the arteries and veins while the central portion of k-space is collected. Note that when enhancing veins overlap the renal artery on a MIP, the artery may appear narrower than its true caliber. To compensate for venous overlap, it is crucial to analyze individual source images as well as multiplanar reformats.

Grading Severity of Occlusive Disease

Since MRA tends to overestimate the severity of renal artery stenosis, it can be difficult to tell the difference between a severe stenosis and renal artery occlusion (Figure 6.22). Clinically, however, it may not be an important distinction.

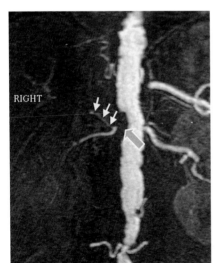

Fig. 6.22. Renal Artery Occlusion. Severely atherosclerotic aorta with aortic plaque overlying renal artery origin causing complete occlusion (*grey arrow*). The occluded right renal artery is reconstituted approximately 1 cm from origin by a small collateral (*arrows*). Also note the asymmetry in renal perfusion with much less enhancement of the right kidney compared to the left.

CHAPTER 7

Mesenteric Arteries

Background

The resolution of 3D contrast MR angiography is sufficient to accurately evaluate the origins of splanchnic arteries, including the celiac axis and superior mesenteric artery (SMA). With fast scanners capable of high resolution imaging during a breath-hold, the inferior mesenteric artery (IMA) may also be evaluated. In patients with complicated anatomy or when the celiac axis and superior mesenteric artery do not arise directly anteriorly from the aorta, the three-dimensional nature of contrast MRA makes it easier to evaluate mesenteric artery origins compared to conventional angiography. Combining 3D contrast MRA with slow measuring techniques allows comprehensive assessment of mesenteric arterial anatomy and function.

Technique

In patients suspected of chronic mesenteric ischemia, patient preparation is not as important for 3D contrast MR angiography as it is for conventional arteriography, computed tomography, or ultrasound. Patients do not need to fast prior to the MR examination. Glucagon (0.5 to 1 mg IV or IM) has been proposed as a means for reducing bowel motion and augmenting celiac flow. However, with a fast scanner capable of high resolution imaging during a breath-hold, arresting bowel motion is not necessary. A high caloric meal prior to the examination can transiently increase splanchnic flow, thereby enhancing visibility of the smaller branch vessels (Figure 7.1). Patients with chronic abdominal symptoms, suspected of acute mesenteric ischemia, should be considered surgical emergencies. MR angiography should only be performed in patients presenting with an acute abdomen under unusual circumstances and only if adequate monitoring is available.

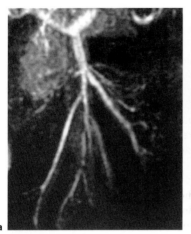 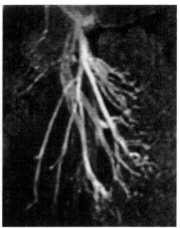

a   b

Fig. 7.1. Increased Mesenteric Flow with Caloric Stimulation.

Clinical Scenario: Normal volunteer.

Technique: Breath-hold 3D contrast MRA with 0.2 mmol/kg gadolinium fasting (**a**) and following caloric stimulation (**b**).

Interpretation: Caloric stimulation increases flow in the splanchnic circulation. Note the improved visualization of superior mesenteric artery branch vessels following caloric stimulation. This phenomenon can be exploited to enhance visualization of splanchnic vasculature on MRA.

Submitted by Jörg F. Debatin, M.D., Essen.

A surgeon should be nearby in the event that the patient rapidly decompensates and requires immediate surgical exploration.

Patients suspected of chronic mesenteric ischemia are often very thin, and thus well-suited to imaging with surface array coils, such as a body array or torso phased array coils. Large patients may be easier to image using the body coil. The patient is placed in the supine position. The arms may be in a comfortable position by the patient's side during the initial localizer sequence but will then need to be elevated over the head for 3D contrast MRA acquisition in the coronal plane. Elevating the arms helps to minimize aliasing and ensures a downhill path for the gadolinium to keep a tight bolus.

Imaging in the coronal plane allows evaluation of the aorta, splanchnic arteries, and portal vein. A partition thickness of 3 or 4 mm or even 5 mm is acceptable if zero padding is available for interpolation. In the absence of an interpolation algorithm, the slice thickness should be kept to less than 3 mm. If the principle clinical question is aimed at determining the presence of stenotic disease involving the proximal mesenteric arteries, then it may be desirable to prescribe the acquisition in the sagittal plane. Aliasing is not as severe for scans in the sagittal plane, so it is possible to prescribe a rectangular field-of-view volume with a high resolution acquisition matrix (e.g. 512×256). Likewise, if a slower magnet is being used, it may be preferable to orient the imaging volume in the sagittal plane so fewer sections are required to cover the aorta, celiac SMA, and IMA. Generally, a short duration breath-hold scan performed in the sagittal plane is superior to a longer duration coronal acquisition that is corrupted by respiratory motion. Imaging parameters should be adjusted to allow for a breath-held data acquisition. Axial imaging may be useful if the primary goal is evaluation of the hepatic arteries, hepatic parenchyma and portal vein (see portal vein chapter). One difficulty with the axial orientation is aliasing in the slice direction, which tends to be severe with the extremely short rf pulses used in 3D contrast MRA. To minimize aliasing, use a coil whose S-I dimension is only slightly larger then the S-I dimension of the imaging volume. Also consider fat saturation or chemically selective fat inversion pulses. This will help minimize unwanted signal from pericardial and abdominal fat wrapping onto the bottom and top of the image volume. A 3D contrast MRA image data set should be collected before, during, and following completion of the IV contrast administration. Pre-contrast images should be checked to be sure the imaging volume is positioned correctly. These images can also be used subsequently for digital subtraction to improve contrast effect.

Proper gadolinium bolus timing is essential for arterial phase acquisitions. This is accomplished with automatic triggering (SmartPrep or care bolus) fluoroscopic triggering (Bolustrak) or with a test bolus to mid abdominal aorta. After arterial phase imaging, a delayed image data set is useful for showing the portal venous and hepatic venous anatomy. If this final data set is corrupted by respiratory motion, it may be useful to have the patient take several deep breaths and repeat an additional breath-held equilibrium phase image data set.

Arterial phase 3D contrast MRA is best analyzed by first performing multiple overlapping MIPs in the coronal plane. Subsequently, reformations and subvolume MIPs can be reconstructed in perpendicular planes through each major abdominal aortic branch vessel, including the celiac trunk, superior mesenteric, and inferior mesenteric arteries. It is also useful to assess the iliac arteries, especially internal iliac arteries, as they may represent an important collateral pathway in patients with chronic mesenteric ischemia. The portal venous and equilibrium phase images are analyzed in a similar manner to evaluate the portal, splenic, superior mesenteric, and hepatic veins. A final consideration is examination of small and large bowel for the expected normal mucosal enhancement following a gadolinium contrast bolus. This will also aid in the identification of more distal, segmental arterial occlusions. In patients suspected of bowel or other mucosal disease, it might be useful to drink diluted barium in advance (e.g. RediCat) to distend and darken the bowel lumen.

Complimentary Sequences

T1- and T2-weighted images covering the liver and upper abdomen may be acquired prior to contrast injection to search for other pathology that might account for the patient's abdominal symptoms. The amount of abdominal intraperitoneal and subcutaneous fat can be assessed on these sequences or on a sagittal T1 or SSFSE locator image. Most patients with mesenteric ischemia will have a scaphoid abdomen and less than 15 mm of subcutaneous fat over the rectus abdominis muscles.

3D contrast MRA provides a morphological analysis of mesenteric arteries. The high incidence of visceral artery stenosis in an asymptomatic population makes it difficult to determine the clinical significance of a morphologic finding. For patients with mesenteric artery stenosis and an equivocal history of mesenteric ischemia (or coexistence of another condition, such as peptic ulcer disease or cholelithiasis, which might account for abdominal symptoms), it may be difficult to predict whether correcting the mesenteric artery stenosis will alleviate symptoms. Functional MR imaging may complement 3D contrast MRA in this regard. Li, et al., used a cine phase contrast sequence to assess blood flow in the superior mesenteric vein (SMV) following caloric stimulation. Post-prandial blood flow is increased within the superior mesenteric vein out of proportion to superior mesenteric artery blood flow with mesenteric ischemia. This effect is due to recruitment of collateral flow. By exploiting the known paramagnetic effect of deoxyhemoglobin, the same investigators also showed close correlation between T2 measurement of blood in the superior mesenteric vein and oxygen saturation in an in-vivo animal model. Identifying low oxygen saturation in the SMV compared to IVC suggests ischemia.

When the celiac and SMA are patent, the possibility of branch vessel stenosis and regional ischemia can be assessed by looking at bowel wall enhancement. Bowel mucosa normally enhances avidly immediately post gadolinium. Regional areas of diminished or delayed bowel enhancement are suggestive of regional ischemia.

The combination of morphologic 3D contrast MRA of the splanchnic vasculature with functional assessment of mesenteric flow holds considerable promise as the emerging modality of choice for evaluation of patients suspected of mesenteric ischemia.

Clinical Applications

Three-dimensional contrast MRA is already capable of displaying the main visceral vessels with excellent diagnostic accuracy (Table 7.1). The spatial resolution achievable with selective catheter angiography remains considerably better for smaller branch vessels. Accordingly, current clinical applications of 3D contrast MRA in the splanchnic circulation focus on clinical situations that require assessment of the proximal celiac axis and SMA, including mesenteric ischemia, visceral artery aneurysms, tumor encasement, anatomic variations, and pre/post liver transplantation (discussed in Chapter 8). Diseases involving primarily the smaller splanchnic branch vessels, including polyarteritis nodosa, lupus, thromboangiitis obliterans, and other forms of vasculitis as well as GI bleeding, are better evaluated by conventional catheter angiography.

Mesenteric Ischemia

Chronic mesenteric ischemia occurs when there is insufficient blood supply to the intestine during periods of high metabolic demand, such as following a meal. It is most commonly caused by severe stenosis or occlusion of at least two of the three main splanchnic arteries (Figure 7.2). Acute mesenteric ischemia occurs when the blood supply to the intestine is so compromised that it is ischemic even during a period of relatively low metabolic demand. This may occur following embolic occlusion of the celiac or superior mesenteric artery. Acute mesenteric ischemia may also occur when there is poor cardiac output, insufficient to perfuse the gut or from acute venous obstruction/thrombosis (see Chapter 8). Vasculitis involving the mesenteric vessels may cause either chronic or acute mesenteric ischemia.

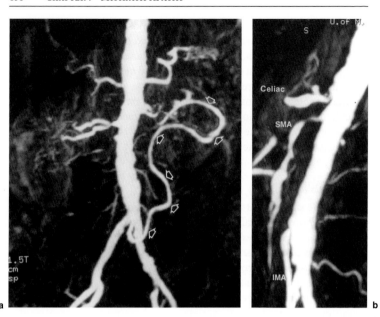

Fig. 7.2. Mesenteric Ischemia.

Clinical Scenario: 55-year-old female with weight loss and post-prandial abdominal pain.

Technique: Coronal Acquisition, TR/TE/Flip = 7.3/2.1/45°, Field-of-View = 360 × 360 × 96 mm, Matrix = 256 × 160 × 34, with zero filling interpolation in the slice direction, Centric Ordering of k-space, Acquisition Time = 28 seconds, 40 ml gadolinium contrast infused at 2 ml/s, and timed with SmartPrep.

Interpretation: Coronal (a) and sagittal (b) MIPs show a diffusely atherosclerotic aorta with severe narrowing of the celiac origin and proximal superior mesenteric artery (SMA) as well as moderate narrowing of the inferior mesenteric artery (IMA) origin. Note that IMA is ectatic distal to the origin and supplies collateral flow to the SMA territory via a prominent arc of Riolan (*arrow*). Also note bilateral renal artery atherosclerotic disease.

Diagnosis: Chronic Mesenteric Ischemia.

Submitted by Ruth Carlos, M.D., Ann Arbor.

Stenoses of the celiac or the superior mesenteric artery are commonly seen in patients with advanced atherosclerotic disease. However, the clinical syndrome of mesenteric ischemia is rare. This is because a rich collateral network in the form of numerous vascular arcades compensate for occlusive disease involving the origin of a single splanchnic artery. Since atherosclerotic disease predominantly affects origins of splanchnic arteries and rarely involves more distal branches, this rich collateral network is rarely compromised. Due to these collaterals, patients generally do not develop chronic mesenteric ischemia unless at least 2 of the 3 splanchnic arteries are severely narrowed or occluded. At this advanced stage patients typically already have atherosclerotic disease elsewhere in their body as well as symptoms characteristic of mesenteric ischemia, including weight loss and post-prandial abdominal pain.

Due to risks associated with arterial catheterization, the diagnosis of mesenteric ischemia is often not made until many other tests have been performed to exclude other possible causes of abdominal pain. In the past, lack of a reliable, non-invasive imaging method to confirm or exclude the diagnosis of chronic mesenteric ischemia has resulted in substantial delays in diagnosis. The reported average time delay between clinical presentation and diagnosis is 18 months for patients with new symptoms and one month for patients with recurrent symptoms. The tendency of mesenteric ischemia symptoms to overlap with or mimic those of more common intestinal disorders, including peptic ulcer disease and chronic cholecystitis, usually results in a plethora of testing prior to arteriography.

Now, with the availability of 3D contrast MRA, the diagnosis can be made safely, reliably, non-invasively and earlier in the course of the disease. Early diagnosis of occlusive disease involving the splanchnic arteries is important because surgical revascularization (Figures 7.3 and 7.4) or transluminal angioplasty of these vessels offers favorable results. Primary technical success rates for revascularization of splanchnic arteries range from 80%–100%, and for long-term clinical improvement, 50%–75%.

MR angiography is also useful post-operatively to evaluate the post-revascularization anatomy in patients who have new or persistent symptoms. Some surgeons like to obtain post-operative 3D contrast MRA examinations routinely in all mesenteric revascularization patients prior to discharge. The relatively large size of the celiac access and proximal SMA make these two vessels readily assessable by 3D contrast MRA, even when performed with older magnets. With state-of-the-art magnets that allow higher-resolution, breath-hold imaging, the smaller size of the inferior mesenteric artery (IMA) is no longer an obstacle to its successful evaluation. Note that the IMA can be challenging to correctly evaluate even by conventional arteriography. It is also possible to evaluate the common and proper hepatic artery post liver transplantation (Figure 7.5).

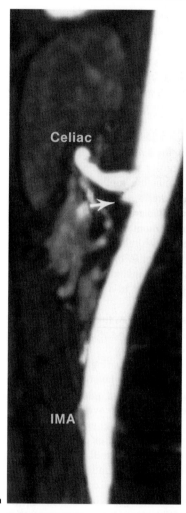

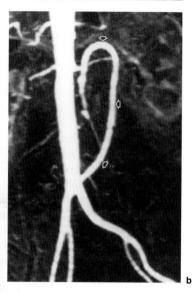

Fig. 7.3. Mesenteric Revascularization.

Clinical Scenario: 57-year-old female who underwent superior mesenteric artery (SMA) revascularization for mesenteric ischemia.

Technique: Coronal Acquisition, TR/TE/Flip = 6.7/1.8/45°, Field-of-View = 300 × 300 × 96 mm, Matrix = 256 × 128 × 32, Sequential Ordering of k-space, Acquisition Time = 28 s, 40 ml gadolinium contrast infused at 2 ml/s, and timed with SmartPrep.

Interpretation: Preoperatively **(a)** a sagittal MIP shows stenosis at the origin of the celiac axis and complete occlusion of the proximal SMA (*arrow*). Following revascularization, **(b)** a coronal oblique MIP shows a graft arising from the distal aorta and supplying the proximal SMA. The graft proximal and distal anastomoses are widely patent.

Diagnosis: Widely patent aorto-SMA graft.

Submitted by Qian Dong, M.D., Ann Arbor.

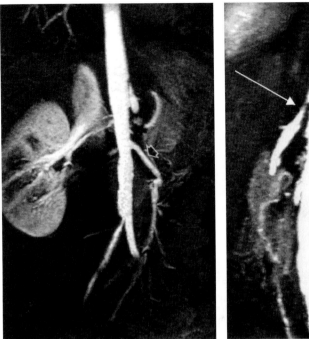
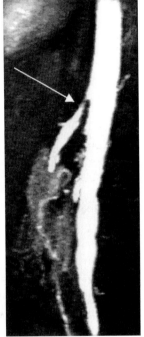

a   b

Fig. 7.4. Celiac Stenosis and Superior Mesenteric Artery (SMA). Revascularization Post-Prandial Flow Measurements.

Clinical Scenario: 35-year-old male having abdominal pain with meals. Patient had a previous inlay graft directly off the aorta to anastomose with the SMA for symptoms of mesenteric ischemia. Patient presented with persistent abdominal pain and weight loss even after revascularization.

Technique: 3D Fast Gradient Echo Coronal Acquisition, TR/TE/Flip = 8.2/1.8/45°, Field-of-View = 360 × 270 × 90 mm, Matrix = 512 × 192 × 60, zero filling, and source subtraction, and 42 ml gadolinium contrast was administered at 2 ml/s. Multiplanar reformats and reprojections were generated from 3D data using MIP and MPVR techniques. In addition, cine cardiac-gated PC flow analysis was performed in the SMA before and 30 minutes following a meal.

Interpretation: The images show the SMA graft to be clearly patent. However, flow measurements demonstrated only a 50 percent increase in SMA blood flow following the meal (normal flow should increase several-fold). These findings suggest small vessel occlusive disease involving the SMA territory. An area of high-grade stenosis noted in the celiac artery proximally (*arrow*).

Diagnosis: Patent SMA inlay graft with flow analysis suggestive of small vessel occlusive disease. Celiac artery stenosis.

Submitted by J. Greg Baden, M.D., Madison.

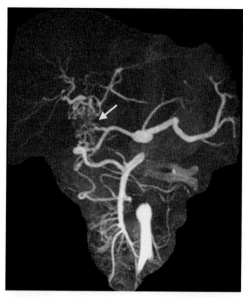

Fig. 7.5. Hepatic Artery Occlusion.

Clinical Scenario: Post Liver Transplantation.

Technique: Coronal acquisition, TR/TE/Flip = 3.2/1.1/25°, Matrix = 512 × 246 × 72 with asymmetric k-space acquisition, Field-of-View = 350 × 290 × 100, 40 ml Gd injected at 2ml/s with a separate test bolus for timing.

Interpretation: Coronal sub-volume MIP, with aorta edited out, shows abrupt occlusion (*arrow*) of proper hepatic artery. There is a network of collaterals which reconstitute the right and left hepatic arteries. SMA is widely patent.

Diagnosis: Segmental occlusion of proper hepatic artery.

Submitted by James Carr, M.D., Chicago.

Table 7.1. Accuracy of 3D contrast MRA for Diagnosing Mesenteric Ischemia

Author	Year	Journal	# of Patients	Sensitivity	Specificity
Prince	1995	Radiology	43	94 %	98 %
Meaney	1997	JMRI	14	100 %	95 %
Carlos	2002	Academic Rad	26	96 %	95 %

Aneurysms

Aneurysmal dilatation of the proximal celiac or SMA can occur in patients with aortic aneurysms. Abdominal aortic aneurysm (AAA) is more commonly associated with iliac, common femoral, and popliteal artery aneurysms. Isolated aneurysms can also involve the splenic (Figure 7.6), hepatic, gastro-duodenal, pancreatico-duodenal, gastric, gastro-epiploic,

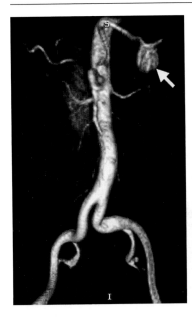

Fig. 7.6. Splenic Artery Aneurysm.
Clinical Scenario: Chronic Pancreatitis.
Technique: Coronal acquisition,
TR/TE/Flip = 6/1.2/30°, Matrix = 512 ×
160 × 32 with 2-fold zero filling in the
slice direction, Field-of-View = 360 × 360
× 83, 30 ml Gd injected by hand with
Smartset and timed using SmartPrep.
Interpretation: Volume rendering shows
tortuous aorta and iliac arteries and a
3 cm splenic artery aneurysm near the
splenic hilum.
Diagnosis: 3cm aneurysm of distal
splenic artery.
Submitted by Martin R. Prince, M.D.,
Ph.D., New York.

and inferior mesenteric arteries. Splenic artery aneurysms are the most common, particularly in post-partum women or secondary to weakening of the splenic artery from pancreatitis. Superior mesenteric artery aneurysms are often mycotic as a result of proximity to the small intestines. Aneurysmal dilatation of the celiac axis may occur secondary to post-stenotic dilatation related to either atherosclerotic narrowing of the origin or narrowing from extrinsic compression by the median arcuate ligament (Figure 7.7).

Tumor Encasement

Tumors may enhance briskly during the arterial phase or, if hypovascular, the tumor may blend in with surrounding tissues making it difficult to identify. Retroperitoneal masses, and particularly pancreatic adenocarcinoma, may surround, encase, and narrow or even occlude the splanchnic arteries and portal venous system (Figures 7.8 and 8.9). Masses arising in the head of the pancreas tend to encase the SMA, SMV and portal vein. Lesions in the body and tail of the pancreas tend to nar-

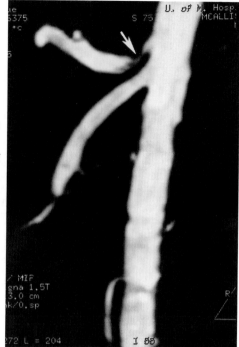

Fig. 7.7. Median Arcuate Ligament.

Clinical Scenario: 53-year-old male with hypertension.

Technique: Sagittal Acquisition, TR/TE/Flip = 7.2/2.1/45°, Field-of-View = 380 × 380 × 83 mm, Matrix = 256 × 160 × 32, with zero filling interpolation to reconstruct 64 slices, Centric Ordering of k-space, Acquisition Time = 26 s, 40 ml gadolinium contrast infused at 2 ml/s, and timed with SmartPrep.

Interpretation: Sagittal MIP shows severe narrowing of the proximal celiac axis secondary to extrinsic compression by the median arcuate ligament. This ligament, which connects the right and left crus, makes an impression along the superior margin of the proximal celiac axis and pulls the celiac axis inferiorly. Note the superior mesenteric artery and inferior mesenteric artery are widely patent and there are no symptoms of mesenteric ischemia.

Diagnosis: Celiac stenosis secondary to median arcuate ligament.

Submitted by Martin R. Prince, M.D., Ph.D., New York.

row the splenic vein. The characteristic serrated lumen of arterial encasement seen with conventional angiography is generally not appreciated on MRA due to its lower resolution. Large masses may also displace the mesenteric arteries without encasement. For example, this displacement may occur with pancreatic pseudocyst, hematoma, or abscess.

Anatomic Variations

Variations in the splanchnic arterial anatomy occur in more than 40% of patients. For this reason, pre-operative planning for hepatic resections,

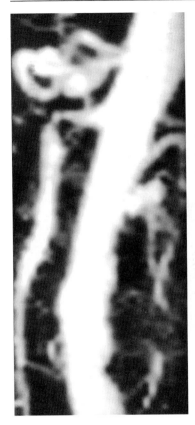

Fig. 7.8. Tumor Encasement of Superior Mesenteric Artery (SMA).

Clinical Scenario: 58-year-old patient with a pancreatic carcinoma referred for MRA of the SMA suspected to be encased by the tumor.

Technique: TR/TE/Flip = 5/2/40°, 40 contiguous 2 mm sections were acquired during a single 26s breath-hold, 15 mmol/kg of Gd-DTPA was administered IV with a power injector at a rate of 2 ml/s beginning 22 s before the start of the acquisition.

Interpretation: Sagittal MIP projection displays the origin of the celiac and SMA from the abdominal aorta. The celiac artery appears normal. A stenosis of the SMA in its proximal portion is demonstrated. The stenotic section of the SMA is elongated rigidly over about 2 cm.

Diagnosis: Encasement of the proximal SMA due to a pancreatic carcinoma.

Submitted by Lars Kopka, M.D., Göttingen.

liver transplantation, resection of retroperitoneal masses, prior to chemo-infusion pump placement, surgical shunting, or other abdominal operations may require mapping of the visceral arterial anatomy. Generally, this is done by conventional angiography for the fine detail necessary to identify variations involving tiny arteries. To evaluate the splanchnic artery origins and major branches, 3D contrast MRA may be sufficient. When patients are undergoing renal revascularization, it is important to know the splanchnic arterial anatomy in case a spleno-renal (Figure 7.9) or hepato-renal bypass must be performed to avoid clamping the aorta. The most common variation is a replaced (17%) or accessory (8%) right

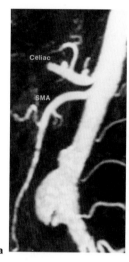

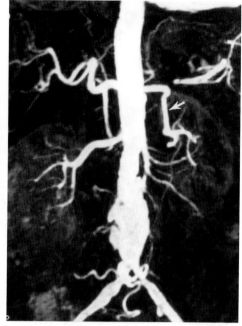

Fig. 7.9. Spleno-Renal bypass graft.

Clinical Scenario: 63-year-old female post left renal revascularization using a spleno-renal bypass.

Technique: Coronal Acquisition, TR/TE/Flip = 7.2/2.1/45°, Field-of-View = 380 × 380 × 83 mm, Matrix = 256 × 160 × 32, with zero filling interpolation to reconstruct 64 slices, Centric Ordering of k-space, Acquisition Time = 26 s, 40 ml gadolinium contrast infused at 2 ml/s, and timed with SmartPrep.

Interpretation: Sagittal (**a**) and coronal (**b**) MIPs show celiac and superior mesenteric arteries (SMA) are widely patent and there is a widely patent graft from the splenic artery to the left renal artery (*arrow*). This type of revascularization is used to avoid having to clamp the aorta in patients with fragile cardiac status. Note also the infrarenal abdominal aortic aneurysm. This aneurysm was not repaired because the patient could not tolerate aortic cross clamping.

Diagnosis: Widely patent spleno-renal graft.

Submitted by Martin R. Prince, M.D., Ph.D., New York.

hepatic artery, most commonly from SMA. Less common variations include the common hepatic artery arising from the SMA (2.5%) or directly from the aorta (2%), left gastric artery arising from the aorta (1%–2%), or a celiaco-mesenteric trunk (<1%) (Figure 7.10).

To maximize image detail for assessing hepatic arterial anatomy it may be useful to acquire 3D data in the axial plane. The quality of source

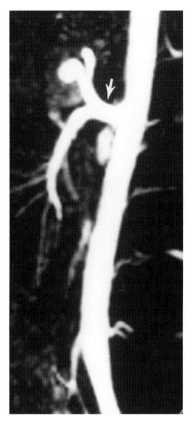

Fig. 7.10. Anatomic Variation.

Clinical Scenario: 30-year-old male with abdominal pain.

Technique: Coronal Acquisition, TR/TE/Flip = 7.2/2.1/45°, Field-of-View = 400 × 400 × 108 mm, Matrix = 256 × 128 × 36, with zero filling interpolation to reconstruct 72 slices, Centric Ordering of k-space, Acquisition Time = 24 s, 40 ml gadolinium contrast infused at 2 ml/s, and timed with SmartPrep.

Interpretation: Sagittal MIP shows a common origin (*arrow*) of the celiac and superior mesenteric artery (SMA), an unusual anatomic variation.

Diagnosis: Common origins of celiac & SMA.

Submitted by Mohammed Neimatallah, M.D., Jiddah.

images is always better than reformations. The axial plane is optimal for tracing each of the hepatic arterial branches and for correlating each portion of liver with its supplying branch.

GI Bleeding

Development of blood pool MR contrast agents is making it possible to replicate the concept of labeled red cell nuclear medicine examinations using 3D Contrast MRA. Although MR blood pool agents are experimental, the higher SNR and resolution of MR compared to nuclear medicine makes this a promising future technique for use in patients suspected of GE bleeding. Arterial and venous mesenteric anatomy can be evaluated during the arterial and venous phases of blood pool contrast agent injection. By periodically re-imaging the patient over time, the accumulation of blood in the GI track can be imaged to identify the site of GI bleeding. Just as with labeled red cells, when bleeding is intermittent, the patient can be scanned periodically, every hour or two until a bleeding episode is detected. The three-dimensional nature of MR imaging makes it easier to identify the specific loop of bowel that is bleeding (Figure 7.11).

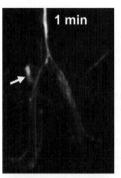 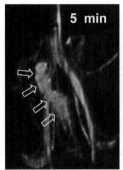 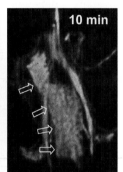

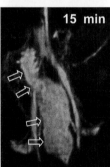

Fig. 7.11. GI Bleeding. 3D Contrast MRA performed at 1, 5, 10 and 15 minutes after initiating a recto-sigmoid bleeding site in an experimental animal model and injecting blood pool contrast agent. At one minute there is a small trace of hemorrhage (arrow) which expands and flows distally (open arrows) at 5, 10 and 15 minutes. Submitted by Stephan Ruehm, M.D., Essen.

Pitfalls

Although 3D contrast MRA is accurate for assessing origins of the celiac axis and superior mesenteric artery, there are a number of important pitfalls.

Celiac Pseudostenosis

A celiac stenosis is commonly caused by extrinsic compression of the celiac axis by the median arcuate ligament (Figure 7.5). Often this has a characteristic appearance where the celiac axis is pulled inferiorly, and there is an impression along the superior margin where the median arcuate ligament joins right and left diaphragmatic crus. This extrinsic compression can vary with respiration, and thus may appear more or less severe, depending on the patient's degree of inspiration or expiration. It is usually asymptomatic, although there are reports of relief of abdominal symptoms following surgical release of a severe extrinsic compression.

Motion Artifact

Respiratory motion may obscure the superior mesenteric artery, particularly along its more distal intraperitoneal course. It may even appear artifactually stenotic at the 90° bend, where the superior mesenteric artery begins to head inferiorly when there is a lot of respiration induced motion. Respiratory motion may also compromise visualization of hepatic and splenic arteries. When the 3D contrast MRA is corrupted by respiratory motion it may be repeated during equilibrium phase. Alternatively, 3D phase contrast MRA (Venc = 40cm/s) acquired post Gd over 5-7 minutes can generally average over sufficient respirations to provide diagnostic evaluation of the celiac and SMA origins.

Surgical Clip Artifacts

Surgical clips, such as those used for a cholecystectomy, may cause signal voids, resulting in poor visualization of neighboring vessels. Clips can generally be recognized by characteristic dark-bright artifacts seen on individual source images. If in doubt, a plain film of the abdomen should be performed to confirm the presence of surgical clips. The extent of clip artifacts is dependent on the underlying material. Increasingly "MR compatible" clips are becoming available. Pointing surgeons to their availability may pay off in better image quality in subsequent post-operative patients. Clip artifact can also be minimized by using the widest possible bandwidth to obtain the shortest possible echo time.

Limited Spatial Resolution

Spatial resolution of 3D contrast MRA is not sufficient to exclude small emboli in distal splanchnic arterial branches. Thus, even though the celiac axis and superior mesenteric artery may be shown to be patent proximally, mesenteric ischemia cannot be absolutely excluded. Small emboli may occlude just a segmental region and cause infarction of a limited segment of bowel. There may also be vasculitis or, rarely, atherosclerotic disease that occurs more distally. Tiny aneurysms of polyarteritis nodosa, thromboangiitis obliterans or other forms of vasculitis are generally not resolved by 3D contrast MRA. However, segmental ischemia of bowel may be detected by identifying absence of the normal mucosal enhancement on delayed images in that segment. Intrinsic resolution limits of MR angiography may also make it difficult to assess the inferior mesenteric artery, particularly on the slower scanners that are not capable of performing high resolution imaging.

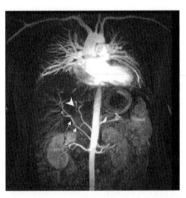

Fig. 7.12. Hepatic Artery Anomaly.
Clinical Scenario: Donor candidate for right lobe liver transplantation.

Technique: Coronal acquisition, TR/TE/Flip = 3.65/1.2/25°, Field-of-View = 450 × 309 × 96 mm, Matrix = 512 × 194 × 32 with zero interpolation to 64 slices, sequential ordering of k-space following injection of 20 ml gadolinium at 2ml/s and timed using a test bolus.

Interpretation: Anomalous right hepatic artery (arrows) arising from superior mesenteric artery, which is favorable for right hepatectomy. Note large middle hepatic artery arising from left hepatic artery supplying segment 4 of the liver (arrowhead).

Diagnosis: Replaced right hepatic artery.

Submitted by Vivian S. Lee, M.D., Ph.D., New York.

CHAPTER 8

Portal Venous System

Background

Portal venous morphology can be depicted during the portal venous and equilibrium phases of abdominal 3D contrast MRA examinations. When imaging the abdominal aorta, renal, or mesenteric arteries in the coronal or axial planes, assessment of the portal vein can be added without the need for additional contrast. The patient merely has to suspend respiration a second time to capture one more 3D image data set following the arterial phase (Figure 8.1). Splenic, hepatic and portal veins are easily resolved on studies optimized for renal and mesenteric arteries as long as the 3D imaging volume is large enough to also encompass the portal venous system.

Technique

There are some technical issues to consider when portal venous system images are needed. By the time extracellular contrast agent reaches the portal vein, it is considerably diluted. This results from contrast extraction at the capillary level for redistribution into the extracellular compartment and Gd extraction in the liver. This dilution must be taken into account when determining the contrast dose. A dose of 0.3 mmol/kg, or at least 40 ml, is recommended for dedicated portal vein imaging. A lower flip angle of 20°–30° may improve visualization of the diluted gadolinium in the portal vein. If, however, it takes more than a few seconds to change the flip angle, it is better to use the same flip angle as used for arterial phase imaging rather than to delay portal venous phase data acquisition.

Imaging plane can be set to either coronal or axial. Coronal imaging has the advantage of including the mesenteric arteries (including IMA) on the arterial phase and also including superior and inferior mesenteric

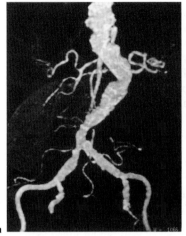

a

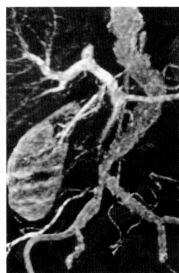

b

Fig. 8.1. Arterial and Portal Venous Phases of Gadolinium Contrast Bolus Injection.

Clinical Scenario: 80-year-old female with hypertension and renal insufficiency.

Technique: Coronal Acquisition, TR/TE/Flip = 7.1/2.1/45°, Field-of-View = 300 × 300 × 70 mm, Matrix = 256 × 128 × 32, Centric Ordering of k-space, Acquisition Time = 29 s, 40 ml gadolinium contrast infused at 2 ml/s, and timed with SmartPrep.

Interpretation: Arterial (**a**) and portal venous (**b**) phases of a contrast bolus can be imaged with two successive breath-holds. The abdominal aorta is diffusely atherosclerotic and ectatic with an occluded left renal artery. Note also the normal splenic, superior mesenteric, and portal veins.

Diagnosis: Diffusely atherosclerotic aorta, occluded left renal artery, and normal portal venous system.

Submitted by Brian Hamilton, M.D., Ann Arbor.

veins and retroperitoneal collaterals. The axial plane has the advantage of imaging the main portal vein and its branches "in-plane", which generally has higher resolution compared to reformations. Axial imaging depicts the entire liver so that hepatic parenchymal enhancement can also be imaged to detect and characterize hepatic tumors. In addition, axial imaging has a smaller FOV without wrap-around artifact since frequency encoding is right-to-left. One limitation of the axial plane is wrap-around in the slice direction (superior to inferior). Bright fat immediately superior or inferior to the imaging volume superimposes on the liver. This problem can be eliminated by utilizing a fat suppression technique and by using an imaging volume that matches the entire volume of coil sensitivity. In this way, tissue above and below the coil will have limited signal to wrap into the image volume.

Axial imaging volumes are readily prescribed from coronal localizers. The axial 3D volume should extend from just above where hepatic veins enter IVC down to well below the spleno-portal confluence. On slower scanners, it may be necessary to use a slice thickness of 5–6 mm to obtain adequate coverage.

If you choose a coronal acquisition volume, extend sufficiently anteriorly to encompass the entire portal and mesenteric venous system. To make sure the coronal positioning is correct, obtain a localizer image on which the portal vein can be readily identified. Usually the main portal vein is depicted well on axial T1, T2 or gradient echo images. Be sure to also identify the anterior extent of right and left portal venous branches so at least their origins can be included in the 3D imaging volume. Extend sufficiently superiorly to include the hepatic venous confluence with the IVC.

High performance gradients and partial Fourier imaging can provide up to 50 imaging sections in a convenient 20 second breath-hold. This makes it easy to encompass the abdominal aorta and portal venous anatomy with 3–4 mm thick slices in nearly all patients. Magnets with inferior gradient performance may require thicker sections of up to 4 or 5 mm, in order to extend far enough anteriorly (for coronal volumes) to include the portal vein and still be fast enough to acquire in a breath-hold.

For portal venous phase imaging the breath-hold interval needs to be kept rather short. A patient who can suspend breathing for 40 seconds during the arterial phase may be too winded for another 40-second breath-hold during the portal venous phase. It is best to keep 3D imaging time under 30 seconds per phase to enable patients to suspend breathing twice in a row with only a few seconds rest in between.

Analysis of the portal venous and equilibrium phase images can be accomplished rapidly by performing a series of overlapping thick MIPs. If about ten MIPs are created each as thick as one-fifth of the imaging volume, there will be 50% overlap. This facilitates tracing vascular structures from one overlapping MIP to the next. Volume rendering may not work as well because of hepatic parenchymal enhancement.

Complementary Sequences

Phase contrast MRA can be used to determine the direction of portal venous blood flow. A single 5–10 mm thick 2D phase contrast image is acquired in an axial or oblique plane, perpendicular to the portal vein. Typical imaging parameters are: TR/TE/Flip = 28/6/45° and Venc = 40 cm/s. On 2D phase contrast images background tissues are gray, while flow perpendicular to the image plane is bright in one direction and black in the other. Flow from superior-to-inferior (S/I), right-to-left (R/L), and anterior-to-posterior (A/P) is bright, whereas flow in the opposite direction is displayed as dark on velocity-encoded 2D phase contrast images. In order to interpret flow data correctly, the orthogonal plane (S/I vs. A/P vs. R/L) coming closest to the scan obliquity needs to be determined. Alternatively, if the portal vein is more vertical than horizontal, a straight axial 2D phase contrast image can be acquired and the flow direction compared to the aorta and inferior vena cava (IVC).

For patients who did not suspend respiration for the portal venous 3D data set, axial 2D gradient echo images can be acquired post-gadolinium with gradient moment nulling (flow compensation) (TR/TE/Flip = 33/8/30°), during either short periods of apnea (5s) or quiet respiration. Paramagnetic contrast within the vascular system enhances time-of-flight image quality allowing use of relatively thick, 5–8 mm slices. For non-breath-held scans a sufficient number of averages (4 NEX), in conjunction with respiratory ordered phase encoding, will usually result in diagnostic image quality. A similar bright vessel effect can be achieved with T1 weighted spin-echo imaging with fat saturation and gradient moment nulling.

Patients with suspected concomitant parenchymal pathology benefit from T1- and T2-weighted spin echo imaging prior to contrast injection. These images aid in identification and subsequent characterization of masses. They can be used as a guide to ensure inclusion of all pathology in 3D contrast MRA data sets. For patients with suspected biliary obstruction or pancreatitis, a HASTE or single shot fast spin echo MRCP-type sequence in coronal or coronal oblique planes is also useful and can generally be performed in a single breath-hold or during quiet respiration.

Clinical Applications

Portal Hypertension

Angiography in patients with portal hypertension is often performed to measure portal venous pressures and the portal-systemic pressure gradient. These measurements cannot be made directly by MR. However, for patients who require a portal-systemic shunt, 3D contrast MRA can be a useful guide for shunt planning. Shunts can be made surgically, percutaneously (e.g., TIPS), or can occur spontaneously (Figure 8.2). Magnetic

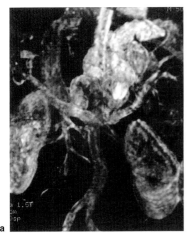

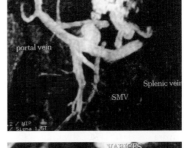

Fig. 8.2. Portal Hypertension.
Clinical Scenario: 50-year-old male alcoholic presenting with upper gastrointestinal bleeding.

Technique: Coronal Acquisition, TR/TE/Flip = 7.9/2.1/45°, Field-of-View = 340 × 340 × 128 mm, Matrix = 256 × 160 × 32, Sequential Ordering of k-space, Acquisition Time = 28 s, 40 ml gadolinium contrast infused at 2 ml/s, and timed empirically.

Interpretation: Coronal MIPs of the entire volume (**a**) and MIPs of narrow subvolume (**b** and **c**) show extensive gastric and esophageal varices in a patient with portal hypertension. A thin MIP limited to the region of the left renal vein (**c**) shows a large spleno-renal shunt.

Diagnosis: Portal hypertension with varices and spleno-renal shunt.
Submitted by Martin R. Prince, M.D., Ph.D., New York.

resonance angiography assesses patency of both spontaneous and surgical shunts (Figure 8.3) as long as metallic clips do not obscure portal venous anatomy. In conjunction with phase contrast techniques, shunt flow volume can be determined non-invasively. TIPS shunts are more difficult to assess due to the metallic stents. Most often, a stainless steel Wall stent is used to bridge the portal and systemic venous systems. Even with the shortest available echo times (<1.0 ms), the lumen of this metal stent cannot be evaluated by MRA.

Liver Transplantation

Imaging proof of a patent portal vein is required for a patient to be placed on the liver transplant waiting list. Ultrasound can image the portal vein but

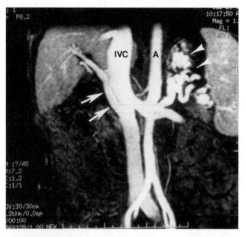

Fig. 8.3. MRA of Portocaval Shunt.

Clinical Scenario: 42-year-old male, status post-portocaval shunt with worsening ascites.

Technique: Coronal Acquisition, TR/TE/Flip = 7.2/1.2/45°, Field-of-View = 300 × 300, Matrix = 256 × 128, Centric Ordering of k-space, Acquisition Time = 32 s, 1 NEX, 40 ml of gadolinium infused at 2 ml/s, and timed empirically.

Interpretation: Coronal subvolume MIP (**a**) and magnification view (**b**) shows a widely patent portocaval shunt (*arrows*). Note also gastric varices (*arrowheads*). During this equilibrium phase image, there is comparable enhancement of the portal vein, IVC, and aorta.

Diagnosis: Patent portocaval shunt.

Submitted by David Stafford-Johnson, M.D., Ann Arbor.

Reprinted with permission from Investigative Radiology. 1998; 33:644-652.

is not 100% reliable. When ultrasound fails to adequately visualize the portal vein, 3D contrast MRA offers a safe, accurate, and comprehensive assessment of portal venous anatomy without requiring iodinated contrast. 3D contrast MRA also evaluates the splenic vein, superior mesenteric vein (SMV), inferior mesenteric vein (IMV), varices (Figure 8.2), and IVC.

Following liver transplantation, rising liver function tests may raise a suspicion of allograft ischemia. Since blood supply to the liver is primarily via the portal vein, this is the most important vessel to evaluate. The most common site of obstruction is at the anastomosis. Usually, anastomoses are easy to identify because of the caliber change between donor and recipient portal veins (Figure 8.4). Stenosis of the transplant arterial anastomosis may be seen on the arterial phase of a portal venous study, but its smaller size and often folded, tortuous course can make it difficult to assess. Generally, it is only possible to ascertain whether it is patent or thrombosed. Occlusion of the transplant artery is important to detect because it results in ischemia to the donor common bile duct and

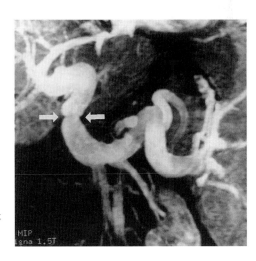

Fig. 8.4. Liver Transplant. *Clinical Scenario:* Status post liver transplant with increased liver function tests.

Technique: Coronal Acquisition, TR/TE/Flip = 7/2.1/45°, Field-of-View = 320 × 320 × 84 mm, Matrix = 256 × 128 × 28, Sequential Ordering of k-space, Acquisition Time = 27 s, 40 ml gadolinium contrast infused at 2 ml/s, and timed empirically.

Interpretation: Coronal oblique subvolume MIP shows widely patent splenic and portal veins. There is minor narrowing (*arrows*) at the site of anastomosis between the native and donor portal veins.

Diagnosis: Widely patent transplant portal vein.

Submitted by Martin R. Prince, M.D., Ph.D., New York.

can lead to biliary strictures and leaks. It is also important to assess the IVC since supra- and infra-hepatic IVC anastomoses may also become narrowed and flow limiting (Figure 8.5).

Hepatic masses, abscesses, and perihepatic post-operative fluid collections are best evaluated on T1- and T2-weighted HASTE or FSE images acquired prior to injection of a contrast agent. Collections with T1 bright signal are likely hemorrhagic, reflecting the paramagnetic effect of methemoglobin. Biliary obstruction may also be evaluated on fast breath-hold HASTE or single shot FSE sequences. Areas of liver infarction are optimally evaluated on post-gadolinium images, i.e. equilibrium phase of the 3D MRA acquisition.

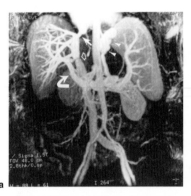 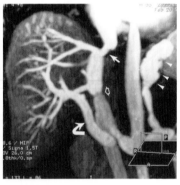

a   b

Fig. 8.5. MRA of Liver Transplant.

Clinical Scenario: 53-year-old male, three weeks post-orthotopic liver transplant with bilateral leg swelling and elevated bilirubin.

Technique: Coronal Acquisition, TR/TE/Flip = 7.2/1.0/45°, Field-of-View = 48 × 48 × 112, Matrix = 256 × 128 × 40, .75 NEX, Sequential Ordering of k-space, Acquisition Time = 30 s, 40 ml of gadolinium contrast infused at 2 ml/s, and timed empirically.

Interpretation: Subvolume MIP demonstrates widely patent portal vein (*curved arrow*). There are infra-hepatic (*straight arrow*) and supra-hepatic (*open arrow*) inferior vena cava (IVC) anastomoses. The supra-hepatic anastomosis (*straight arrow*) is moderately stenotic and explains the patient's leg swelling. Also note large gastric varices (*arrowheads*).

Diagnosis: Anastomotic stenosis of supra-hepatic IVC.

Submitted by David Stafford-Johnson, M.D., Ann Arbor. Reprinted with permission from Radiology 1998; 207:153-160.

Portal Vein Thrombosis and Cavernous Transformation

3D contrast MRA accurately detects portal vein thrombosis (Table 8.1). A variety of etiologies have been implicated as causes of portal venous thrombosis (Figure 8.6). These include local infection, appendicitis, pancreatitis or other intra-abdominal inflammatory disease, portal venous stasis (i.e. portal hypertension), trauma, including iatrogenic trauma (e.g., TIPS), malignancy (Figure 8.7), and coagulopathy. The acutely thrombosed, portal vein is expanded with thrombus and contains no flow (Figure 8.6). It is usually best seen on minimum intensity projection images. There may be perivascular enhancement from the inflammatory response associated with acute thrombosis. Portal flow to the liver is substantially diminished, resulting in delayed and patchy liver parenchymal enhancement. Over time, a network of small collateral vessels develops to bypass the portal venous occlusion. This network of collaterals, known as cavernous transformation, is identified by its characteristic enhancement pattern in the hepatic hilum during portal venous and equilibrium phases of 3D contrast MRA (Figure 8.8).

Table 8.1. Accuracy of 3D Contrast MR Portography

Author	Year	Journal	# of Patients	Sensitivity	Specificity
Stafford-Johnson	1998	Radiology	13	100 %	100 %
Wilson	1998	Invest Radiol	27	86 %	100 %
Kopka	1999	Radiology	140 (60*)	100 %	100 %
Kreft	2000	Radiology	36	100 %	98 %
Glockner	2000	AJR	34 (20*)	100 %	94 %
Ernst	2000	AJR	33	100 %	100 %
Haliloglu	2000	JMRI	3	100 %	
Cheng	2001	Transplantation	38	100 %	100 %
Squillaci	2001	Radiol Med	28	100 %	97.3 %

* Number with angiography or surgical correlation

Tumor Encasement

Adenocarcinoma of the pancreas and other pancreatic and retroperitoneal masses may surround, encase, narrow, and eventually occlude the portal vein (Figure 8.9). Invasion of the portal vein makes tumor resection with clear margins nearly impossible, thus, removing the patient as a surgical candidate. Tumors in the pancreatic head may encase the SMV, portal vein, and medial splenic vein. These tumors are also more likely

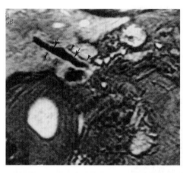

Fig. 8.6. Portal Vein Thrombosis.

Clinical Scenario: 21-year-old female with post-partum abdominal pain.

Technique: Coronal Acquisition, TR/TE/Flip = 7/1.2/45°, Field-of-View = 320 × 320 × 84 mm, Matrix = 256 × 128 × 28, Sequential Ordering of k-space, Acquisition Time = 28 s, 40 ml gadolinium contrast infused at 2 ml/s, and timed empirically.

Interpretation: Coronal MIP shows acutely thrombosed portal vein (*arrows*) distended by the thrombus. There is a thin rim of perivascular enhancement (*arrowheads*), representing the typical perivascular inflammatory response to an acute venous thrombosis.

Diagnosis: Acute thrombosis of the portal vein.

Submitted by Martin R. Prince, M.D., Ph.D., New York.

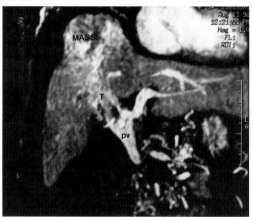

Fig. 8.7. Hepatoma.

Clinical Scenario: 54-year-old female with abdominal pain and elevated AFP.

Technique: Coronal Acquisition, TR/TE/Flip = 8.1/2.1/45°, Field-of-View = 320 × 320 × 96 mm, Matrix 256 × 160 × 32, Centric Ordering of k-space, Acquisition Time = 29 s, 40 ml gadolinium contrast infused at 2 ml/s, and timed empirically.

Interpretation: A coronal MIP from the portal venous-phase of the contrast bolus shows an enhancing mass in the dome of the liver with heterogeneously enhancing tumor invading the right portal vein and extending down to the confluence of right and left portal veins. The main and left portal veins are widely patent.

Diagnosis: Hepatoma with invasion of right portal vein.

Submitted by Martin R. Prince, M.D., Ph.D., New York.

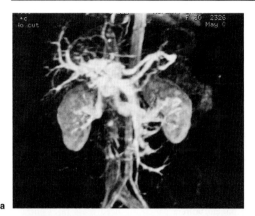

a

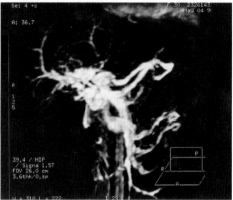

b

Fig. 8.8. Cavernous Transformation.

Clinical Scenario: 30-year-old female with Lupus and a long history of abdominal pain.

Technique: Coronal Acquisition, TR/TE/Flip = 7/2.1/45°, Field-of-View = 360 × 360 mm, Matrix = 256 × 160, Zero Filling Interpolation in the slice direction, Centric Ordering of k-space, Acquisition Time = 30 s, 40 ml gadolinium contrast infused at 2 ml/s, and imaged during the portal-venous phase of the bolus.

Interpretation: Coronal MIP of entire volume of data (**a**) and of a subvolume encompassing just the expected region of the portal vein (**b**) shows a network of numerous enhancing serpiginous vascular channels.

Diagnosis: Chronic portal vein occlusion with cavernous transformation.

Submitted by Qian Dong, M.D., Ann Arbor.

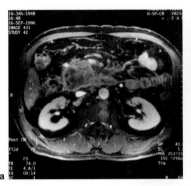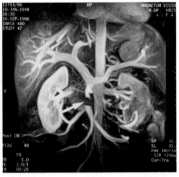

Fig. 8.9. Tumor Encasement of Portal Vein.

Clinical Scenario: 48-year-old patient with a pancreatic head mass (**a**). Contrast-enhanced 3D-MRA (**b**) was performed to evaluate local resectability.

Technique: 3D-MRA (TR/TE/Flip = 5/2/40°), 40 contiguous 2 mm sections were acquired breath-held over 29 s. Gadolinium-DTPA (0.2 mmol/kg) was manually administered over 15 s followed by a 20 cc saline flush. The sequence was started 45 s after the beginning of contrast injection (portal venous phase).

Interpretation: MIP of the entire 3D volume shows infiltration of superior mesenteric vein (*arrow*). Splenic and portal vein are unremarkable. There is residual contrast within the aorta.

Diagnosis: Unresectable adenocarcinoma of the head of the pancreas with infiltration of the superior mesenteric vein.

Submitted by Jochen Gaa, M.D., Mannheim.

to be detected early because they cause biliary obstruction, and thereby may be more likely to be resectable. Tumors in the body and tail of the pancreas may become larger before being detected and more commonly occlude the splenic vein. Splenic vein occlusion has a tendency to produce short gastric varices serving as venous collaterals that enhance on delayed images.

Budd Chiari

Hepatic vein thrombosis (Budd Chiari) is difficult to diagnose by any method. Conventional arteriography requires selective canalization and injection of each heptic vein to look for the characteristic spider web appearance. However, on equilibrium phase 3D contrast MRA, Budd Chiari can be diagnosed by observing absence of hepatic veins (Figure 8.10) together with a constellation of peripheral hepatic

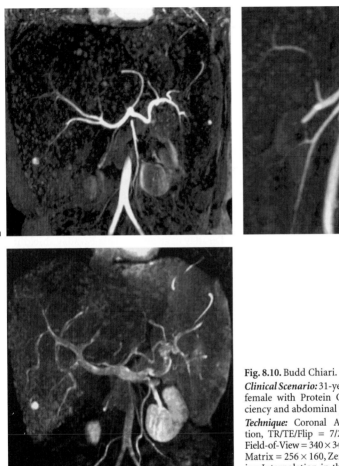

Fig. 8.10. Budd Chiari.

Clinical Scenario: 31-year-old female with Protein C deficiency and abdominal pain.

Technique: Coronal Acquisition, TR/TE/Flip = 7/2.1/45°, Field-of-View = 340 × 340 mm, Matrix = 256 × 160, Zero Filling Interpolation in the slice direction, Elliptical centric ordering of k-space, Acquisition Time = 30 s, 40 ml gadolinium contrast infused at 2 ml/s, and imaged during the arterial and portal-venous phases of the Gd bolus.

Interpretation: Arterial phase coronal MIP (**a**) and Sagittal MIP (**b**) show normal aorta, splenic, hepatic, left gastric and gastro-duodenal arteries. Portal venous phase (**b**) shows normal splenic and portal veins but there are no hepatic veins. The liver shows numerous enhancing nodules which can occur late in the course of chronically occluded hepatic veins.

Diagnosis: Budd Chiari.

Submitted by Martin Prince, M.D., Ph.D., New York.

changes that spare the central liver. Peripheral liver is brighter on T2 and has more heterogenous enhancement while the central liver will have normal signal and eventually will hypertrophy. In advanced cases the periperhal liver develops numerous hepatic nodules.

Pitfalls

Clip and Stent Artifacts

Surgical clips are commonly present around the hepatic hilum due to their widespread use in cholecystectomy. These metal clips as well as Wallstents, used in TIPS, create susceptibility artifact that may obscure visualization of the portal vein and IVC. These artifacts can be minimized by using the shortest possible echo time (TE). Newer stents made of non-magnetic material such as nitinol or platinum may still be difficult to see inside due to the Faraday cage effect. This Faraday shielding effect may be at least partially overcome by using a large flip angle.

Blurring

Breath-holding twice in a row to capture both the arterial and portal venous phases is difficult for many patients. It is therefore essential to keep the exam time short and stress the importance of breath-holding for each phase of the contrast bolus to the patient. Oxygen, 2L by nasal connulae, can help lengthen a patient's breath-hold capacity.

Insufficient Enhancement of the Portal Vein

There is considerable dilution and extraction of the paramagnetic contrast by the time it reaches the portal venous circulation. For these reasons, it may be necessary to use a larger contrast dose than what is ordinarily used for arterial imaging in order to ensure adequate portal venous enhancement. The lower concentration of Gd also requires a smaller flip angle compared to the same dose used for arterial imaging.

CHAPTER 9

Peripheral Arteries

Background

Peripheral vascular disease (PVD) is caused by the generalized systemic process of atherosclerosis, and is frequently associated with coronary, renal, and carotid arterial disease. Patients with peripheral vascular disease may present with an acute limb threatening event, a chronically threatened limb (i.e., rest pain, tissue loss, cellulitis or ulceration), or merely claudication. Although the atherosclerotic disease process is diffuse, patients can benefit if the disease site of greatest severity is dilated or bypassed. Sometimes, the disease site of greatest severity can be determined by the location of symptoms. Aortic, common or internal, iliac artery stenosis (i.e. inflow disease) may primarily cause buttock claudication. External iliac, common femoral and profunda femoral artery disease results in thigh claudication. Lastly, SFA, popliteal and trifurcation disease causes calf claudication.

Atherosclerotic lesions frequently occur at sites of complex flow (e.g. branching points) and sites of mechanical stress on the vessel. For this reason, the adductor canal, popliteal artery, aortic bifurcation and common iliac bifurcation are common sites for atherosclerosis. Vascular disease distribution can also depend upon features specific to an individual patient. For example, isolated aorto-iliac disease is often seen in 40-60 year old smokers, and distal disease is predominantly found in patients with adult onset diabetes and/or renal insufficiency. With the advent of improved surgical and angioplasty techniques for the treatment of PVD, accurate diagnosis and characterization of atherosclerotic lesions have become more important for all of these sites.

Diagnosing PVD is usually a two-step process. First, patients undergo non-invasive tests, which include segmental pressure measurements and Doppler or Plethysmographic analysis of flow. These studies measure the severity of the disease and help localize the pathology to general anatomic regions. Non-invasive data is used to classify patients into suspected "inflow" (aorto-iliac) or "outflow" (femoro-popliteal) disease groups. If non-invasive tests indicate that symptoms are in fact caused by hemodynamically significant vascular disease, the patient goes on to the next level of investigation, which typically involves obtaining an arteriogram. Arteriography precisely defines the location and extent of occlusive disease and provides a "road map" for planning therapy. Taking into consideration the risks and cost of contrast arteriography, this method is usually reserved for patients who are candidates for percutaneous intervention or surgery. Information regarding the exact anatomic location of occlusive disease, as well as the length of pathologic segments, helps to stratify patients into those who are eligible for percutaneous transluminal angioplasty and those who require an operative procedure. The angiogram road map also shows the surgeon where to locate anastomoses for bypass grafts and the status of inflow and distal runoff vessels (outflow); all of which help to predict the probability of a graft or angioplasty site staying open.

A minimally invasive approach for direct anatomic imaging of peripheral vasculature had been elusive until the advent of 3D Contrast MRA. Historically, axial 2D time-of-flight (2D TOF) has been the standard technique for acquiring peripheral MR angiograms. 2D TOF methods have been shown to be accurate for the assessment of infra-inguinal disease. However, several practical problems complicate using 2D TOF for a survey of peripheral arteries. First and foremost, 2D TOF data acquisition times are prohibitively long. Second, flow in peripheral arteries is highly pulsatile. Typical velocities in the popliteal artery are 50 cm/s in systole, but only 5 cm/s throughout the cardiac cycle. During diastole, there may be flow reversal, which can cause artifacts and reduce the net forward flow. When saturation pulses are used, the reversal of flow during diastole will degrade arterial signal unless there is a sufficient gap between the imaging slice and band of saturation. Third, collateral vessel formation may reverse arterial flow direction, further complicating the use of spatial presaturation for eliminating venous signal. This causes occlusive disease to falsely appear more extensive.

Technique

Peripheral vascular 3D contrast MRA can be performed at one or more anatomic stations. Several approaches to multi-station 3D contrast MRA have been proposed. All of these approaches have some merit, and no single technique has yet emerged as the clear method of choice in every case. A multi-station 3D contrast MRA examination can be performed using a single contrast injection and a series of 3D acquisitions that chase the bolus down the legs. This technique is known as floating table or bolus chase 3D contrast MRA (Figure 9.1). It can be performed with a single, slow infusion of Gd contrast followed by a series of 30-45 second images at three different stations (Figure 9.2) or with a faster injection with faster imaging and faster table motion in between stations for greater sharing of the bolus between stations. Finally, peripheral MRA can be performed as a series of separate, low-dose contrast injections using image subtraction to eliminate effects of Gd accumulation from preceding injections (Figure 9.3).

The patient is placed supine in the MR scanner, and positioned with arms either above the head or crossed over the chest. It is important to position the patient's legs horizontally in order to limit the A/P extent of the 3D volume that is required. The most anterior position of lower extremity arteries occurs where the common femoral arteries pass anterior to the femoral head. The greatest posterior extent typically occurs as the popliteal arteries pass posterior to the knee. Therefore, the knees and ankles are positioned on a bolster in order to flex the leg slightly at the hip so that the patella is positioned a couple of inches higher than the femoral head. The magnet alignment light can be used to verify that the thigh and calf are reasonably horizontal with knees slightly flexed following placement of cushions under the knees and ankles. This places the patient's arteries in a favorable horizontal position to allow thinner partitions in the 3D contrast MRA acquisition. Images may be acquired with the body coil or preferably with a dedicated phased-array lower extremity coil. Particularly, small distal vessels benefit from dedicated, phased array coils (Figure 9.4). However, the entire exam benefits from coil assembly such as AngioSURF, which permits translating the patient through a phased array coil (Figure 2.18).

Axial 2D TOF scout images may be acquired at 20–30 cm intervals along the pelvis, thighs, and lower legs. These images are used to determine the location of peripheral arteries for prescribing pre-contrast coronal 3D mask images used for image subtraction. Most proposed methods use image subtraction in order to reduce background signal and improve vessel-to-background contrast (Figure 1.13), which is especially useful for small vessels. Likewise, during multi-station examinations, image subtraction may be used to cancel signal from contrast

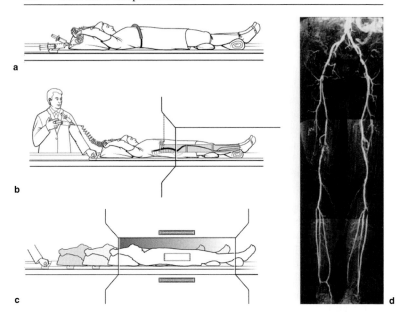

Fig. 9.1. Floating Table Exam for Peripheral Vascular Disease.

Clinical Scenario: 58-year-old male with claudication.

Technique: Floating Table Coronal Acquisition, TR/TE/Flip = 9/2.3/40°, 1 NEX, Field-of-View = 400 × 320 × 100mm, Matrix = 512 × 160, with zero filling in the slice direction to create 50 slices, Sequential Ordering of k-space, Acquisition Time = 30 s/station (total imaging time for angio sequence = 3 minutes), 40 ml Gd injected at 0.5 ml/s, and timed empirically (30 second delay from start of injection to start of scanning). Three stations (calf, thigh, and pelvis) acquired pre-contast, and then rapidly in sequence post-contrast to chase the contrast bolus down the legs. Note that the patient is positioned supine (**a**) with bolsters under the knees and ankles to make the legs as horizontal as possible. Coronal 3D acquisition was acquired (**b**) prior to injecting contrast for three stations, beginning with the calf, then the thighs, and finally the pelvis. Injection of contrast was then initiated, and the 3D coronal data was acquired during the bolus arterial phase, beginning with the pelvis, then the thighs, and finally the calf, with rapid manual repositioning of the table (**c**) to chase the bolus down the legs. Finally, the pre-contrast data was subtracted from the arterial phase data to produce (**d**) a digital subtraction arteriogram of the peripheral arteries.

Interpretation: Coronal MIPs of digitally subtracted arterial phase data shows an ectatic infrarenal abdominal aorta, mild stenosis of the right common iliac artery origin, and focal occlusion of the right superficial femoral artery at the level of the adductor canal.

Diagnosis: Peripheral vascular disease.

Submitted by James F.M. Meaney, M.D., Dublin.

Fig. 9.2. Early approach to MRA in Patient With Bilateral Iliac Occlusion.

Clinical Scenario: 67-year-old male patient with history of bilateral calf claudication with a free walking distance of 30 meters. Referred for MRA after unsuccessful attempt at conventional angiography.

Technique: A multi-channel quadrature/phased array peripheral vascular coil, extending from the aortic bifurcation to the ankle, is used for imaging. In a total acquisition time of 70 seconds, the pelvic and thigh arteries are imaged over the first 30 seconds, followed by a 10 second imaging break, during which time the MR table is manually repositioned to the center of the lower imaging volume. The second data set containing the lower thigh and lower limb arteries is again collected over 30 seconds. The 3D EFGRE sequence employed the following parameters: TR/TE/Flip = 5.2/1.5/30°, TI 28 ms, 2.4 mm slice thickness, 48 sections, 480×360 mm Field-of-View, combined with a 256×192 matrix, renders a spatial res-

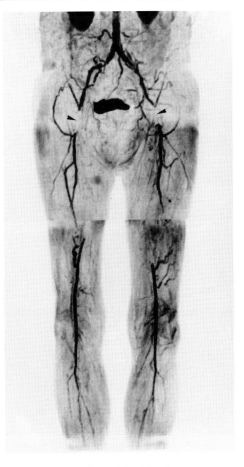

olution of $1.8 \times 2.5 \times 1.2$ mm. For determination of scan-delay following contrast bolus injection, axial multiphase GRE images were collected at the lower thigh level following injection of a 2 ml Gd-DTPA test bolus. A dose of 0.3 mmol/kg Gd-DTPA is injected intravenously using an automated injector over 70 seconds. The administered rate varies between 0.5 and 0.8 ml/s, depending on patient weight.

Interpretation: Image interpretation is performed by viewing source images and combined MIP images.

Diagnosis: Significant stenosis of the common iliac artery on the right side. Bilateral occlusions of the common (*arrowhead*) and superficial femoral arteries with extensive collateralization.

Submitted by Thomas F. Hany, M.D., Zurich.

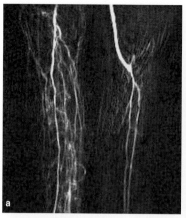
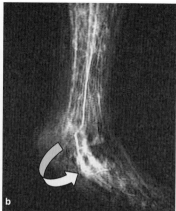
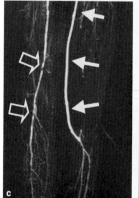
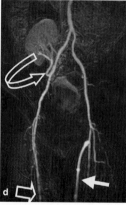

Fig. 9.3. Separate Injections for Each Station.

Clinical Scenario: Diabetic with right leg claudication.

Technique: Time-resolved 2D Projection MRA of calf (**a**), right foot (**b**), followed by 3D Contrast MRA of thigh-upper calf (**c**) and abdomen-pelvis (**d**) with escalating Gd doses. For the time-resolved imaging, 5ml Gd was injected per acquisition. For the thigh, 15 ml Gd was injected at 1ml/s using timing information from the time-resolved 2D Projection MRA and mapping k-space linearly in a high resolution 48 cm FOV, 512 × 256 Matrix acquisition lasting 45 s. Finally the abdomen-pelvis was imaged with 20 ml Gd, sequential mapping of k-space at 512 × 160 Matrix with a 30 second breath-hold.

Interpretation: Left proximal SFA to below knee popliteal artery graft is widely patent (*arrows*). Transplant renal artery in right pelvis is widely patent (*curved open arrow*). Multiple stenoses along right SFA and popliteal artery are present (*open block arrows*). Right foot is supplied by a single run-off vessel which terminates in a region of vigorous early enhancement at the LisFranc joint indicating a developing Charcot foot (*curved solid arrow*).

Diagnosis: Multiple right SFA and Popliteal artery stenoses with runoff via the peroneal artery (single vessel) and a developing charcot foot. Renal transplant artery and left SFA to below knee Popliteal artery graft are widely patent.

Submitted by Martin R. Prince, M.D., Ph.D., New York.

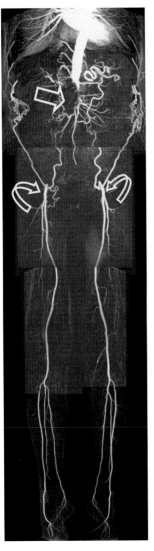

Fig. 9.4. Bolus chase MRA with coil array. Higher SNR with improved depiction of vascular detail is possible with a coil array that covers the region of interest. A switching mechanism allows selection of the coil elements appropriate for each station as the patient slides through the magnet during bolus chase MRA. Note the infrarenal aortic (*open arrow*) and bilateral iliac artery occlusions with reconstitusion of common femoral arteries (*curved arrows*) and normal runoff.

Submitted by Tim Leiner, M.D. and K.Y.J.A.M. Ho, M.D., Maastricht. Reprinted from Radiol Clin North Am 202;40:835-846.

accumulated in the veins or surrounding stationary tissues from prior injections.

Following a non-enhanced scout image, a 3D exam is acquired during the infusion of contrast. Selection of a specific acquisition technique depends upon the available MR scanner technology as well as clinical goals of the examination. 3D contrast MRA techniques have been shown to be accurate for the aorto-iliac and superficial femoral arteries. More recent results suggest that 3D contrast MRA is also accurate for imaging distal runoff vessels of the lower extremities, particularly when performed at higher spatial resolution or ASA time-resolved acquisition. If there are extra-anatomic axillary-to-femoral artery grafts, then the first station should begin in the chest (Figure 9.5).

Three-dimensional contrast MRA of peripheral arteries requires three or four stations in order to image from distal aorta to the ankle. For scanners that do not have special "moving table" technology, it is possible to perform two acquisitions covering the

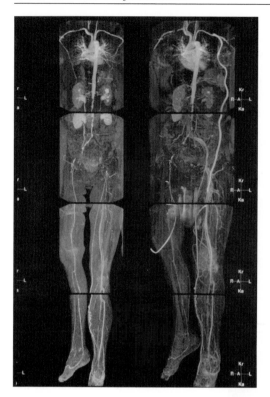

Fig. 9.5. Total Body MRA for Evaluation of Axillary-Femoral Bypass Graft.

Clinical Scenario: 70-year-old female patient with chronic LeRiche syndrome and ulcers of the fourth toe on the left foot. Pelvic radiotherapy of a cervix carcinoma 30 years prior to the vascular occlusion. Translumbar digital subtraction angiography (DSA) confirmed an occlusion of the left common iliac and right external iliac artery. MRA was performed for pre-operative planning.

Technique: Acquisition consists of a series of four 3D MRA datasets (TR/TE/Flip = 7.1/1.0/50°, 1 NSA - 54 contiguous 2 mm sections) with delays of 4 s for manual table displacement. 50 ml of Gd contrast was injected during acquisition of the first 1.5 k-space volumes.

Interpretation: Prior to surgery, MRA demonstrates high-grade, tandem stenoses of the infrarenal aorta and iliac occlusions as seen with DSA. In addition, a normally perfused subclavian artery and a left superficial femoral artery are demonstrated, with only slight atherosclerotic changes. After axillo-femoral graft surgery, a significant increase in perfusion of the left leg via a patent bypass is seen.

Diagnosis: Aortic occlusion treated with an axillary-femoral graft.

Submitted by PD Dr.med. K.U. Wenz, Winterthur.

aorto-iliac and superficial femoral arteries only. In these cases, it is important to image the distal runoff vessels in the lower leg and foot prior to the abdomen-pelvis and thigh-calf stations. Distal vessels can be imaged with 2D TOF (prior to contrast injection) using an inferior saturation pulse with ~10 mm sat. gap to eliminate venous signal.

Typical acquisition parameters for the peripheral vascular 3D contrast MRA methods include: Coronal acquisition, TR<7 ms, TE<2.5 ms, flip = 30–40°, field-of-view = 360 to 480 mm, and a $512 \times 192 \times 24$ acquisition matrix that is reconstructed to $512 \times 512 \times 48$ slices using zero padding. Use of a rectangular field-of-view helps match the imaging volume to the anatomy of interest since extended regions of the anatomy need to be covered only in the cranio-caudad direction.

The continuous infusion method uses a prolonged infusion of Gd contrast in conjunction with rapid movement of the MR scanner table to obtain images over the entire lower extremity (Figures 9.1 and 9.2). Images are obtained using 3D contrast MRA acquisitions during a slow (39 ml volume at 0.3–0.5 ml/s) infusion of paramagnetic contrast. Enhancement of the veins does not occur because the Gd chelate is extracted into the extracellular space during the first pass of contrast agent through the capillary bed. The fast imaging approach collects two or three 48 cm data sets over <60 seconds. This approach permits faster administration of paramagnetic contrast at rates of 1–2 ml/s and seeks to share the bolus between stations. In the faster scanning approach, venous enhancement is avoided by using elliptical centric encoding of k-space on the distal stations and acquiring at least the center of k-space before contrast reaches the veins.

Alternatively, a time-resolved 3D TRICKS or 2D projection MRA can be performed with a small Gd injection, typically 5–6 ml. Time-resolved imaging of the foot can serve as a bolus timing run for planning subsequent bolus chase 3D contrast MRA. The time-resolved acquisition will show when contrast arrives in the distal calf arteries as well as the distal veins. If the flow is very fast with early venous enhancement, then the bolus chase has to be accelerated. If it takes less than 20 seconds for contrast to reach the calf, it will be impossible for bolus chase MRA to keep up with the flow. In this instance, it may be preferable to perform each additional proximal station with a separate injection (Figure 9.3). Alternatively, tourniquets can be applied to slow down flow.

The slow infusion with long imaging times per station work because extraction of contrast capillaries reduces venous enhancement. However, this requires a long infusion with minimal sharing of the bolus between stations. Optimal sharing of the bolus between multiple stations of a bolus chase examination occurs when the 3D MR angiography and table movement is fast enough to keep up with the flow of contrast down the legs. This is challenging because the rate at which contrast flows down the legs is about 5–6 seconds per station. Extremely fast imaging and fast table motion is necessary to accomplish both within 6 seconds per station. Several approaches to accelerating MRA to begin to approach this goal have been described as follows:

Shoot and Scoot:

This approach to accelerating bolus chase MRA for greater bolus sharing takes advantage of the fact that the central k-space data dominates image contrast. After obtaining pre-contrast mask data, Gd is injected and an initial, fast bolus chase is performed collecting only central k-space data during the arterial phase. Then a second, slower pass collects peripheral k-space data to increase MRA image resolution. Finally, all the data is post-processed to subtract background and combine central with peripheral k-space data to create the optimized high resolution arterial phase multi-station image (Figure 9.6).

Continuous Table Motion:

Since there are only 5-6 seconds available to collect data per station and time used for table motion is precious, many investigators prefer to manually move the table as it is faster than the automatic table movement. Indeed manual table motion may take 1–2 seconds while automatic table motion may be 4-8 seconds, depending upon the manufacturer. An alternative solution is to collect MRA data while the table is continuously moving. This approach, somewhat analogous to spiral CTA, completely eliminates the table motion time penalty although it introduces new challenges. In particular, gradient warp effects change as the table moves. Motion correction and other reconstruction artifacts need to be resolved. Several strategies for continuous motion data acquisition have been advocated. One strategy is to image with an axial volume acquisition that is continuously translating with the table. Another is to use a coronal volume with FOV smaller than magnet FOV so that it remains stationary with respect to the patient and then jumps forward when it reaches the limit of the magnet FOV.

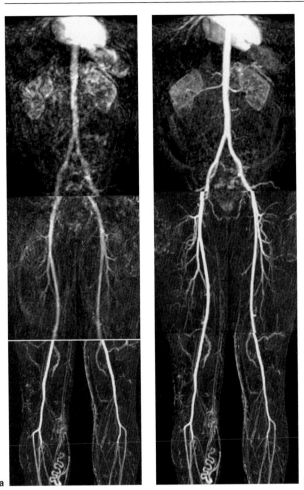

a   b

Fig 9.6. Shoot and Scoot. (**a**) An initial bolus chase collects only the central k-space data in the proximal (abdomen-pelvis) and middle (thigh) stations in order to reach the calf station as quickly as possible. After completing a full, high-resolution data acquisition of the calf, the table reverses direction to finish collecting peripheral k-space data for middle and proximal stations (**b**). Note after the center of k-space (**a**) MRA shows contrast but does not reveal image detail. But after the peripheral k-space data are collected (**b**) there is more detail with preservation of arterial phase contrast. Reprinted from Aksit P, Frigo FJ, Polzin J, Choyke P, Ho VB, Hood MN, Hess S, Montequin M, Foo T. Shoot and Scoot: A segmented Volume Acquisition Method for High-Resolution Multi-station Imaging of peripheral Vasculature (abst.) ISMRM 10th Scientific Meeting and Exhibition program. Berkeley CA 2002;208. (18-24 May 2002; Honolulu, Hawaii).

Wakitrak:

This approach to accelerating data acquisition utilizes parallel imaging so that scanning can keep up with the contrast bolus. SENSE is used, in combination with a body array coil, to accelerate data acquisition for the abdomen-pelvis 2-fold down to 10 seconds (Figure 2.16). A relatively low resolution coronal scan of the thighs is obtained with the body coil in 10 seconds. Finally, a third station covering calf and feet in the sagittal plane is acquired with the spine array coil with elliptical centric encoding of k-space and an extended acquisition of 77 seconds to obtain sub-millimeter resolution. This approach has the advantages of being fast in the upper stations for maximum bolus sharing and avoiding venous contamination. It is also high resolution in the calf and feet for resolving atherosclerotic stenoses in tiny tibial and pedal arteries.

Time-Resolved Peripheral MRA:

The time-resolved 3D MR digital subtraction angiography (DSA) method uses the separate injections at three different anatomic stations. This has the advantage of demonstrating temporal enhancements such as delayed filling of arteries distal to occlusive disease (Figure 9.7). Three injections are typically administered in escalating doses (e.g. 0.075, 0.1, and 0.125 mmol/kg or 5–10, 10–15, and 15–20 ml) in order to compensate for deterioration in image quality that occurs as contrast accumulates in the tissues and veins. Images are reconstructed with a 512×512 matrix every few seconds in order to isolate an arterial phase of contrast passage at each station. Higher resolution temporal MRA can be obtained with 2D Projection MRA but with only a single projection. With 3D TRICKS and VIPR, images are reconstructed with lower temporal resolution (typically every 7 seconds) with the advantage of having 3D data that can be reconstructed into any obliquity with MIP or volume rendering post-processing techniques.

Time-Resolved and Bolus Chase MRA:

Because of the merits of both time-resolved MRA (particularly for infrapopliteal arteries) and the bolus chase technique (for abdominal aorta, iliac, femoral and popliteal arteries), the most useful combination is a time-resolved 3D-TRICKS or 2D projection MRA of the calf and feet, followed by a bolus chase MRA of abdomen, pelvis, thigh and trifurcation (Figure 9.8).

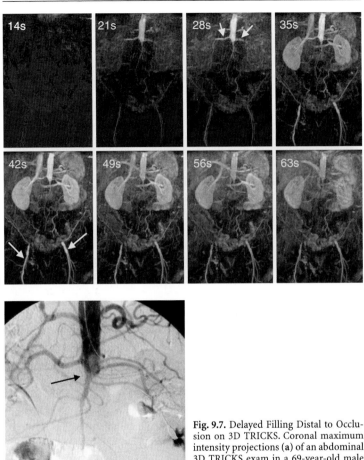

Fig. 9.7. Delayed Filling Distal to Occlusion on 3D TRICKS. Coronal maximum intensity projections (**a**) of an abdominal 3D TRICKS exam in a 69-year-old male patient with complete aortic occlusion. The advantages of a time-resolved acquisition are reflected in the peak arterial filling of the aorto-renal arteries just above the occlusion at 28 seconds (*short arrows*) and the maximum signal from the common femoral arteries at 42 seconds (*long arrows*). The time-resolved method allows demonstration of vessels distal to occlusions that may be otherwise difficult to see on digital subtraction angiography (**b**) or single-phase MRA exams. (Reprinted from Swan JS, Carroll TJ, Kennell TW, Heisey DM, Korosec FR, Frayne R, Mistretta CA, Grist TM. Time-resolved 3D contrast-enhanced MRA of the peripheral vessels. Radiology, 2002)

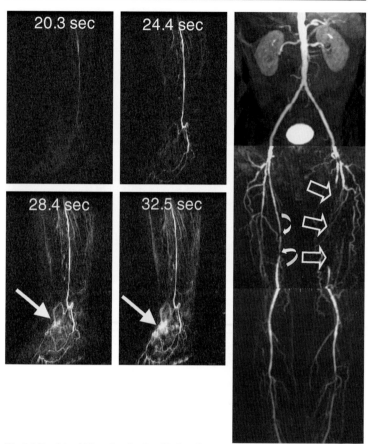

Fig. 9.8. Combined Time-Resolved and Bolus Chase MRA.

Clinical Scenario: Diabetic with non-healing left toe ulcer.

Technique: 2D time-resolved Projection MRA of left calf and foot with 5ml Gd injected by hand as a bolus followed by 3D bolus chase MRA with 40 ml Gd injected by hand at 2ml/s. Timing information from time-resolved calf imaging is used to plan the 3D bolus chase timing.

Interpretation/Diagnosis: Left long SFA occlusion (*open arrows*) with single vessel runoff via peroneal artery that reconstitutes plantar arch. Early enhancement in left Lisfranc joint (*arrow*) indicates early Charcot changes. Multiple Right SFA severe stenoses (*curved arrows*).

Submitted by Martin Prince, M.D., Ph.D., Priscilla Winchester, M.D., Neil Khilnani, M.D., New York.

Complimentary Sequences

As described above, 2D TOF imaging of the lower extremities has been effective for the infra-inguinal vessels. Typical 2D TOF parameters include: TR = 30-45 ms, TE = 6.9 ms with gradient moment nulling, flip = 60°, field-of-view = 240 to 320 mm, and a 256 × 128 acquisition matrix. For the SFA and popliteal arteries, 3 mm slice-spacing is used with 4 mm thick overlapping slices. For distal runoff vessels, it is desirable to reduce the slice thickness and increase spatial resolution in order to resolve small arteries of the lower leg. Typical acquisition parameters for distal vessels include 2 mm slice thickness and spacing and in-plane resolution of 0.8 × 0.8 mm. These higher resolution parameters for imaging small distal vessels require a high signal-to-noise coil such as extremity coil, knee coil or head coil. Smaller, extremity coils give higher SNR for higher quality MRA but they require several coil placements per leg and can only image one leg at a time. The larger head coil can usually image both feet simultaneously, and requires only 2 coil placements to cover trifurcation down to mid foot, but the SNR is only half that of the extremity coil. If the clinical indication focuses on just one leg, it is better to use the extremity coil for the higher SNR.

Due to triphasic flow in peripheral vessels, it is desirable to synchronize the 2D TOF acquisition with the cardiac cycle, thereby reducing the effects of retrograde flow. To remove venous signal, a spatial presaturation slab is placed inferior to the slice, and is programmed to move concurrently (concatenated saturation) with the slice. The gap between the spatial presaturation pulse and the acquisition slice is typically set to 10 mm. A smaller gap can result in saturation of arterial flow during the portion of the cardiac cycle in which the flow is reversed. A larger saturation gap, on the other hand, may insufficiently suppress venous flow. In the foot, slow venous flow in some patients may require selection of a saturation gap of 5 mm.

Clinical Indications

Peripheral Vascular Disease (PVD)

Three-dimensional contrast MRA is useful for evaluating PVD. It can be used to augment 2D TOF methods. At most centers, 3D contrast MRA has eclipsed the entire 2D TOF exam since the 3D contrast enhanced methods can markedly reduce examination time and improve image quality. Additionally, 3D contrast MRA techniques are inherently more accurate for determining the length of an occluded segment than 2D TOF methods since there are no saturation pulses applied. Table 9.1 summarizes papers reporting on the diagnostic accuracy of 3D contrast MRA and several recent meta analyses are summarized in Table 9.2.

Table 9.1. Diagnostic Accuracy of 3D Contrast MRA of Peripheral Arteries

Author	Year	Journal	# of Patients	Sensitivity	Specificity
Prince	1995	Radiology	43	94 %	98 %
Snidow	1996	Radiology	32	100 %	98 %
Hany	1997	Radiology	39	93–96 %	96–100 %
Poon	1997	Radiology	15	100 %	100 %
Rofsky	1997	Radiology	15	97 %	96 %
Quinn	1997	JMRI	30	100 %	99 %
Perrier	1998	J Radiol	23	92 %	93 %
Yamashita	1998	JMRI	15	96 %	83 %
Ho	1998	Radiology	43	93 %	98 %
Ho	1998	Radiology	28	94 %	93 %
Maspes	1999	Radiol Med	47 (11**)	100 %	87.5 %
Lenhart	1999	RoFo	22 (17*)	82–96 %	87–99 %
Oberholzer	1999	RoFo	8	89 %	100 %
Link	1999	Radiology	67	100 %	83 %
Meaney	1999	Radiology	20	81–94 %	91–97 %
Mitsuzaki	2000	Radiology	22	91 %	89 %
Bourlet	2000	J Radiol	22	96 %	80 %
Wikstrom	2000	Eur J Vasc Endovasc Surg	30	86 %	88 %
Lundin	2000	Acta Radiol	39	81–94 %	81-94 %
Lenhart	2000	RoFo	45 (20*)	87.5–100 %	96.8–100 %
Huber	2000	AJR	24	100 %	94–98 %
Sueyoshi	2000	Acta Radiol	13	100 %	96.5 %
Ruehm	2000	AJR	61	92.3 %	99.4 %
Ruehm	2001	JMRI	23	90 %	95 %
Brillet	2001	J Mal Vasc	15	kappa = 0.75 %	
Di Cesare	2001	Radiol Med	45	97–100 %	84.8–89 %
Reid	2001	J Vasc Interv Radiol	13	100 %	
Ruehm	2001	Lancet	6	91–94 %	90–93 %
Winterer	2002	EJR	43	84 %	60 %
Carriero	2002	CIR	11	94.1 %	99.2 %
Khilnani	2002	Radiology	30	91–95 % agreement with DSA	
Goyen	2002	Radiology	10	95.3 %	95.2 %
Schoenberg	2002	Invest Radiol	41	78–97 %	75–96 %
Swan	2002	Radiology	69	89 %	91 %

Table 9.2. Peripheral MRA Meta Analyses

	N	Sensitivity	Specificity
Nelmans Radiology 2000, 217: 105-114			
GD MRA (8 Papers)	253	92-100 %	91-99 %
2D TOF (11 Papers)	344	64-100 %	68-96 %
Visser & Hunick Radiology 2000, 216: 67-77			
GD MRA (9 Papers)	216	97.5 %	96.2 %
Duplex US (18 Papers)	1059	87.6 %	94.7 %
Koelemay et al. JAMA 2001, 285: 1338-45			
3D GD MRA	475	94 %	94 %
2D TOF & PC	615	90 %	90 %

Aorto-Iliac (Inflow) Vessels

The advent of 3D contrast MRA methods has significantly improved the accuracy of MRA in assessing the pelvic arterial system of patients with aorto-iliac disease. Two-dimensional TOF methods have limited accuracy in the pelvis due to tortuosity of iliac vessels, pulsatile blood flow, as well as bowel and respiratory motion artifacts and bowel gas susceptibility artifact. 3D contrast MRA is flow-insensitive, and therefore not affected by these artifacts (Figure 1.2). The short TE of 3D contrast MRA helps to eliminate susceptibility artifact from bowel gas or any surgical clips. The 3D contrast MRA method can more accurately determine the length of the stenotic or occluded segment than 2D TOF, therefore identifying whether the patient will need percutaneous angioplasty or surgical intervention.

Distal (Runoff) Vessels

Contrast MRA is more complicated to perform on distal lower extremity vessels due to substantial variations in contrast travel time, especially in patients with occlusive disease. Although this problem may be overcome by using a time-resolved acquisition or a long continuous infusion, these methods still need to be validated in large-scale clinical trials. Early results, however, are encouraging (Figures 9.1–9.2, Table 9.1).

Bypass Graft Patency

Accuracy of 2D TOF methods for surveillance of graft patency has been demonstrated. However, several pitfalls exist. They include retrograde flow in vessels just proximal to distal graft anastomoses, arteriovenous fistulas associated with the graft, and artifacts associated with metal clips that can mimic a stenosis on 2D TOF. The pitfalls of surgical clip artifact, in-plane flow in tortuous grafts, turbulent flow at anastomoses are largely eliminated on 3D contrast MRA due to a shorter TE (Figure 9.5). For these reasons, 3D contrast MRA is increasingly utilized for evaluating bypass grafts (Figure 9.9).

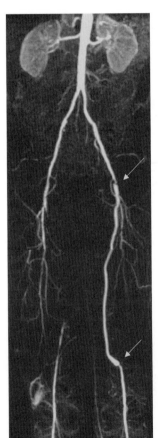

Fig 9.9. Fem-Pop Bypass Graft with Anastomotic Stenoses.

Clinical Scenario: Elevated velocities at bypass graft anastomoses on routine surveillance doppler ultrasound.

Technique: Bolus chase peripheral MRA.

Interpretation: MRA show left femoral to popliteal artery bypass graft with severe stenoses at both proximal and distal anastomoses. Also note right SFA long occlusion.

Diagnosis: Severe anastomotic stenoses on left femoral to popliteal artery bypass graft.

Submitted by Thomas M. Grist, M.D., Madison.

Table 9.3. Accuracy of 3D Contrast MRA for Peripheral Bypass Grafts

Author	Year	Journal	# of Patients	Sensitivity	Specificity
Bendib	1997	J Vasc Surg	23	91 %	92 %
Loewe	2000	Eur Radiol	35	100 %	91.3 %
Bertschinger	2001	AJR	39 (30*)	100 %	100 %
Dronbeck	2002	Invest Radiol	15	100 %	90 %

Arteriovenous Malformations (AVM)

Arteriovenous malformations are benign, soft tissue neoplasms that can cause complications due to local extension. Three-dimensional contrast MRA can detect arteriovenous malformations or fistulas of the upper or lower extremities. It is helpful to obtain a multi-phase exam in order to demonstrate early filling of the draining veins (Figure 9.10 and 9.11).

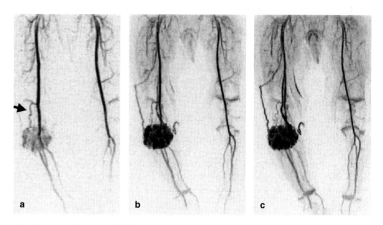

Fig. 9.10. Arteriovenous Malformation in Leg.

Clinical Scenario: 2-month-old child with leg mass.

Technique: Time-resolved imaging. Sequential 3D volumes were reconstructed every 2 seconds using the 3D TRICKS technique. Images show early arterial filling of the vascular malformation (**a**) from geniculate vessels (*arrow*), followed by the blush (**b**), and then the venous drainage is demonstrated. Time resolved imaging allowed the use of a small 2 cc bolus in this infant, without a timing scan.

Interpretation: Rapidly enhancing mass with venous shunting.

Diagnosis: Arterio-venous malformation.

(Reprinted with permission form Carroll TJ and Grist TM. Technical developments in MR angiography, Radiol Clin N Am 40 (2002) 921-951).

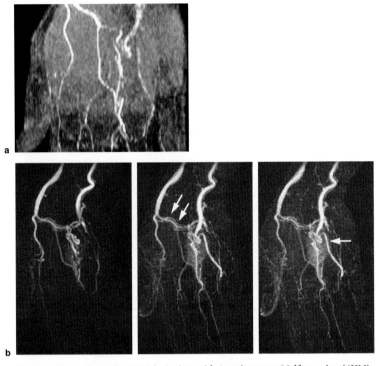

Fig. 9.11. Upper Extremity MRA in Patient with Arteriovenous Malformation (AVM).
Clinical Scenario: 37-year-old male with a known arteriovenous malformation of the left hand previously treated with radiation therapy and surgery in 1993.

Technique: Exam was performed with the patient's arm in a transmit/receive extremity coil. (**a**) 2D TOF axial acquisition was initially used for diagnosis, TR/TE/Flip = 45/6.9/45°, 3 mm slice thickness, 60 slices, Field-of-View = 160 × 160 mm, Matrix = 256 × 160. (**b**) Three separate 3D fast gradient echo coronal acquisitions were acquired with a TR/TE/Flip = 6.3/1.7/45°, Field-of-View = 200 × 150 × 60 mm, Matrix = 256 × 256 × 60, zero filling, with source image subtraction. A 20 ml bolus of intravenous gadolinium contrast was administered at 1.0 ml/s. Multiplanar reformats and reprojections were generated from the resulting data using MIP and MPVR techniques.

Interpretation: Images demonstrate some residual blush and vascularity in the AVM, but no significant progression in lesion size since the prior study. 3D contrast MRA more clearly demonstrates the palmer arch and feeding vessels of the AVM due to the lack of in-plane flow saturation artifact. In addition, the contrast technique is inherently more sensitive for demonstrating (*arrows*) the blush associated with soft tissue neoplasm (*arrow*).

Diagnosis: Left hand AVM.

Submitted by J. Greg Baden, M.D., Madison.

This allows discrimination of "fast flow" AVMs from the hemangioma and capillary malformations with slow flow. It is beneficial to use a dedicated extremity coil for evaluation of the AVM to obtain the highest resolution images. A smaller field-of-view can be prescribed with extremity coils to stay within the coil sensitivity region.

Dialysis Fistulas

Dialysis shunts are created using graft material interposed between upper extremity arteries and the adjacent vein or a direct arterial-venous anastomosis. Alternatively a dialysis fistula is created by directly anastomosing an upper extremity artery to a vein and allowing time for the vein to "mature" into a site suitable for dialysis access. Complications of dialysis shunts and fistulas include restenosis, thrombosis, occlusion, and aneurysm formation. In addition, the fistula can create a steal phenomenon that reduces flow to the distal arm and hand or leg if the fistula is in the lower extremity. Three-dimensional contrast MRA can identify these complications associated with upper extremity arteriovenous shunts for dialysis access (Figure 9.12). The examination may be performed using the body coil and a large field-of-view if a survey is desired, or a local coil and a small field-of-view for a high resolution scan at the anastomosis. Inflation of a blood pressure cuff at moment of the Gd bolus arterial phase may allow imaging for a longer period of time to obtain higher resolution images.

Peripheral MRA in Children

Despite improved techniques and smaller catheters, conventional angiography has a higher complication rate in children relative to adults. In addition, complications resulting in lower extremity occlusive disease may result in long-term adverse sequela, including like limb length discrepancy. Three-dimensional contrast MRA represents an ideal non-invasive alternative for evaluating the pediatric population (Figure 9.10 and 9.13). In the pediatric population, 3D contrast MRA needs to be modified to use slower injection rates of the paramagnetic contrast agent in order to account for the differences in patient weight, central blood volume, and cardiac output. The general principal of matching the injection time (with physiologic dispersion) to the image acquisition time results in high quality images. However, the tendency for faster flow

Fig. 9.12. Upper Extremity MRA in Dialysis Fistula.

Clinical Scenario: 48-year-old female presents with poorly functioning dialysis fistula.

Technique: Coronal 3D contrast MRA, Body Coil, TR/TE/Flip = 10/2.3/45-60°, Field-of-View = $360 \times 360 \times 88$ mm, Matrix = $512 \times 160 \times 44$, zero filling, with source image subtraction. A 40 ml bolus of intravenous gadolinium contrast was administered at 1.4 ml/s.

Interpretation: The dialysis fistula is patent, but a severe stenosis is present in the venous outflow limb. There is also aneurysmal dilatation of the draining vein distal to the stenosis.

Diagnosis: Patent dialysis fistula with severe stenosis of outflow.

Submitted by Thomas M. Grist, M.D., Madison.

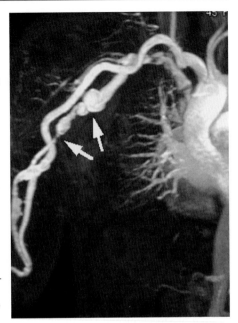

in children favors use of time-resolved 3D MRA (Figure 9.10). For time-resolved acquisitions, a bolus injection at the fastest reasonable rate is acceptable because there is always some physiological dispersion of the bolus as it passes through the heart and lungs. It is important to account for the dead space in the IV tubing since the tubing becomes a substantial factor in determining time delay between injection and arrival of contrast in the imaging region in the patient.

Non-Atherosclerotic Peripheral Vascular Disease

It is important to realize that atherosclerosis is not the only cause of arterial stenoses and occlusions. Since atherosclerosis tends to be symmetrical, asymmetrical disease should always raise the suspicion of an alternative pathology. Emboli tend to lodge at branch points such as aortic bifurcations, common femoral bifurcation or the trifurcation (Figure 9.14). An

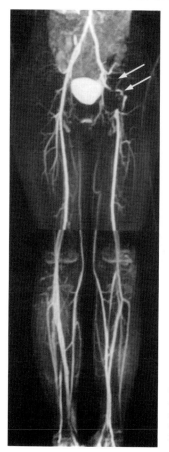

Fig. 9.13. Pediatric Lower Extremity MRA.

Clinical Scenario: 8-year-old boy with intermittent complaints of claudication in the left leg. In early childhood, he underwent dilation of the aortic valve because of a congenital aortic stenosis. Access of intervention was the common femoral artery in the left groin.

Technique: A 3D MRA strategy (3D spoiled gradient echo sequence, TR/TE/Flip = 5.2/1.5/30°, TI 28 ms, 0.5 NEX) combining a dedicated vascular coil with a single injection was applied. Two 3D acquisitions, each consisting of 46 continuous sections with a section thickness of 2.4 mm, were collected over 30 seconds. The first covered the pelvis and thighs while the second covered the popliteal and trifurcation vessels. Gadolinium contrast agent (0.3 mmol/kg) was administered through an iv with a power injector at a rate of 0.6 ml/s.

Interpretation: The 3D MR angiographic MIP image shows an occlusion of the left external iliac artery (*arrows*) due to a post-interventional complication after catheter insertion. Collateral vessels originating from the left internal iliac artery are well visualized.

Diagnosis: Occlusion of the left external iliac artery.

Submitted by Stefan G. Ruehm, Essen.

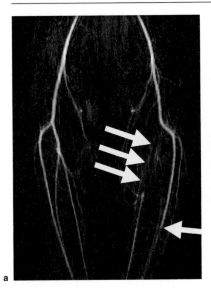

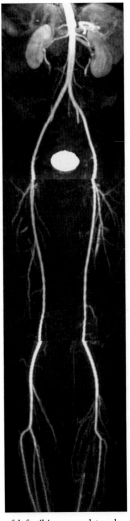

Fig. 9.14. Embolus to Trifurcation.

Clinical Scenario: 36-year-old oncology patient with left calf claudication.

Technique: Time-resolved 2D Projection MRA (**a**) of calf followed by bolus chase MRA (**b**).

Interpretation: time-resolved (**a**) and bolus chase (**b**) MRA show assymetrical occlusive disease isolated to left calf. Abrupt occlusion of left tibioperoneal trunk, peroneal artery and upper posterior tibial artery (*3 arrows*) with reconstitution of posterior tibial artery at mid-calf via geniculate collaterals. A second site of abrupt arterial cut-off noted in mid-anterior tibial artery (*arrow*).

Diagnosis: Embolus to trifurcation.

Submitted by Martin R. Prince, M.D., Ph.D., New York.

anatomic variant in gastrocnemius tendon insertion on the femoral condyle can pinch the popliteal artery during plantar flexion causing entrapment syndrome (Figure 9.15). Another rare condition that narrows the popliteal artery is cystic adventitial disease in which gelatinous cysts in the wall of the artery cause extrinsic compression during flexion of the knee (Figure 9.16).

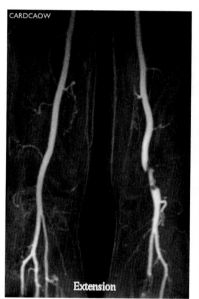
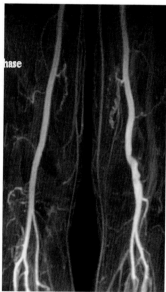

a   b

Fig. 9.15. Popliteal Entrapment.

Clinical Scenario: 52-year-old male with unilateral intermittent claudication.

Technique: Dose timing was performed with 1cc Gadolinium through a peripheral IV at 0.8 cc/s to determine arrival time in the popliteal artery. Subsequent coronal non-elliptical 3D fat-suppressed SPGR (TI 21/TR 4/TE 1.6/29°) was obtained with acquisition time of 24 s. One dynamic series was obtained with injection of 13 ml Gd during active plantar-flexion followed by a brief muscle rest period, then another series in dorsi-flexion with additional injection of 17 ml Gd contrast.

Interpretation: MRA that shows narrowing and medial deviation of popliteal artery during plantar-flexion (**a**) by extrinsic compression from a fibrous band mimicking thrombus which is relieved with dorsi-flexion. Also note post-stenotic dilatation causing focal popliteal aneurysm.

Diagnosis: Popliteal Entrapment: confirmed at surgery.

Submitted by Kris Pillai, M.D. and Thomas Grist M.D., Madison.

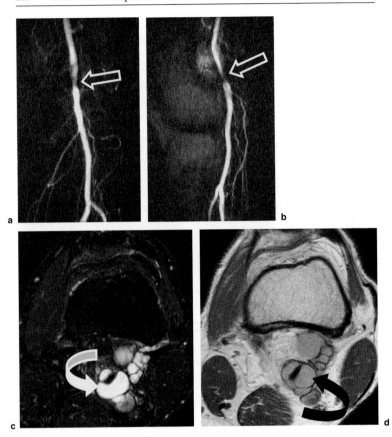

Fig 9.16. Cystic Adventitial Disease.

Clinical Scenario: 44-year-old male with unilateral claudication climbing stairs.

Technique: 2D Projection MRA in extremity coil, TR/TE/Flip = 7/1.2/60, Field-of-View = 240 × 240 × 50, Matrix = 256 × 192 × 1, 5ml Gd injected by hand as fast as possible (~5ml/s) twice for coronal and then sagittal acquisitions. Fourier data were post-processed to perform complex subtraction of multiple masks from the sum of multiple arterial phases using AutoDSA.

Interpretation: Coronal (a) and Sagittal (b) peak arterial phase images show focal smooth narrowing in popliteal artery at the top of the femoral condyle (*open arrows*). Axial STIR (c) and proton density (d) images show cysts within the popliteal artery adventia (*curved arrows*) which are pinching the lumen. At surgery, these cysts were aspirated to restore normal popliteal artery caliber.

Diagnosis: Popliteal artery stenosis by cystic adventitial disease.

Submitted by Hale Ersoy Erel, M.D. and Sanjay Rajagopalan, M.D., New York. Reprinted from Vascular Medicine 2002;7:55.

Pitfalls

Timing of Vessel Opacification

One issue affecting all forms of 3D contrast MRA is of particular relevance when considering the peripheral arteries: timing of image acquisition relative to arrival of contrast. This problem is also encountered with conventional angiography of the peripheral vasculature. Substantial delays in contrast arrival can occur for vessel segments distal to an occlusion. These delays are neither predictable nor symmetric. Timing should be based on the "slower" extremity or the symptomatic extremity. Multiphase or time-resolved MRA acquisitions obviate the need for timing altogether, even in highly complex cases involving distal runoff where delays and variations in contrast arrival time can be substantial. Alternatively, methods that use a long, slow infusion of contrast may circumvent the problem of delayed enhancement of vessels distal to an occlusion as well as due to the prolonged dispersion of the arterial contrast.

Metal Clip and Stent Artifacts

Metallic surgical clips placed near vascular bypass grafts can create artifacts that simulate stenoses. Artifact is caused by susceptibility effects of the metal, which causes signal dropout in the clip region. The metal artifact can be identified due to the signal void that has a characteristic bright build-up of signal on one side of the void. These artifacts are minimized, but not completely eliminated, using short TE sequences of 3D contrast MRA (Figure 9.17). To get the shortest possible TE, use the widest bandwidth available on your imaging system. Intravascular stents may be particularly problematic depending upon stent composition. The most MR compatible stents are nitinol or platinum, which are totally non-magnetic (see Table 1.1). Even non-magnetic stents may obscure the artery lumen by attenuating the rf signal. This can be at least partially overcome in platinum and nitinol stents using a higher flip angle (e.g. 60°–120°).

Pseudo-Occlusion from Inadvertent Exclusion of Arteries

It is critical to include the arteries within the 3D contrast MRA imaging volume. It is tempting to use a narrow volume to be able to have a fast scan with high resolution by using a small number of narrow slices.

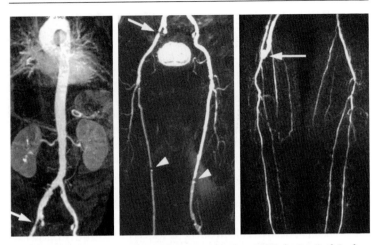

Fig. 9.17. Metallic Clip Artifact on 3D MR DSA in Patient with Infra-Inguinal Grafts.

Clinical Scenario: 68-year-old with right leg claudication two years following surgical revascularization.

Technique: A 3D fast gradient echo acquisition was used with a Coronal Acquisition, TR/TE/Flip = 10/12.3/60°, Field-of-View = 480 × 360 × 66 mm, Matrix = 512 × 256 × 44, zero filling, with source image subtraction, 3D TRICKS Acquisition Sequence, with a 3D volume reconstructed every 7 seconds. A 16 ml bolus of iv gadolinium contrast was administered in three sequential doses at a rate of 2 ml/s.

Interpretation: This multi-station peripheral MRA exam demonstrates a right iliac stenosis (*arrow*) and bilateral femoral-popliteal bypass grafts. The bypass grafts are patent although small focal areas of signal loss are seen at the location of metallic clips (*arrowheads*) placed at the time of surgery. The characteristic appearance of susceptibility artifact is shown, as demonstrated by the focal area of signal loss with adjacent bright signal.

Diagnosis: Right iliac stenosis and patent bilateral femoral-to-popliteal bypass grafts with clip artifacts.

Submitted by Thomas M. Grist, M.D., Madison.

However, if the tolerance is too tight, a small error in positioning or movement of the patient may result in part of an artery drifting out of the FOV. Vessels most susceptible to this problem include tortuous common iliac arteries, common femoral arteries (Figure 9.18) and popliteal arteries.

Aneurysm May Be Larger Than Lumen

Since MRA shows the vessel lumen, the true vessel diameter is not displayed well on 3D contrast MRA. Whenever an aneurysm is suspected,

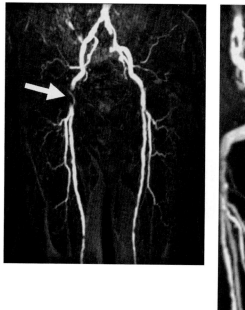

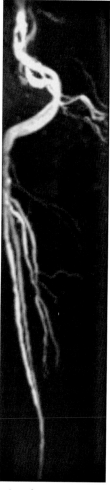

Fig. 9.18. Common Femoral Artery Inadvertently Excluded. Coronal MIP (**a**) shows a focal occlusion of the right common femoral artery (*arrow*). However, sagittal MIP (**b**) reveals that the common femoral arteries are not completely contained within the 3D imaging volume. Thus the appearance of common femoral artery occlusion may be false and the patient must be called back to repeat the study with more anterior positioning of the imaging volume. To prevent this error, meticulous attention must be paid to the location of common femoral arteries on an axial TOF localizer. Submitted by Martin R. Prince, M.D., Ph.D., New York.

the possibility that the aneurysm is lined with thrombus should be considered. This can be assessed on post-Gd Axial TOF or T1 flow compensated images (Figure 9.19).

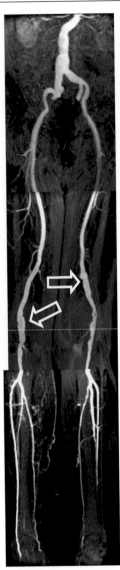

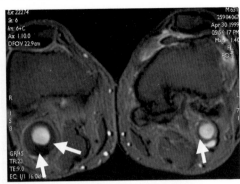

Fig. 9.19. Popliteal Artery Aneurysm. Bolus chase MRA (**a**) shows ectatic vessels with mildly aneurysmal popliteal arteries bilaterally (*arrows*). However a post gadolinium axial 2D TOF (**b**) obtained at the level of dashed line in (**a**) with 5 mm thick slices using the head coil shows the aneurysms are lined with thrombus (*arrows*). Thus the aneurysms are larger than the size apparent on bolus chase MRA. Submitted by Martin Prince, M.D., Ph.D., New York.

Osseous Landmarks

Although MRA may show the site of pathology, it may be difficult to determine where a stenosis or aneurysm is located relative to standard bony landmarks. This makes it difficult for a surgeon to determine where to make the incision. One solution is to film a coronal MIP and a corresponding coronal T1 weighted image side by side. Alternatively, a representative coronal T1 weighted image can be partially added to the arterial MIP (Figure 9.20).

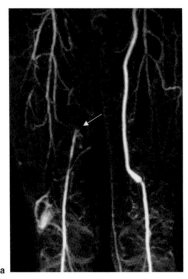 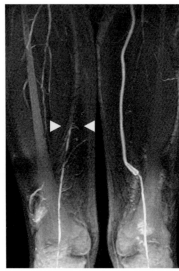

a   b

Fig. 9.20. Osseous Landmarks.

Clinical Scenario: 65-year-old with history of PVD presented with right non-healing ulcer.

Technique: The figure shows images from the thigh station in a three station peripheral vascular MRA exam using 40 cc gadolinium contrast agent. The arterial phase image (a) is obtained by acquiring the contrast-enhanced image and subtracting the unenhanced mask. However, surgical landmarks are not well seen in the subtracted image. Therefore, the subtracted image is added back to a scaled down version of the un-enhanced image to generate a composite image (b) that contains the osseous landmarks. This approach is preferred over simply performing a MIP display of the arterial phase image, because background fat signal often overwhelms the signal available from the contrast-enhanced vessels.

Interpretation: Occlusion of right superficial femoral artery (*arrow*) with reconstitution at the adductor canal (*arrowheads*).

Diagnosis: Right SFA occlusion.

Submitted by Thomas Grist, M.D., Madison.

CHAPTER 10

Extracranial Carotid Arteries and Arch Vessels

Background

Catheter-based angiographic techniques, including digital subtraction angiography (DSA), have been the gold standard for diagnosis of carotid bulb disease. These projection images of the carotid bulb were the sole basis for treatment decisions in the NASCET and ESCT trials. DSA has several limitations, however, foremost of which is an approximately 4% incidence of transient ischemic attack and 1% incidence of disabling stroke caused by selective arterial catheterization. In addition, the DSA method is primarily implemented as a projection of the vascular lumen. Due to eccentric disease, the measurement of percent stenosis may vary by projection. Projection variation combined with substantial observer variability reduces the accuracy of conventional DSA. Nevertheless, accurate depiction of carotid stenosis is critical. Misclassification of the degree of a stenosis may result in unnecessary surgery. Since surgery is also associated with an estimated 1% incidence of disabling stroke or death, it is paramount that any diagnostic technique is accurate for differentiating surgical and non-surgical disease.

These issues have motivated the development of less invasive cross-sectional methods for imaging the carotid bifurcation using MRA. Several non-contrast-enhanced MRA techniques evaluating extracranial carotid arterial disease include 2D TOF and single or multiple slab 3D TOF. Accuracy of these methods has been evaluated in a number of clinical trials. Since 2D TOF and 3D TOF methods have complementary imaging characteristics, it is important to use a combination of these techniques in order to accurately diagnose stenotic disease. These TOF methods require 5 to 10 minutes of imaging time for each sequence, are compromised by motion artifacts, and yield images that have a physical basis different than conventional angiography. Non-contrast techniques are inherently flow sensitive, and therefore are prone to pitfalls associated with slow flow or turbulence.

In addition, recent re-analysis of the NASCET data reveals that a significant number of strokes are caused by disease outside the carotid bifurcation. Furthermore, surgery may be contra-indicated if significant tandem lesions are present in the proximal or distal carotid circulation. Therefore, it is desirable to image the carotid circulation from aortic arch through Circle of Willis, which is difficult to accomplish without using Gd contrast enhancement.

By virtue of its insensitivity to flow artifacts, 3D contrast MRA is an ideal method to more precisely depict the arterial morphology in extracranial carotid stenotic disease. The paramagnetic contrast agent increases vascular signal and reduces signal loss from in-plane saturation or intra-voxel phase dispersion (Figure 10.1). Furthermore, data can be acquired in either the coronal or sagittal planes, thereby reducing the acquisition volume required to depict carotid arteries. This also reduces data acquisition time permitting collection of time-resolved, subtracted image sets capable of isolating the contrast bolus arterial phase. Finally, 3D contrast MRA images represent a luminogram free of dephasing artifacts for accurate determination of true vessel lumen diameters even in high-grade stenoses. It is important to note, however, that spatial resolution must be high in order to accurately depict the degree of stenosis on MR angiograms, even in the presence of gadolinium contrast agents. For example, in a carotid artery that measures 6 mm, a 70% stenosis results in a 1.8 mm diameter lumen. Partial volume effects may cause significant under-estimation of the degree of stenosis if the voxel size exceeds $1 \times 1 \times 1.5$ mm. Therefore, meticulous attention to detail is required to insure that the maximum possible spatial resolution is achieved for carotid MRA.

Three-dimensional contrast MRA also has a significant advantage over conventional catheter angiography. The three-dimensional nature of the data permits data-reformation into any plane, and thus virtually eliminates the potential of projection related errors in the estimation of stenosis severity. There are also safety advantages of eliminating nephrotoxicity, ionizing radiation, and the risk of stroke associated with conventional catheter angiography.

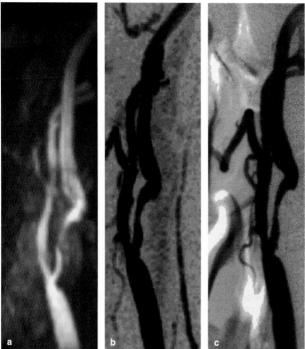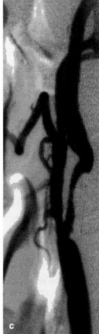

Fig. 10.1. 3D Contrast MRA eliminates intravoxel dephasing. 3D TOF (**a**) shows internal carotid artery stenosis but the precise degree of narrowing is difficult to assess due to intravoxel dephasing. 3D Contrast MRA (**b**) depicts the stenosis more accurately and similar to convention DSA (**c**). The short echo time of 3D contrast MRA reduces the time for phase dispersion to occur at sites of high-velocity, jet-like flow in severe stenoses. This allows 3D contrast MRA to more accurately depict the true lumen dimensions.
Submitted by Pat Turski, M.D. and Frank Korosec, Ph.D., Madison.

Technique

Three-dimensional contrast MRA of carotid arteries is uniquely challenging because the arterial venous recirculation time is very short in the brain and the blood-brain barrier prevents extraction of the Gd chelate. For these reasons, it is difficult to avoid jugular venous enhancement. Unfortunately, jugular venous signal can obscure visualization of the adjacent carotid artery. This problem can be resolved by acquiring precisely timed, or a time-resolved, sequence so that images from the arterial phase are acquired before venous enhancement occurs. If image data sets are collected using a time-resolved exam at 5-second intervals, only one set of images will depict the arterial phase. More recently, investigators have demonstrated that a precisely timed, elliptically centric encoded acquisition may be satisfactory for eliminating venous enhancement. The advantage of this method is that an extended acquisition may be used (up to 1–2 minutes) to improve spatial resolution and SNR. Even further improvement is obtained by recessing the absolute center of k-space a few seconds in from the very beginning of the scan to be able to take advantage of the leading edge of the Gd bolus. In addition, post-processing methods may be used to reconstruct individual partitions, depicting only the carotid artery.

Three-dimensional contrast MRA images may be acquired in the coronal or sagittal planes. A coronal acquisition containing both carotid arteries following administration of a single contrast dose is generally preferred. Spatial resolution in the slice encoding direction (A/P) must be maximized to obtain sufficient resolution on sagittal oblique projections, which are important for opening up the carotid bifurcations. Coronal oblique projections are also important as they demonstrate great vessel origins arising from the aortic arch. In fact, the ability of the contrast-enhanced MRA technique to demonstrate the carotid circulation from aortic arch origin to Circle of Willis is a major advantage of the contrast-enhanced techniques over TOF MRA.

A sagittal acquisition, limited to just one carotid artery, can be used to reduce the number of acquired sections and reduce FOV without wrap-around. This improves in-plane spatial resolution in the lateral projection. However, this approach does not image the aortic arch. Furthermore, residual contrast agent from the first injection reduces image quality somewhat for the second injection, which is required to depict the contra-lateral carotid artery.

Typical parameters for a 3D contrast MRA carotid acquisition include TR < 5 ms, TE < 2 ms, Flip = 30 to 45°, Field-of-View = 280 × 280 × 80 mm, Matrix = 512 × 256 × 48 for sub-millimeter spatial resolution and an estimated 60 second acquisition. The preferred acquisition technique for carotid MRA uses an elliptically centric encoded acquisition that is precisely timed to the arrival of contrast agent in the carotid arteries to maintain venous suppression (Figure 10.2). It can also be useful to recess the absolute center of k-space a few seconds from the beginning of the scan to avoid ringing artifacts from inadvertent early initiation of scanning.

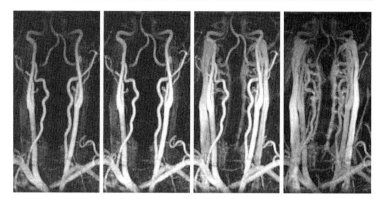

Fig. 10.2. Normal Carotid Artery.

Clinical Scenario: Asymptomatic 35-year-old male.

Technique: Coronal Acquisition, Neck Coil, TR/TE/Flip = 10/2.3/60°, Field-of-View = 240 × 120 × 24 mm, Matrix = 512 × 256 × 24, 3D TRICKS technique with reconstruction of a 3D data set every 3 seconds, and 30 ml Gd injection at 2ml/s. The 3D TRICKS acquisition is prescribed in the coronal plane after a sagittal thick-slab 2D phase contrast acquisition with flow encoding in the S/I direction. This allows the coronal volume to be precisely positioned to maximize spatial resolution in the slice A/P direction, while ensuring adequate coverage to include the entire carotid artery.

Interpretation: A time series of coronal MIP projections through the carotid bifurcation are shown. Note the distinct arterial and venous phases of contrast enhancement in this patient. High temporal resolution is required (3 seconds/frame) in order to separate the arterial and venous phases of contrast enhancement and to eliminate overlap artifact from signal in the jugular vein.

Diagnosis: Normal carotid artery: time-resolved 3D MR DSA exam using 3D.

Submitted by Timothy Carroll, Ph.D. and Frank R. Korosec, Ph.D., Madison.

3D TRICKS may be used to reconstruct multiple time frames. 3D TRICKS acquisition parameters can be manipulated to result in a reconstructed frame rate of one 3D volume every 3 or 4 seconds. An example of a time-resolved 3D MR DSA exam in a normal carotid artery is shown in Figure 10.2. Images were reconstructed every 3 seconds. Note the distinct arterial and venous phases of contrast enhancement. If the TR is short enough, it is possible to perform a time-resolved acquisition without the need for view sharing and temporal interpolation (Figure 10.3). Short, fast acquisition time sequences are simply repeated quickly enough to isolate an arterial phase of contrast enhancement. Early results suggest that an acqui-

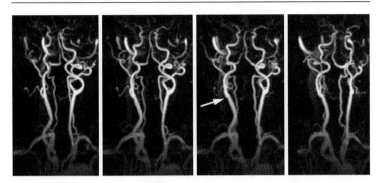

Fig. 10.3. Ultrashort Repetition Time (TR) Time-Resolved Acquisition.
Clinical Scenario: Cerebrovascular symptoms.
Technique: Coronal Acquisition, Neck Coil, TR/TE/Flip = 3.2/1.3/30°, Matrix = 256 × 128 × 48, ultra-fast 3D flash technique with acquisition time of 10.6 s.
Interpretation: Coronal oblique MIP through the arch and carotid arteries shows some venous enhancement is seen with this 10.6 second acquisition time, the venous signal does not obscure arterial detail. Mild atherosclerotic narrowing is seen in the right distal common carotid artery (*arrow*), but no significant stenosis is identified.
Diagnosis: No significant stenosis, mild right common carotid disease.
Submitted by T. S. Chung, M.D., Yonsei Yongdong University Hospital, Seoul, and Daisy Chien, Ph.D., Erlangen.

sition time of 10 seconds may be sufficient to minimize venous contamination in most cases. However, the limited spatial resolution of the short acquisition may create misclassification of stenosis as described above.

For longer non-time-resolved acquisitions, it is necessary to perform a dose timing scan, a "SmartPrep" acquisition, or a fluoroscopically-triggered acquisition to sense the arrival of contrast at the imaging region. With these approaches, a coronal acquisition with a single Gd contrast agent bolus is preferred (Figure 10.4). In addition, an acquisition with elliptical centric k-space weighting or slightly recessed elliptical centric weighting is effective at eliminating jugular venous contamination. Elliptical centric encoding concentrates the center of k-space at the beginning of the scan so that longer scans with higher resolution are possible without jugular venous contamination (Figure 10.5). A recessed elliptical centric 3D contrast MRA approach allows acquisition to begin before bolus peak to take advantage of the rising leading edge of the Gd bolus for more effective venous suppression.

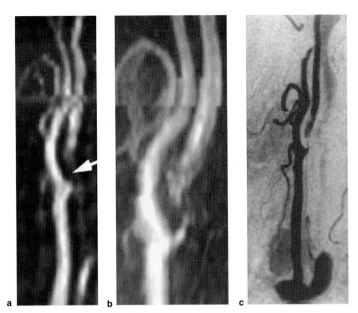

a   b   c

Fig. 10.4. Comparison of 2D TOF, 3D TOF, and 3D contrast MRA in severe carotid stenosis.

Clinical Scenario: 68-year-old male with symptoms of left brain transient ischemic attacks.

Technique: Standard 2D TOF and 3D TOF MOTSA protocols (see text), 3D contrast MRA performed using 3D TRICKS technique and Sagittal Acquisition, TR/TE/Flip = 10/2.3/60°, Field-of-View = 200 × 100 × 24 mm, Matrix = 512 × 256 × 24, 3D TRICKS with reconstruction of a 3D data set every 3 seconds, 15 ml Gd injection at 2ml/s.

Interpretation: The 2D TOF exam (**a**) shows the stenosis as an area of complete signal void at and distal to the stenosis (*arrow*). The 3D TOF study (**b**) demonstrates signal within the stenosis; however, flow in the internal carotid artery distal to the stenosis is poorly visualized due to saturation. This could result in underestimation of the stenotic lumen, depending upon where the observer measures the "normal" segment of the distal internal carotid artery. Note the limited imaging volume of non-enhanced 3D TOF exam, which is due to saturation of signal in the distal carotid. In contrast, the 3D contrast MRA exam demonstrates flow in the distal internal carotid artery, while at the same time the signal at the stenosis is preserved due to the short TE and small voxel size (**c**). As seen in this example, the contrast MRA method eliminates some pitfalls of non-enhanced techniques, and therefore can be used to increase observer confidence and resolve findings that can be observed in discordant MRA and Doppler ultrasound studies. Note also that the carotid artery is demonstrated from its origin at the aortic arch and the imaging volume includes the distal carotid at the siphon. Improved imaging at the arch is due to greater blood signal available, and therefore areas that are relatively signal poor on 2D TOF imaging can be seen.

Diagnosis: Severely stenotic carotid artery in a patient with symptomatic carotid arterial disease.

Submitted by Thomas M. Grist, M.D., Madison.

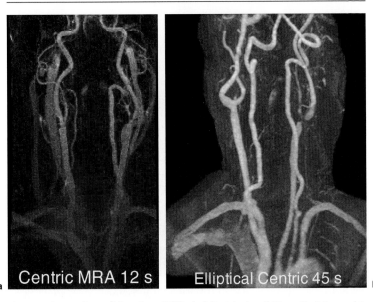

Fig. 10.5. Comparison of Centric and Elliptical Centric Acquisition. Centric acquisition (**a**) obtained in 12 seconds has jugular venous enhancement obscuring the carotid arteries. Elliptical centric acquisition (**b**) eliminates jugular venous enhancement even though the scan time is longer. This is because elliptical centric acquisition concentrates the center of k-space at the beginning of the scan before jugular vein enhancement occurs.

Submitted by Kevin Demarco, M.D., New Brunswick.

Post-processing carotid 3D contrast MRA data relies on several techniques, including image subtraction, MIP display, volume rendering, and reformatting individual sections. Subtraction of pre-contrast images from post-contrast images is helpful to reduce signal from background stationary tissues and fat. In addition, subtraction helps to improve fidelity of MIP displays at stenoses. Since an element of thresholding is performed in MIP displays, subtraction helps to improve conspicuity of signals at a stenosis relative to background signals. Nineteen MIP images are typically constructed at 10° intervals in order to demonstrate the carotid arteries at multiple angles. In addition to MIP displays, source images that encompass the carotid arteries are filmed, and images are reformatted at oblique angles as needed to demonstrate carotid bifurcations.

Complimentary Sequences

Conventional unenhanced 2D and 3D TOF MRA sequences currently are the mainstay of carotid MRA. Two-dimensional time-of-flight is sensitive to slow blood flow and may be the only non-contrast-enhanced method that reliably detects the "string sign" distal to a severe stenosis. However, 2D TOF methods cannot directly measure the stenotic lumen because flow disturbances create intra-voxel signal loss at the stenosis. Typically, thin (1.5 mm) axial sections are acquired and reformatted at multiple angles. 2D TOF can also serve as a localizer sequence to allow precise positioning of the 3D Gd MRA image volume so the slices can be made as thin as possible for maximum spatial resolution.

Due to a shorter echo time and a smaller voxel size resulting in less signal dephasing within a stenosis, the 3D TOF method predicts severity of a carotid lesion more accurately than 2D TOF methods. Three-dimensional time-of-flight is limited, however, by artifacts associated with saturation of slow, in-plane and retrograde flow, as well as turbulent flow distal to a high-grade stenosis.

In an attempt to combine advantages of 2D and 3D TOF MRA, a hybrid method based on multiple overlapping thin slab acquisition (MOTSA) was developed by Dennis Parker. This hybrid technique maintains the high spatial resolution of 3D TOF while simultaneously retaining some sensitivity to slow flow, which is characteristic of 2D TOF acquisitions. A clever refinement known as SLINKY eliminates venetian blind artifact occurring at slab overlap zones. A limitation of this method, however, is that it requires a longer acquisition time, and therefore is more susceptible to artifacts associated with patient motion.

Clinical Indications

Carotid Bifurcation Disease

Carotid bulb disease is the leading cause of stroke and consequently causes considerable morbidity and mortality. The NASCET and ESCT multi-center outcome studies have documented a measurable benefit of carotid endarterectomy in symptomatic patients with carotid stenosis of 70% or greater. In addition, ESCT showed no benefit of carotid endarterectomy for stenoses less than 30%. Further stratification of the NASCET trial patients with 70% to 99% stenoses also revealed a correlation between post-surgical risk of stroke and degree of stenosis. Thus, both studies have shown convincing evidence that therapy decisions should be based on the degree of stenosis. Therefore, accurate measures of stenosis severity are important in determining the need for therapy. Although only recently implemented for imaging carotid arteries, 3D contrast MRA has yielded promising results. By virtue of high signal, reduced sensitivity to slow artifacts, and comprehensive coverage from great vessel origins to Circle of Willis, 3D contrast MRA is the ideal method for obtaining an exact delineation of the stenotic lumen in patients with carotid bulb disease.

Table 10.1. Accuracy of 3D Contrast MRA for Carotid Disease

Author	Year	Journal	# of Patients	Sensitivity (%)	Specificity (%)	Accuracy (%)
Carotid Artery Stenosis >70%						
Leclerc	1998	AJNR	27	100	98	
Remonda	1998	Radiology	21 (44*, 18**)			94
Wintersperger	2000	Radiology	14	100	100	
Barbier	2001	JR	29	94–95	89–91	64–74
Oberholzer	2001	RoFo	55	97.7	94	
Huston III	2001	Radiology	50	90	95.5	93.8
Randoux	2001	Radiology	22	93	100	
Remonda	2002	AJNR	120 (73**)			93
String Sign (Pseudo-oclusion)						
Remonda	1998	Radiology	21 (44*, 3**)			100
Huston III	2001	Radiology	50 (6**)			83.31
Remonda	2002	AJNR	120 (9**)			77.7
Carotid Artery Occlusion						
Leclerc	1998	AJNR	27 (54*, 6**)			100
Remonda	1998	Radiology	21 (44*, 7**)			100
Sardanelli	1999	JCAT	30 (114*, 6**)		100	
Kollias	1999	Neuroradiology	20 (40*, 3**)			100
Serfaty	2000	JR	44 (63*, 2**)			100
Phan	2001	Stroke	422 (6**)			100
Remonda	2002	AJNR	120 (28**)			100
Internal Carotid Artery Aneurysm						
Kollias	1999	Neuroradiology	20 (40*, 2**)			100
Ulcerated Plaque						
Leclerc	1998	AJNR	27 (108*, 1**)		100	
Kollias	1999	Neuroradiology	20 (40*, 3**)			100
Serfaty	2000	AJR	44 (63*, 3**)			100
Catalano	2001	RM	37 (74*, 12**)		100	
Randoux	2001	Radiology	22 (44*, 8**)	100	88.9	

* Number with angiography or surgical correlation   ** Number of lesions

At this time, indications for carotid contrast MRA at our institutions include:

1. Discordant Doppler ultrasound and non-contrast MRA examinations,
2. Delineation of the stenosis in patients with 50–70% stenosis
3. Poor image quality of non-contrast MRA due to motion artifact or low signal to noise,
4. Detection or confirmation of a "string sign", demonstrating patency of an internal carotid artery distal to a high-grade stenosis (Figure 10.6),
5. Demonstration of complex stenosis morphology, e.g., deep ulceration (Figure 10.7), and
6. Assessment of tandem lesions at the arch origin vessels or at the carotid siphon (Figure 10.8).

Arch Vessel Disease

MR angiography had little to contribute to evaluation of arch vessel disease until the introduction of 3D contrast MRA. Atherosclerotic disease involving the proximal aortic arch vessels is infrequent, but an important cause of cerebrovascular pathology. The left subclavian artery is more commonly involved than the right, and stenotic disease also tends to involve the vertebral origins. Subclavian steal syndrome arises when a proximal left subclavian stenosis causes hypoperfusion of the arm. The resultant pressure differential creates a pattern of retrograde flow through the left vertebral artery to provide blood flow to the left arm, especially during exercise. Three-dimensional contrast MRA can effectively demonstrate the underlying stenotic disease involving the subclavian artery (Figure 10.8). Additional phase contrast velocity measurements or time-resolved contrast MRA may demonstrate retrograde flow in the vertebral artery. 3D contrast MRA also depicts bypass graft anatomy (Figure 10.9).

It is now possible to simultaneously visualize the carotid bifurcation and arch origin vessels using 3D contrast MRA. Because of the possibility of synchroneous lesions, routine 3D contrast MRA should include both arch vessel origins as well as carotid bifurcation.

Vertebral Artery Disease

MRA of vertebral arteries has been limited in the era of TOF because of flow artifacts. The tortuous course of the vertebrals particularly at C1-2 causes in-plane saturation making it impossible to adequately assess for

a

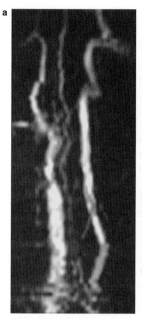

b

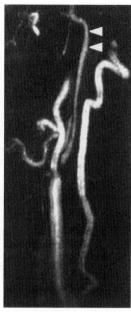

Fig. 10.6. Capability of the 3D contrast MRA Method to Detect a "String Sign" Associated with Slow Flow in the Internal Carotid Artery Distal to a High Grade Stenosis.

Clinical Scenario: Patient with cerebrovascular symptoms and equivocal non-contrast MRA for demonstrating patency of the distal internal carotid artery.

Technique: Standard 2D TOF and 3D TOF MOTSA protocols (see text), 3D Contrast MRA performed using 3D TRICKS, Sagittal Acquisition, TR/TE/Flip = 10/2.3/60°, Field-of-View = $200 \times 100 \times 24$ mm, Matrix = $512 \times 256 \times 24$, 3D TRICKS with reconstruction of a 3D data set every 3 seconds, and 15 ml Gd injection at 2 ml/s.

Interpretation: The 2D TOF exam (**a**) shows questionable signal in the distal internal carotid artery. No signal was identified on the 3D TOF MRA exam. On the other hand, the time-resolved exam demonstrated signal in the distal internal carotid that confirmed patency of the vessel (**b**, *arrowheads*). Identification of this signal is important since demonstration of patency of the distal vessel suggests carotid endarterectomy is appropriate since the carotid is patent.

Diagnosis: Severe internal carotid artery stenosis with "string sign", showing patency of the distal internal carotid on 3D contrast MRA.

Submitted by Donald Willig, M.D., Madison.

occlusive disease. In addition, respiratory motion at the thoracic inlet causes artifact that obscures vertebral artery origins. However, these difficiencies with TOF are eliminated with 3D contrast MRA. Data on accuracy for assessing vertebral arteries is presented in Table 10.2.

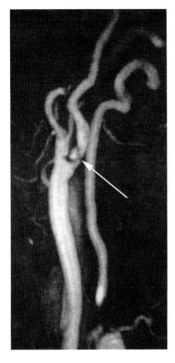

Fig. 10.7. 3D Contrast MRA Shows Complex Plaque Morphology.

Clinical Scenario: 58-year-old female with symptoms of transient ischemic attack.

Technique: 3D Contrast MRA performed using 3D TRICKS, Sagittal Acquisition, TR/TE/Flip = 10/2.3/60°, Field-of-View = 200 × 100 × 24 mm, Matrix = 512 × 256 × 24, 3D TRICKS with reconstruction of a 3D data set every 3 seconds, and 20 ml Gd injection at 2ml/s.

Interpretation: Sagittal MRA demonstrates a deep ulceration of the plaque at the proximal internal carotid artery (*arrow*). The ulceration was not well seen on the non-contrast techniques due to complex flow that caused dephasing and signal saturation at the ulceration.

Diagnosis: Ulcerating stenosis, internal carotid artery.

Submitted by Patrick Turski, M.D., Madison.

Table 10.2. Accuracy of 3D Gd-MRA for Vertebral Arteries

Author	Year	Journal	# of Patients	Accuracy
Vertebral Artery Stenosis >50%				
Leclerc	1998	AJNR	27 (50*, 3**)	98 %
Phan	2001	Stroke	422 (44**)	100 %
Vertebral Artery Occlusion				
Leclerc	1998	AJNR	27 (50*, 1**)	100 %
Pahn	2001	Stroke	422 (3**)	100 %
Carotid and Vertebral Artery Dissection				
Phan	2001	Stroke	422 (56*, 14**)	85.7 %
Leclerc	1999	AJNR	16 (32*, 2**)†	100 %
Subclavian Steal Syndrome				
Van Grimberg	2000	JMRI	2	100 %

* Number of vessels with correlation   ** Number of lesions

† Pseudoaneurysm

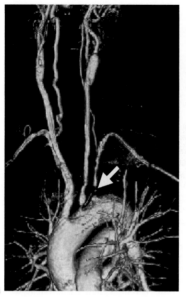

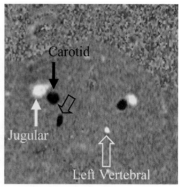

Fig 10.8. Subclavian steal: Role of Phase Contrast. Volume rendered 3D contrast MRA (**a**) shows patulous internal carotid arteries post-endarterectomy, severe stenosis of left common carotid artery origin and near occlusion of proximal left subclavian artery. Vertebral arteries are widely patent. Axial 2D phase contrast MRA encoding flow in the superior to inferior direction shows dark signal in common carotid arteries (*black arrow*), bright signal in jugular veins (*white arrow*) and bright signal in left vertebral artery (*open white arrow*) indicating that the vertebral artery flow is superior to inferior. Note that the flow in the other vertebral artery is in the normal inferior-to-superior direction (*black open arrow*) indicated by the dark signal. Submitted by Samer Suleiman, M.D. and Thomas M. Grist, M.D., Madison.

Pitfalls

Intraluminal Artifacts Due to k-space Weighting

Since arterial-venous transit time is quite short in carotid arteries, the signals may be strongly modulated by the rapidly changing contrast curve. A rapidly changing contrast curve can result in intraluminal stripe or ringing artifacts that may simulate dissection or other pathology. An example of this pitfall in the common carotid artery is shown in Figure 10.6. Perfect bolus timing and recessing the absolute center of k-space a few seconds in from the beginning of the elliptical centric scan helps to minimize this artifact.

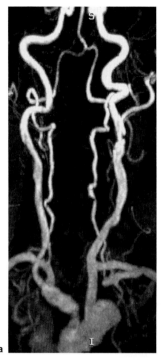

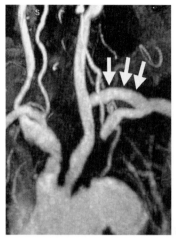

Fig 10.9. Carotid-Subclavian Bypass Graft.

Clinical Scenario: Post-op bypass graft, Evaluate patency.

Technique: Coronal Acquisition, TR/TE/Flip = 7/1.2/30°, Field-of-View = 280 × 168 × 64, Matrix = 512 × 150 × 32 with 2-fold zero interpolation in the slice direction, 20 ml Gd injected by hand using the Smartset timed with fluoroscopic triggering and recessing the center of k-space by 3 seconds.

Interpretation: Coronal MIP (**a**) and magnified oblique subvolume MIP show atherosclerotic disease in great vessel origins with occluded left subclavian artery which is reconstituted by a left common carotid to left subclavian bypass graft (*arrows*). Also note atherosclerotic disease causing mild narrowing of proximal left common carotid and innominate arteries.

Diagnosis: Widely patent carotid-to-subclavian bypass graft.

Submitted by Hale Ersoy Erel, M.D., New York.

Coil Drop Out

In patients with a low aortic arch or elevated shoulders, coil sensitivity may begin to drop off in the region of the aortic arch. This can impair evaluation of great vessel origins. Fortunately, new head-neck neurovascular coils are available which provide better upper thorax and arch coverage of the neck and arch, yet still have high signal-to-noise ratio.

Venous Susceptibility Artifact

When a paramagnetic agent is rapidly injected into an arm vein, it remains highly concentrated in the ipsilateral subclavian and innominate veins. Highly concentrated paramagnetic contrast creates susceptibility artifacts, obscuring signal in adjacent arteries, thereby simulating the presence of a stenosis or even an occlusion (Figure 10.10). To avoid susceptibility artifact in the region of the left brachiocephalic vein, inject a right arm vein. It is also useful to follow the contrast injection with a large volume of saline flush (at least 20 ml) and to elevate the arm being injected to clear contrast from the veins as quickly as possible. This artifact may also be reduced by using the shortest possible echo time or diluting the contrast agent before injecting.

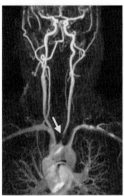

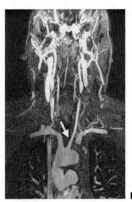

a   b

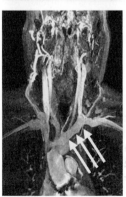

c

Fig. 10.10. Susceptibility Artifact from Left Arm Injection. Arterial phase (**a**) MIP from arch-carotid MRA performed with left arm venous injection show apparent stenosis of the proximal left common carotid artery (*arrow*). A subvolume MIP from the equilibrium phase (**b**) shows the same region of left common carotid (*arrow*) to be widely patent. A full MIP of the equilibrium phase (**c**) shows the apparent stenosis corresponds with the path of the left brachiocephalic vein (*long arrows*). This artifactual signal dropout in the left common carotid falsely simulating a stenosis is caused by highly concentrated Gd in the left subclavian and brachiocephalic vein during injection. The artifact can be completely eliminated by injecting the right arm. It may be reduced by injecting dilute gadolinium at a higher rate. Submitted by Thomas M. Grist, M.D., Madison.

CHAPTER 11

3D Contrast MR Venography

Background

Veins are easier to image on MR as compared to arteries because of their larger size, slower flow, and more homogeneous flow profiles. Venous pathology also tends to be more extensive, so high resolution is not essential. For example, the high resolution required for grading the severity of focal arterial stenoses is not necessary for diagnosing venous thrombosis, which typically completely occludes the vein. Conventional TOF and phase contrast MR venography, which do not require paramagnetic contrast agent injection, have evolved into reliable and clinically accepted methods for the assessment of the deep venous system. The techniques are of limited use, however, in the presence of inordinately slow flow, tortuous venous anatomy or visualization of small circuitous collateral channels. Time-of-flight and phase contrast MRA are also time consuming. In order to overcome these limitations, the use of 3D contrast MR venography has been suggested for the assessment of the peripheral venous system. There are two principle approaches to 3D contrast MR venography: indirect and direct.

3D Contrast MR Venography Techniques

Indirect Venography

The indirect approach images the veins during the equilibrium contrast phase following the injection of paramagnetic contrast into the antecubital vein (Figures 8.1–8.10, 9.12 and 11.1). The advantage of the indirect approach is two-fold: it does not require cannulation of the veins in the affected extremity and it is often easy to obtain venous access in the contralateral arm vein. One disadvantage is the large dose required, typically

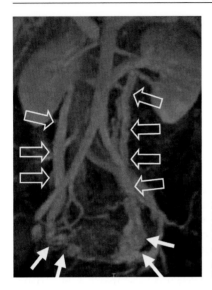

Fig. 11.1. Pelvic Congestion Syndrome. Early venous phase of 3D contrast MRA shows prominent pelvic varices (*arrows*) on either side of the uterus with bilateral enormous dilated gonadal vein (*block arrows*). Submitted by Barry Stein, M.D., Hartford.

0.3 mmol/kg; This is because the contrast is considerably diluted and partially extracted as it passes through the lungs, arteries, systemic capillary beds, and finally reaches the veins.

Imaging must be performed during the early equilibrium phase before the Gd has had a chance to substantially redistribute into the extracellular fluid compartment. This redistribution has a time constant of approximately 11 minutes for extracellular Gd contrast agents that are currently available. Thus, there is only a very short window of opportunity immediately following injection of Gd during which optimal MR venography imaging can be achieved. For indirect venous enhancement, the injection rate should be slightly slower than a typical injection for arterial imaging (1 ml/s). This has the effect of prolonging the period of time that demonstrates maximum venous enhancement.

Image quality in the legs or arms can be substantially improved by obtaining pre-contrast image data in order to subtract from contrast-enhanced 3D image sets. Subtraction does not work as well in the abdomen and chest where breath-holding is required. Spatial misregistration of pre- and post-contrast data sets can result in the reduction of image quality.

Because of the relatively large caliber of veins as compared to arteries, the collection of thicker partitions is acceptable. Typically, a 3–5 mm partition thickness with 256 × 160 or 192 matrix is appropriate for a field-of-view less than 320 mm. For a larger field-of-view, it is helpful to image using a 512 acquisition matrix in order to obtain optimal higher resolution.

Direct Venography

Direct MR venography requires continuous intravenous infusion of dilute paramagnetic contrast upstream from the vein of interest. For example, direct injection of the antecubital vein to image the subclavian or innominate veins (Figures 11.2, 11.3), injection of hand veins to image veins of the entire arm (Figure 11.4) or direct injection of the dorsal foot vein to image calf, thigh and pelvic veins (Figures 11.5). This approach requires considerably less paramagnetic contrast but is diluted into a

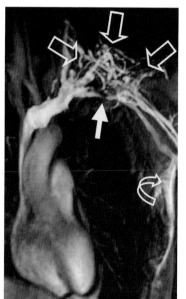

Fig. 11.2. Direct MR Venography: Left Subclavian Stenosis.

Clinical Scenario: Left arm swelling for several months.

Technique: Coronal Acquisition, TR/TE/Flip = 6/1.2/40°, Field of View = 400 × 400 × 90, Matrix = 512 × 160 × 30 with zero filling to 60 slices, 10 ml Gd diluted into 120 ml normal saline injected by hand with Smartset at 3ml/s. 3D data acquisition with sequential ordering of k-space initiated at midpoint of injection with breath-holding.

Interpretation: Subvolume Coronal MIP shows left subclavian thrombosis with partial recanalization (*solid arrow*). Numerous collateral vessels fill with contrast (*open arrows*) indicating the subclavian venous obstruction is hemodynamically significant. Bright signal overlying the left arm (*curved arrow*) is wraparound artifact from the right arm due to FOV smaller than width of patient. This artifact can be avoided by elevating the right arm over the head during data acquisition.

Diagnosis: Chronic left subclavian vein thrombosis with partial recanalization.
Submitted by Hale Ersoy Erel, M.D., Ankara.

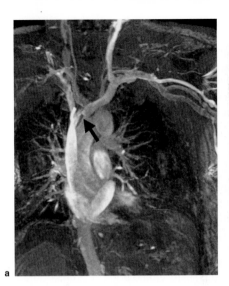 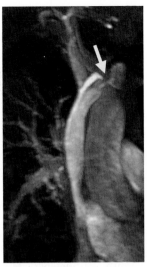

a b

Fig. 11.3. Direct Venography: Left Innominant Stenosis. Coronal MIP (**a**) and subvolume MIP (**b**) show contrast filling predominantly via the left cephalic vein and subclavian vein with a left Innominant venous stenosis (*arrow*). 3D data are acquired with sequential ordering of k-space during a breath-hold beginning half-way through injection of 120 ml dilute Gd (20:1 dilution into normal saline). Because the stenosis only mildly impedes flow, contrast has reached into pulmonary arteries and aorta.

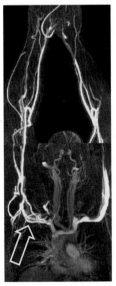

Fig. 11.4. Direct Venography of the Arms.
Clinical Scenario: Right arm swelling.
Technique: Direct MR venography of upper extremities with simultaneous hand injection of distal arm vein.
Interpretation: Contrast fills the left arm veins normally. On the right, the axillary and subclavian veins are occluded and there are prominent collateral veins (*open arrow*).
Diagnosis: Right axillary and subclavian vein occlusion.
Submitted by Stephan G. Ruehm, M.D., Essen.

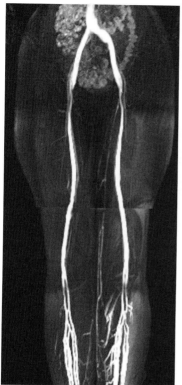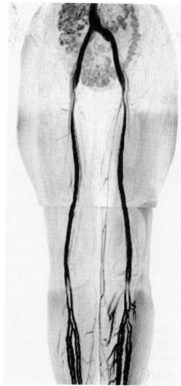

a   b

Fig. 11.5. MR Venography by Pedal Injection of Dilute Contrast.

Clinical Scenario: 35-year-old woman with swelling and pain in the left lower leg after a 14 hour flight. Due to known allergies against iodinated contrast media, an MR-venogram was performed.

Technique: 3D Coronal Acquisition TR/TE/Flip 5.2/1.5/30°, TI = 28 ms, 0.5 NEX. Following placement of a dedicated lower extremity vascular coil application, 80ml of diluted (1:20) paramagnetic contrast were manually injected into both feet at a rate of 1ml/s. Two 3D acquisitions, each consisting of 46 contiguous sections with a thickness of 2.4 mm were collected over 30 s – the first covering the pelvis and thighs, the second covering the popliteal and trifurcation vessels.

Interpretation: Normal morphology of the deep venous system bilaterally is displayed on the MIP venogram in the conventional (**a**) as well as the "inverse video" (**b**) mode. No evidence of DVT.

Diagnosis: Normal deep venous system.

Submitted by Stephan G. Ruehm M.D., Essen.

large volume to keep the vein distended by contrast injection for the entire period of imaging. To avoid T2-shortening effects, the extracellular contrast agent (0.5 molar) must be diluted into normal saline by a factor of about 20:1. One simple dilution approach is to inject the contents of a 15 ml vial of paramagnetic contrast into a 250 ml bag of normal saline. This 17:1 dilution is loaded into several 60 ml syringes, which can be used for injecting over a substantial period of time. It is important to mix the solution well prior to injection in order to ensure that the Gd has not settled-out dependently in the syringe prior to injection.

This direct injection method also employs a 3D spoiled gradient echo pulse sequence. Pre-contrast data are acquired for subtraction purposes. The partitions can be 3–5 mm thick; zero interpolation is recommended. Use the shortest TR and TE and a flip of about 40°. To ensure a continuous contrast bolus, a tubing set that allows simultaneous attachment of two 60 ml syringes of dilute contrast can be helpful (SmartSet, Topspins, Inc.). Imaging should begin following the injection of the first 30–60 ml of dilute contrast agent. The injection should continue during imaging with sequential mapping of k-space so that the center of k-space is acquired in the middle of the acquisition. This produces the least k-space artifact and allows more time for collateral filling in the event of venous occlusion.

While the contrast is being administered intravenously, the 3D spoiled gradient echo pulse sequence can be repeated multiple times. This is especially useful for patients with suspected venous obstruction downstream from the injection site because there may be a considerable delay due to the filling of collaterals and reconstitution of flow beyond the site of occlusion.

To depict the venous system in a single extremity, it is sufficient to inject only a single ipsilateral intravenous site. For visualization of the more central veins, such as the superior vena cava (SVC) or pelvic veins, it is better to simultaneously inject both the right and left extremities so there is symmetric introduction of dilute contrast material (Figure 11.6). As the contrast bolus reaches central veins, dilution from merging venous tributaries causes a reduction of the very bright signal. Thus, for depicting central veins, it is better to have slightly less dilution of the Gd (e.g. 10:1 dilution).

Although frequently more cumbersome from a patient handling point of view, the direct imaging approach results in superior contrast-to-noise when compared to the "indirect" equilibrium images. This translates into better image quality and a more detailed depiction of the venous anatomy.

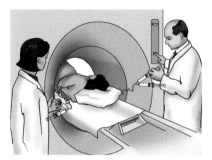

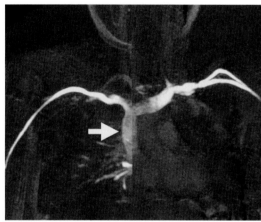

Fig. 11.6. Simultaneous Injection of Both Arms to Image SVC. Gd is diluted by injecting 15 ml into a 250 ml bag of normal saline. This dilute mixture is loaded into four 60ml syringes, two for each arm. Both arms are simultaneously injected by hand as fast as possible to rapidly fill and distend the veins. Imaging is initiated after 50 ml is injected using Coronal 3D spoiled gradient echo pulse sequence during breath-holding. Note that both subclavian veins are widely patent but the SVC (*arrow*) is not as bright because of further dilution of the contrast by blood. Submitted by Martin Prince, M.D., Ph.D., New York.

Complementary Sequences

Conventional TOF or phase contrast techniques are well suited for most forms of venous imaging and can either complement 3D Gd venography or be used as a back-up in the event of failure to achieve high quality direct or indirect images. The quality of TOF imaging can be maximized by orienting the image acquisition plane perpendicular to the direction of blood flow. Usually, this is the axial plane since most veins flow in the S/I orientation. The sagittal plane is optimal for subclavian veins, renal veins, or transverse sinus because they are more horizontal. It is also useful for slices to be as thin as possible to allow complete inflow refreshment of unsaturated spins within the TR interval. Using a longer TR also allows more time for fresh inflow of unsaturated spins, which further enhances image quality, particularly in veins with slow flow. Spatial saturation bands can be employed to eliminate arterial signal although typically they are not necessary.

Paramagnetic contrast in the vascular system improves 2D TOF image quality; however, elimination of arterial signal with spatial pre-saturation will not be possible. Hence, complimentary 2D TOF sequences are ideally performed after the Gd enhanced acquisition. Phase contrast techniques can be useful in differentiating very slow flow from thrombus, in determining blood flow direction, and in quantifying blood flow through a particular vessel. Phase contrast MRA also tends to improve when performed post-contrast agent injection.

Clinical Applications

3D contrast MR venography has not yet found its way into mainstream clinical imaging. Rather, it is being performed predominantly on a research basis. Nevertheless, several clinical applications are emerging.

Upper Extremity Veins

Contrast-enhanced MR venography is a particularly well-suited technique to the evaluation of axillary, subclavian, innominate veins, and SVC. For bilateral subclavian venous evaluation, simultaneous injection of both right and left arm antecubital veins is necessary (Figure 11.7). This usually requires two operators for injecting contrast, each with two 50-60 ml syringes of Gd. The injection should be coordinated so that both operators complete injection of the first syringe at approximately the same time, and both will be in the midst of injecting the contents of the second syringe during acquisition of the image data. Alternatively, the SVC can be imaged with the indirect approach (Figures 11.8 and 11.9).

This can be especially useful in patients who are approaching dialysis, in whom iodinated contrast may carry unacceptable risks. It may also be useful for patients who already have a dialysis shunt or fistula, in whom mapping of the fistula luminal anatomy is desired. The fistula can either be injected directly with dilute Gd, or one can inject the contralateral arm and image during the equilibrium phase to see both the arterial and venous shunt anastomoses (Figure 9.12).

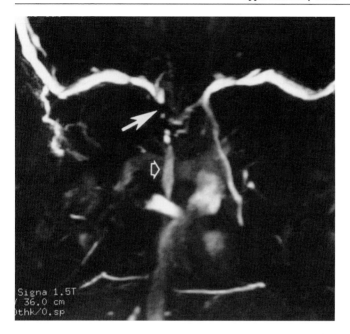

Fig. 11.7. Superior Vena Cava (SVC) Occlusion.

Clinical Scenario: 44-year-old male with cystic fibrosis, multiple past Hickman lines for antibiotic therapy and new upper extremity and facial swelling.

Technique: Coronal Acquisition, TR/TE/Flip = 6.8/2.1/45°, Field-of-View = 360 × 360 × 98 mm, Matrix = 256 × 128 × 24, with zero filling interpolation to reconstruct 48 slices, Sequential Ordering of k-space, Acquisition Time = 16 s, 20 ml Gd contrast diluted into 250 ml normal saline and infused simultaneously via right and left antecubital vein at 2 ml/s, and timed empirically.

Interpretation: Coronal MIP shows right and left subclavian veins are widely patent but the SVC is occluded superiorly (*arrow*) at the venous brachiocephalic. The SVC reconstitutes closer to the heart (*open arrow*).

Diagnosis: Superior Vena Cava occlusion.

Submitted by Martin R. Prince, M.D., Ph.D., New York.

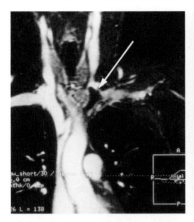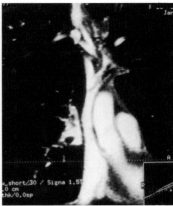

Fig. 11.8. Upper Extremity Venous Magnetic Resonance Angiography (MRA).

Clinical Scenario: 48-year-old female with left upper extremity swelling.

Technique: Coronal Acquisition, Body Coil, TR/TE/Flip = 8/2.1/60°, Field-of-View = 380 × 380 × 88 mm, Matrix = 512 × 160 × 44, 1 NEX, zero filling interpolation of slices, Sequential Phase Encoding Order, Acquisition Time = 32 s, 40 ml Gd was injected at 0.8 ml/s. IV access was obtained in the contralateral normal arm because the upper extremity swelling prevented cannulation of the ipsilateral hand vein. Two images were acquired; an arterial phase that was initiated 10 seconds after the injection, as well as a venous phase that was acquired beginning 55 seconds following the start of injection.

Interpretation: The source images demonstrate a low signal filling defect in the left brachiocephalic vein (*arrow*) that extends into the jugular vein and SVC.

Diagnosis: Left brachiocephalic venous thrombosis.

Submitted by Thomas M. Grist, M.D., Madison.

Table 11.1. Accuracy of 3D Contrast Venography for Central Venous Pathology

Author	Year	Journal	# of Patients	Sensitivity	Specificity
Central Veins					
Stafford-Johnson	1998	Radiology	13	100 %	100 %
Shinde	1999	Radiology	15(9*)	100 %	100 %
Thornton	1999	AJR	37	100 %	100 %
Kroencke	2001	Chest	16(3*)	100 %	100 %
Aslam Sohaib	2002	J Urol	12	100 %	98 %

*   Correlation available

Lower Extremity Venous Pathology

Often, 2D TOF without contrast provides adequate visualization of iliofemoral and popliteal veins for diagnosis of deep venous thrombosis.

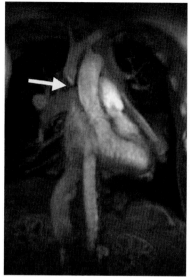 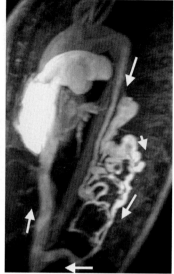

a   b

Fig. 11.9. SVC Obstruction.

Clinical Scenario: Recurrent left pleural effusion.

Technique: Coronal contrast-enhanced venous phase image from a multi-phase exam. Images were obtained after 30 ml Gd injection.

Interpretation: (**a**) Demonstrates severe abrupt stenosis involving the superior vena cava (*arrow*). (**b**) Shows extensive collateral pathways, with retrograde flow into the azygous system, then into the IVC (*arrows*).

Diagnosis: Chronic SVC obstruction.

Submitted by Frank Thornton, M.D. and Samer Suleiman, M.D., Madison.

However, if higher resolution is required, direct injection of dilute Gd into a foot vein can be performed (Figure 11.5). Tourniquets may be applied at the ankle to maximize filling of the deep venous system. A tourniquet may also be applied at the upper thigh to distend veins and prevent too rapid washout of the contrast. If the patient is carefully positioned to make the leg horizontal, it is possible to slide the table during the acquisition of coronal volumes of imaging data in order to capture in sequence the calf, the thigh, and finally the pelvis with a single injection of contrast. With 3D spoiled gradient echo coronal volume imaging, 30-40 sections, each 3–5 mm thick, and a 40–48 cm field-of-view will be appropriate. If available, interpolation with zero filling should be implemented in the slice direction to increase the number of sections to 60–80 for improved reformations and MIPs. An initial data acquisition is performed at each station of interest, prior to injection of contrast, for subtraction of background tissue signal. If only a single station of data is required, i.e., only the calf, then higher resolution and image quality can be achieved by using a surface array coil or a head coil.

When imaging primarily pelvic veins, the indirect, early equilibrium phase imaging of a larger contrast dose is preferable (Figures 11.1 and 11.10).

Table 11.2. Accuracy of 3D Contrast Venography for Pelvic and Peripheral Veins

Author	Year	Journal	# of Patients	Sensitivity	Specificity
Hoshi	1999	NIHGZ	70** (46*)	100 %	92 %
Ruehm	2000	Radiology	25 (35**)	94–100 %	92–98 %

*   Correlation available
**   Number of Legs

Pitfalls

For indirect imaging, potential pitfalls are similar to those discussed previously. Timing 3D data acquisition must ensure the center of k-space coincides with the venous phase of the contrast bolus. To assure adequate image quality, a large contrast dose (0.3 mmol/kg) is generally required. Furthermore, acquisition of a pre-contrast data set for image subtraction should be considered. For direct 3D contrast MR venography, several other potential pitfalls need to be taken into account as follows:

Insufficient Dilution of the Paramagnetic Contrast Agent

Insufficient dilution of the contrast agent will cause T2- and T2* shortening which may render the venous system completely dark. Standard 0.5 molar, extracellular contrast formulations should be diluted at least 10-fold to avoid this problem.

Delayed Venous Filling

In cases of venous occlusion, the infusion may not last long enough to completely fill collateral veins and reconstitute the major vein beyond an

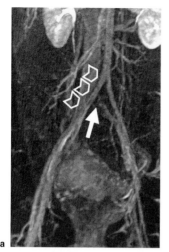

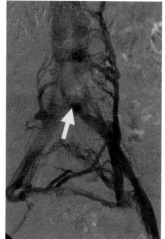

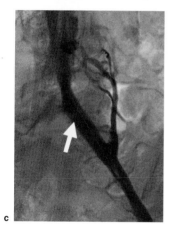

Fig. 11.10. May-Thurner Syndrome.   Early venous phase MIP (**a**) from 3D contrast MRA of the abdomen-pelvis shows compression of the left common iliac vein (*arrow*) by the right common iliac artery (*arrowheads*). At venography (**b**) injection of contrast via the left common femoral vein shows narrowing of the common iliac vein (*arrow*) and extensive filling of trans-sacral and paralumbar collateral veins, bypassing the obstruction indicating the magnitude of hemodynamic significance. Following angioplasty and stent (**c**), the normal caliber is restored and collaterals are no longer filling. Submitted by Barry Stein, M.D., Hartford.

occlusion. In this event, an image may be largely blank. To avoid this pitfall, several acquisitions should be collected during and immediately following infusion of contrast agent. If images are inadequate, consider repeating the scan utilizing a longer and larger infusion.

Incomplete Coverage

Images may be incomplete if the imaging volume is misplaced or not large enough to encompass the entire venous anatomy. Venous anatomy may be less predictable and thus may require longer and thicker imaging volumes to be sure that all the veins are included. Collateral veins are especially unpredictable. This pitfall can also be avoided by collecting a pre-contrast image set and analyzing the source images carefully to be sure that all veins are included before injecting contrast. For upper extremity imaging, consider placing a cushion under the arm to bring the forearm veins to a similar A/P position as the subclavian vein and SVC. When positioning the arm, note the location of the clavicle, which marks the most anterior part of the subclavian vein.

Glossary of Technical Terms

3D Contrast MRA: Three dimensional contrast-enhanced magnetic resonance angiography. A general term encompassing the variety of MRA techniques described in this book.

3D MR DSA: The method of obtaining a series of contrast-enhanced 3D MRA data sets and subtracting pre-contrast, unenhanced images from subsequent contrast-enhanced images that follow to achieve greater suppression of background tissues.

3D TRICKS: Acronym for 3D Time-Resolved Imaging of Contrast Kinetics. An MR pulse sequence that acquires a series of 3D volume images during the passage of a MR contrast agent by over sampling the center of k-space and sharing peripheral k-space data between temporal phases.

Acquisition Matrix: The number of data points acquired in the frequency and phase-encoding directions. This corresponds to the number of pixels in the image. The spatial resolution of the acquired images becomes better as the size of the acquisition matrix increases, but the time required for the acquisition increases simultaneously. The acquisition matrix has the dimensions $X \times Y \times Z$, where X is the number of pixels along the frequency encoding axis (typically 256-512), Y is the number of pixels along the phase encoding axis (typically 128-256), and Z corresponds to the number of pixels along the slice encoding axis (typically 30-60). Note that with 3D acquisitions the edge slices in an acquisition are often discarded, and therefore only 28 slices from 3D volume with an acquired slice matrix size of 32 may be displayed.

Artifacts: False features in the image produced by the imaging process. Random fluctuation of intensity due to noise can be considered separately from artifacts.

Bolus: A concentrated mass of pharmaceutical preparation given all at once intravenously, typically for diagnostic or medicinal purposes, e.g., an opaque contrast medium or radioactive isotope.

Bolus-Chase MRA: The technique, used to image peripheral vasculature, where a bolus of gadolinium contrast agent is sequentially imaged in a succession of image volumes as the bolus moves from abdomen-pelvis to thigh-calf.

Centric Encoding: The order in which the MR scanner collects Fourier data. Centric encoding acquires the data at the center of k-space (i.e. low spatial frequency data) first. Therefore, image contrast in a centric 3D acquisition is determined primarily by the signals at the beginning of the acquisition. As the scan progresses, higher spatial resolution k-space data is acquired that determines detail in the image.

Coil: Single or multiple loops of wire (or other electrical conductor, such as tubing, copper foil, etc.) designed either to produce a magnetic field from current flowing through the wire, or to detect MR signals.

Contrast: In conventional radiography, contrast is defined as the difference of signal intensities divided by average signal intensity in two adjacent regions. In a general sense, we can consider image contrast, where relative strength of image intensity in adjacent regions of the image is compared, or object contrast, where relative values of a parameter affecting the image (such as spin density or relaxation time) in corresponding adjacent regions is present. Object contrast is more difficult in MR imaging than in conventional radiography, as there are more object parameters affecting the image and their relative contributions are dependent on the particular imaging technique used. As in other kinds of imaging, image contrast in MRI will also depend on region size, as reflected through the modulation transfer function (MTF) characteristics. The contrast between object (e.g., lesion) and background will also depend on the particular choice of designated background (e.g., fat, muscle, etc.).

Contrast Agent: Substance administered to subject being imaged in order to selectively alter image intensity of a particular anatomical or functional region. In the case of MRA, contrast agents are primarily used to reduce the blood T1-relaxation time, so that the blood signal appears bright in the image. MR contrast agents also generally decrease $T2^*$ and, in the case of pulse sequences with long echo times, may cause signal loss. Approved agents consist of chelated gadolinium molecules (e.g., Gd-DTPA), as well as chelated manganese and iron oxide.

Elliptical-Centric: The technique using a k-space acquisition scheme where low spatial frequency signals which dominate image contrast are acquired at the beginning of the scan. This technique concentrates the center of k-space into a shorter period of time at the beginning of the acquisition compared to standard "centric" k- space encoding. This technique has significant value for improving suppression of venous enhancement, isolating signals to arteries, minimizing ringing and reducing respiratory and other motion artifacts. A further refinement in the elliptical centric encoding method is to recess the absolute center of k-space a few seconds from the beginning to avoid ringing artifact produced by the rising leading edge of the bolus.

Field-of-View: Dimensions of the area that is imaged.

Fluoro-triggered MRA: This technique uses a thick slab, low resolution 2D acquisition to image and reconstruct, in real time, the region of interest. Arrival of the leading edge of the gadolinium bolus is observed on this 2D (fluoro) technique so that the operator knows when to trigger acquisition of the 3D contrast MRA study.

Fractional Echo: MR acquisition technique in which only a portion of the MR signal (or echo) is read out. Normally, at least 60% of the echo is acquired. Typically the first 1/3 of the echo is eliminated so as to begin reading out closer to echo peak. This substantially shortens echo time and helps suppress flow and suceptibility artifacts.

Fractional NEX: A scheme where only a fraction of the phase encodings along one direction (normally ky) are acquired. In general, slightly more than 50% of the encodings are collected so it speeds up the scan by almost, but not quite, a factor of 2.

Fourier Transform (FT): A mathematical procedure to separate out the spatial frequency components of a signal from its amplitudes as a function of time, or vice versa. The Fourier transform is essential to virtually all MR imaging techniques. The FT can also be thought of as a mathematical transform between the spatial-frequency domain and the image domain. A series of MR images are formed (or reconstructed) by taking the Fourier transform of the k-space (Fourier) data. The Fourier transform can be generalized to multiple dimensions. Planar and volume images are reconstructed by a 2D FT or a 3D FT, respectively.

Gadolinium: Lanthanide element that is paramagnetic in its trivalent state. It is used as the active component in most MR contrast agents because it shortens T1 relaxation times of tissues in which it distributes. Although toxic by itself, it can be given safely in a chelated form such as Gd-DTPA.

Gradient: The amount and direction of change in space of some quantity, such as magnetic field strength. Commonly used to refer to magnetic field gradient.

Gradient coil: Loop of wire or other type of electrical conductor which can alter the magnetic field to produce the main magnetic field gradient. Typically there are three gradient coils- one for each direction, x,y, and z. These may also be referred to as slice encoding gradient, frequency encoding gradient and phase encoding gradient.

Gradient Echo: Spin echo produced by reversing direction, or applying balanced pulses, of magnetic field gradient before and after a refocusing RF pulse so as to cancel out the position-dependent phase shifts that have accumulated due to the gradient. In the latter case, the gradient echo is generally adjusted to coincide with the RF spin echo. When the RF and gradient echoes are not coincident, the time of the gradient echo is denoted TE and the difference in time between the echoes is denoted TD, while TER refers to the time of the RF spin echo.

Image Acquisition Time: Time required to collect the Fourier data necessary to produce an MR image. Image acquisition time equals the product of the repetition time (TR), the number of signals averaged (NSA), and the number of phase encoding steps (i.e. pixels of resolution in the phase encoding direction).

k-space - Fourier space: An array of data representing the Fourier transform of an object. It is generally characterized as having low spatial frequency data (center of k-space) which dominates image contrast and high spatial frequency data (periphery of k-space) which dominates image detail. Most MR imaging techniques collect data in this domain. Images are then reconstructed by performing the Fourier transform. By convention, data along kx is frequency encoded (and collected during a single MR echo); Data along ky or kz is phase-encoded and collected using multiple echoes.

Magnetic Resonance Angiography (MRA):   A form of selectively displaying vascular morphology with MR techniques.

Magnetic Resonance Imaging (MRI):   A form of imaging in a magnetic field and using radio frequency waves at the appropriate resonant frequency to rotate some of the protons in the subject. These protons then emit a signal from which an image can be formed.

Mask Image: A pre-contrast image that can be subtracted from contrast-enhanced images in order to suppress or reduce an undesired image component, such as background tissue signal.

Maximum Intensity Projection (or MIP):	An image processing technique for reducing 3D data to a 2D projection. MIP images are formed by projecting along parallel rays, through the volume data, and recording the maximum pixel intensity encountered along each ray.
Moving Table MRA:	The technique used for peripheral vascular imaging, where the MR scanning table is rapidly repositioned during the acquisition to acquire multiple 3D contrast MRA data sets at different locations following the contrast bolus passage down the arteries. The technique has also been called "floating" table MRA or bolus-chase MRA and has been expanded to cover the entire body, "whole-body MRA".
Paramagnetic:	A property of materials whereby a magnetic field is increased in strength in the presence of the material. For example, gadolinium, melanin, methemoglobin are paramagnetic. Iron may be so strongly paramagnetic, it is referred to as superparamagnetic.
Paramagnetic Contrast Agent:	A paramagnetic substance (e.g. gadolinium chelates) which increases the magnetic field locally around individual contrast agent molecules creating field gradients which facilitate T1 relaxation and cause tissues to become brighter on T1 weighted images.
Phantom:	Object that simulates a person for purposes of testing, calibrating or teaching MRI pulse sequences and procedures.
Phase Encoding:	The process where gradients before the readout are used to encode spatial location. Normally phase encoding is used for ky and kz directions and frequency encoding is used for kx.
Phased Array Coil:	MR coil with multiple elements to improve SNR and optimize field-of-view. Multiple individual coils are each electronically connected to separate preamplifiers, and images are reconstructed for each individual coil, then combined to yield one large field-of-view image with higher SNR typical of smaller coils.
Projection Reconstruction MRA:	A reconstruction technique for performing MR angiography that does not require Fourier (spin-warp) imaging in all 3 directions. The technique is analogous to computed tomography, where images are reconstructed using a series of angular projections of the data, followed by filtered backprojection processing. With this technique, reconstructed spatial resolution is largely independent of acquisition time or the number of views obtained.

Pulse Sequence: Computer program that instructs the MRI system in how to give radio frequency pulses at the appropriate frequency and duration and how to optimally adjust magnetic field gradients to acquire images with appropriate contrast, resolution, field-of-view, location, etc.

Read Out (or Frequency Encoding):   The acquisition of the MR signal concurrent with a constant gradient. Results in a line of k-space data, which by convention is parallel to kx.

Recessed Centric: A k-space data acquisition encoding scheme in which central k-space data are acquired at the beginning of the scan (centric) but the absolute center of k-space is recessed a few seconds into the scan. This helps to prevent ringing artifact caused by collecting the absolute center of k-space as the contrast bolus is arriving.

Reconstruction Matrix: Number of pixels of resolution in the final image in each dimension after reconstructing the acquired raw k-space data. Because of zero-filling and/or homodyne reconstruction, as well as projection reconstruction techniques, dimensions of the reconstructed matrix may be larger than corresponding dimensions of the acquisition matrix.

Sequential k-space Acquisition: A data acquisition scheme in which MR k-space data are acquired sequentially beginning at the periphery of k-space, $k = 0$. Central k-space data are acquired in the middle. Additional peripheral k-space data are acquired at the end. Signals measured during the middle of the acquisition, corresponding to central k-space, determine image contrast. For a 30-second 3D contrast MRA exam, image contrast will be primarily determined by data acquired 10-20 seconds following initiation of the scan.

SmartPrep: A contrast bolus timing technique that repeatedly samples a single large voxel placed on the aorta to sense the arrival of contrast and automatically trigger data acquisition beginning with the center of k-space. Typically, the sampling voxel completely encompass a section of a large vessel, e.g., the aorta. By detecting the leading edge of the bolus, there will be about 6-8 seconds of image acquisition delay before bolus peak. During this image acquistion delay, the patient is instructed to "take in a deep breath" and then "stop breathing."

Spiral MRA: MR data acquisition technique using a spiral sampling of k-space, rather than standard rectilinear sampling of k-space in Fourier imaging. Since data acquisition spirals start at the center of k-space the echo time is near zero which may help reduce flow and susceptibility artifacts. Each spiral collects more k-space coefficients than each horizontal line of a rectilinear scan. Thus, spiral data acquisition is inherently faster but it may introduce off-resonance effects and other artifacts.

T1:

Spin-lattice or longitudinal relaxation time; the characteristic time constant for spins to align with the external magnetic field. Starting from zero, magnetization will grow $1/e$ (~63%) of its final maximum value in a time T1. Typical T1 values are for fat = 270ms, muscle = 650 ms, liver = 400ms, brain = 800 ms.

T2:

Spin-spin or transverse relaxation time; the characteristic time constant for loss of phase coherence among spins oriented at an angle to the static magnetic field which occurs in a magnetic field of perfect homogeneity. Loss of phase coherence is due to interactions between the spins, with resulting loss of transverse magnetization and NMR signal. Transverse magnetization will decay so that it loses $1/e$ (63%) of its initial value in a time, T2, if relaxation is characterized by a simple single exponential decay. Typical T2 value are for CSF = 2000ms, tumor = 100ms, liver = 50 ms, muscle = 40ms, cortical bone < 1ms.

T2*:

The actual observed loss of MR signal phase coherence which tends to be less than the intrinsic tissue T2 because of inevitable inhomogenieties in the magnetic field.

TE - Echo time:

The time between the middle of an exciting (e.g., 90°) RF pulse and the peak of the spin echo or gradient echo signal. In general, the longer this period becomes, the greater MR signal loss due to T2*-decay or fast blood flow.

TR - Repetition time:

The period of time between successive MR primary excitation pulses.

Time-of-Flight:

MRA technique where the local magnetization of fluid is selectively altered in a region, e.g., by selective excitation, such that it will carry the altered magnetization with it when it moves, thus tagging the selected region. This is the source of several flow effects.

VIPR – Vastly under-sampled Isotropic Projection Reconstruction:

A k-space data acquisition scheme in which k-space is traversed with multiple radial lines instead of the standard rectilinear scheme in which k-space is traversed horizontally. This technique allows higher resolution imaging and larger FOV for short data acquisition periods. When performed in 3D, it provides isotropic resolution.

Zero-Filling: An interpolation scheme where extra zeroes are added to the k-space data array prior to Fourier transformation (FT). These extra data points cause the FT to automatically reconstruct more voxels which are interpolated between the acquired voxels. This is better than most interpolation schemes because it utilizes both phase and magnitude data to increase resolution of the final magnitude image.

Bibliography

Basic Concepts

Alley MT, Shifrin RY, Pelc NJ, Herfkens RJ. Ultrafast contrast-enhanced three-dimensional MR angiography: state of the art. Radiographics 1998; 18(2):273-285.

Anderson CM, Edelman RR, Turski PA. Clinical Magnetic Resonance Angiography. New York, NY; Raven Press; 1993.

Barger AV, Block WF, Toropov Y, Grist TM, Mistretta CA. Time-resolved contrast-enhanced imaging with isotropic resolution and broad coverage using an undersampled 3D projection trajectory. Magn Reson Med 2002;48:297-305.

Bernstein MA, Huston J 3rd, Lin C, Gibbs GF, Felmlee JP. High-resolution intracranial and cervical MRA at 3.0T: technical considerations and initial experience. Magn Reson Med. 2001 Nov;46(5):955-62.

Debatin JF, Hany TF. MR-based assessment of vascular morphology and function. Eur J Radiol 1998; 8:528-539.

Douek P, Revel D, Amiel M. Angiographie par resonance magnetique. Revue du Praticien 1996; 46:835-841.

Finn JP, Baskaran V, Carr JC, McCarthy RM, Pereles FS, Kroeker R, Laub GA. Thorax: Low-Dose Contrast-enhanced Three-dimensional MR Angiography with Subsecond Temporal Resolution Initial Results. Radiology. 2002;224(3):896-904.

Goede SC, Goyen M, Forsting M, Debatin JF: Preventative Imaging without Radiation – Introducing an MR-based Screening Strategy. Radiologe 2002; 42: 622-629.

Goldfarb JW, Edelman RR. Coronary arteries: breath-hold, gadolinium-enhanced, three-dimensional MR angiography. Radiology 1998; 206:830-834.

Goyen M, Quick HH, Debatin JF, Ladd ME, Barkhausen J, Herborn CU, Bosk S, Kuehl H, Schlepütz M, Ruehm SG. Whole Body 3D MR Angiography Using A Rolling Table Platform: Initial Clinical Experience. Radiologe 2002; 224: 270-277.

Goyen M, Ruehm SG, Debatin JF: Arterial Disease Screening Using Whole-Body 3D MR-Angiography. Med Klin 2002; 97(5):285-289.

Goyen M, Herborn CU, Kröger K, Lauenstein TC, Debatin JF, Ruehm SG: Detection of Atherosclerosis: Systemic Imaging for a Systemic Disease Using Whole Body 3D MR-Angiography – Initial Experience Radiology (in press).

Goyen M, Herborn CU, Kröger K, Vogt FM, Verhagen R, Yang Y, Bosk S, Debatin JF, Ruehm SG. Using a 1 M Gd-Chelate (Gadobutrol) For Total-Body Three-dimensional MR Angiography Preliminary Experience JMRI (under review).

Goyen M, Goehde SC, Herborn CU, et al. MR-based Full Body Imaging for Disease Screening -Technique and Preliminary Experience Radiology (under review).

Hany TF, Schmidt M, Steiner P, Debatin JF. Optimization of contrast dosage for gadolinium-enhanced 3D MRA of the pulmonary and renal arteries. Magn Reson Imaging 1998.

Hany TF, Schmidt M, Leung DA, Debatin JF. Wertigkeit der kontrastverstärkten 3D MR-angiographie der nierenarteriesn. Radiologe 1997; 37:547-553.

Ho VB, Foo TK, Czum JM, Marcos H, Choyke PL, Knopp MV. Contrast-enhanced magnetic resonance angiography: technical considerations for optimized clinical implementation. Top Magn Reson Imaging. 2001;12(4):283-99.

Higgins CB. Essentials of Cardiac Radiology and Imaging. Philadelphia, PA; J.P. Lippincott Company; 1992.

Krebs TL, Daly B, Wong JJ, Chow CC, Bartlett ST. Vascular complications of pancreatic transplantation: MR evaluation. Radiology 1995; 196:793-798.

Leung DA, Hany TF, Debatin JF. Three-dimensional contrast-enhanced magnetic resonance angiography of the abdominal arterial system. Cardiovasc Intervent Radiol 1998; 21:1-10.

Leung DA, McKinnon GC, Davis CP, Pfammatter T, Krestin GP, Debatin JF. Breath-hold, contrast-enhanced, three-dimensional MR angiography. Radiology 1996; 200:569-571.

Maki JH, Chenevert TL, Prince MR. Three-dimensional contrast-enhanced MR angiography. Top Magn Reson Imaging 1996; 8:322-344.

Omary RA, Frayne R, Unal O, Grist TM, Strother CM. Intra-arterial gadolinium-enhanced 2D and 3D magnetic resonance angiography: A preliminary study. JVIR, 1999;10:1315-1321.

Omary RA, Frayne R, Unal O, Warner T, Korosec FR, Mistretta CA, Strother CM, Grist TM. MR-guided angioplasty of renal artery stenosis in a pig model: A feasibility study. JVIR 2000;11(3):373-381.

Omary RA, Unal O, Koscielski DS, Frayne R, Korosec FR, Mistretta CA, Strother CM, Grist TM. Real-time MR imaging-guided passive catheter tracking with use of gadolinium-filled catheters. JVIR 2000;11:1079-1085.

Omary RA, Henseler KP, Unal O, Smith RJ, Ryu RK, Resnick SA, Saker MB, Chrisman HB, Frayne R, Finn JP, Li D, Grist TM. Validation of injection parameters for catheter-directed intraarterial gadolinium-enhanced MR angiography. Acad Radiol 2002;9:172-185.

Potchen JE, Haacke EM, Siebert JE, Gottschalk A. Magnetic Resonance Angiography: Concepts and Applications. St. Louis, MO; Mosby, 1993.

Prince MR. Contrast-enhanced MR angiography: theory and optimization. MRI Clin N Am 1998; 6:257-267.

Prince MR. Gadolinium-enhanced MR aortography. Radiology 1994; 191:155-164.

Prince MR, Yucel EK, Kaufman JA, Harrison DC, Geller SC. Dynamic gadolinium-enhanced three-dimensional abdominal MR arteriography. J Magn Reson Imaging 1993; 3:877-881.

Ruehm SG, Goyen M, Barkhausen J, Kröger K, Bosk S, Ladd ME, Debatin JF. Whole Body 3D MRA: 5 Steps And a Single Injection in 72 s. LANCET 2001; 357: 1086-1091.

Ruehm SG, Schroeder T, Debatin JF. Interstitial MR lymphography with gadoterate meglumine: initial experience in humans. Radiology 2001; 220: 816-821.

Ruehm SG, Goyen M, Debatin JF. MR-Angiography – First Choice For The Assessment Of The Arterial Vasculature RoFo Fortschr Geb Rontgenstr Neuen Bildgeb Verfahr 2002; 174(5): 551-561.

Ruehm SG, Goyen M, Quick HH, Schleputz M, Schleputz H, Bosk S, Barkhausen J, Ladd ME, Debatin JF. Whole-body MRA on a rolling table platform (AngioSURF). RoFo ROFO Fortschr Geb Rontgenstr Neuen Bildgeb Verfahr 2000; 172: 670-674.

Runge VM, Kirsch JE, Lee C. Contrast-enhanced MR angiography. J Magn Reson Imaging 1993; 3:233-239.

Wiesner W, Pfammatter T, Krestin GK, Debatin JF. MRT und MRA von Nierentransplantaten - Gefäss- und Perfusionsbeurteilung. RöFo 1998 (in press).

Yano T, Kodama T, Suzuki Y, Watanabe K. Gadolinium-enhanced 3D time-of-flight MR angiography. Experimental and clinical evaluation. Acta Radiologica 1997; 38:47-54.

Yucel EK, Anderson CM, Edelman RR, Grist TM, Baum RA, Manning WJ, Culebras A, Pearce W. (AHA Scientific Statement) Magnetic resonance angiography: Update on applications for extracranial arteries. Circulation 1999;100:2284-2301.

Yucel EK. Magnetic Resonance Angiography. A Practical Approach. New York, NY; McGraw-Hill, Incorporated; 1995.

K-Space Effects and Technical Details

Amann M, Bock M, Floemer F, Schoenberg SO, Schad LR. Three-dimensional spiral MR imaging: Application to renal multiphase contrast-enhanced angiography. Magn Reson Med. 2002 Aug;48(2):290-6.

Fain SB, Riederer SJ, Huston J 3rd, King BF. Embedded MR fluoroscopy: high temporal resolution real-time imaging during high spatial resolution 3D MRA acquisition. Magn Reson Med. 2001 Oct;46(4):690-8.

Fain SB, Riederer SJ, Bernstein MA, Huston J 3rd. Theoretical limits of spatial resolution in elliptical-centric contrast-enhanced 3D-MRA. Magn Reson Med. 1999 Dec;42(6):1106-16.

Foo TK, Ho VB, Hood MN, Marcos HB, Hess SL, Choyke PL. High-spatial-resolution multistation MR imaging of lower-extremity peripheral vasculature with segmented volume acquisition: feasibility study. Radiology. 2001 Jun;219(3):835-41.

Goyen M, Lauenstein TC, Herborn CU, Debatin JF, Bosk S, Ruehm SG. 0.5 M Gd-Chelate (Magnevist) vs. 1.0 M Gd-Chelate (Gadovist): Dose-independent Effect on Image Quality of Pelvic 3D MRA. J Magn Res Imaging 2001; 14: 602-607.

Goyen M, Herborn CU, Lauenstein TC, Debatin JF, Bosk S, Ruehm SG. Optimization of Contrast Dosage For Gadobenate Dimeglumine-Enhanced High-Resolution Whole Body 3D MR Angiography. Iinvest Radiol 2002; 37: 263-268.

Herborn CU, Lauenstein TC, Ruehm SG, Bosk S, Debatin JF, Goyen M: Intraindividual Comparison of Gadopentetate Dimeglumine, Gadobenate Dimeglumine, and Gadobutrol for Pelvic 3D MR-Angiography. Iinvest Radiol (in press).

Kopka L, Vosshenrich R, Rodenwaldt J, Grabbe E. Differences in injection rates on contrast-enhanced breath-hold three-dimensional MR angiography. AJR Am J Roentgenol 1998; 170:345-348.

Maki JH, Chenevert TL, Prince MR. The effects of incomplete breath-holding on 3D MR image quality. J Magn Reson Imaging 1997; 7:1132-1139.

Maki JH, Prince MR, Londy FJ, Chenevert TL. The effects of time varying intravascular signal intensity and k-space acquisition order on three-dimensional MR angiography image quality. J Magn Reson Imaging 1996; 6:642-651.

Maki JH, Wilson GJ, Eubank WB, Hoogeveen RM. Utilizing SENSE to achieve lower station sub-millimeter isotropic resolution and minimal venous enhancement in peripheral MR angiography. J Magn Reson Imaging. 2002 Apr;15(4):484-91.

Peters DC, Korosec FR, Grist TM, Block WF, Holden JE, Vigen KK, Mistretta CA. Undersampled projection reconstruction applied to MR angiography. Magn Reson Med 2000;43:91-101.

Prince MR, Chenevert TL, Foo TK, Londy FJ, Ward JS, Maki JH. Contrast-enhanced abdominal MR angiography: optimization of imaging delay time by automating the detection of contrast material arrival in the aorta. Radiology 1997; 203:109-214.

Vigen KK, Peters DC, Grist TM, Block WF, Mistretta CA. Undersampled projection-reconstruction imaging for time-resolved contrast-enhanced imaging. Magn Reson Med 2000;43:170-176. Radiologica 1997; 38:173-175.

Watts R, Wang Y, Prince MR, Winchester PA, Khilnani NM, Kent KC. Anatomically tailored k-space sampling for bolus-chase three-dimensional MR digital subtraction angiography. Radiology. 2001;218(3):899-904.

Wilman AH, Yep TC, Al-Kwifi O. Quantitative evaluation of nonrepetitive phase-encoding orders for first-pass, 3D contrast-enhanced MR angiography. Magn Reson Med. 2001 Sep;46(3):541-7.

Wilman AH, Riederer SJ. On the cause of increased aliasing in the slice-select direction in 3D contrast-enhanced magnetic resonance angiography. Magn Reson Med. 2000 Aug;44(2):336-8.

Wilman AH, Riederer SJ, King BF, Debbins JP, Rossman PJ, Ehman RL. Fluoroscopically triggered contrast-enhanced three-dimensional MR angiography with elliptical centric view order: application to the renal arteries. Radiology 1997; 205:137-146.

Wilman AH, Riederer SJ. Performance of an elliptical centric view order for signal enhancement and motion artifact suppression in breath-hold three-dimensional gradient echo imaging. Magn Reson Med 1997; 38:793-802.

Timing Strategies

Carroll TJ, Korosec FR, Swan JS, Hany TF, Grist TM, Mistretta CA. The effect of injection rate on time resolved contrast-enhanced peripheral MRA. J Magn Reson Imag 2001; 14:401-410.

Earls JP, Rofsky NM, Decorato DR, Krinsky GA, Weinreb JC. Hepatic arterial-phase dynamic gadolinium-enhanced MR imaging: optimization with a test examination and a power injector. Radiology 1997; 202:268-273.

Foo TKF, Saranathan M, Prince MR, Chenevert TL. Automated detection of bolus arrival time and initiation of data acquisition in fast, three-dimensional, gadolinium-enhanced MR angiography. Radiology 1997; 203:275-280.

Hany TF, McKinnon GC, Prammatter T, Debatin JF. Optimization of contrast timing for breath hold three-dimensional MR angiography. J Magn Reson Imaging 1997; 7:551-556.

Korosec FR, Frayne R, Grist TM, Mistretta CA. Time-resolved contrast-enhanced 3D MR angiography. Magn Reson Med 1996; 36:345-351.

Prince MR, Chenevert TL, Foo TKF, Londy FJ, Ward JS, Maki JH. Contrast-enhanced abdominal MR angiography: optimization of imaging delay time by automating the detection of contrast material arrival in the aorta. Radiology 1997; 203:109-114.

Prince, MR, Narasimham DL, Londy FJ, Pfammatter T, Akhavan R. A simple MR-compatible infusion pump. Magn Reson Imaging 1996; 14:121-128.

Riederer SJ, Tasciyan T, Farzaneh F, Lee JN, Wright RC, Herfkens RJ. MR fluoroscopy: technical feasibility. Magn Reson Med 1988; 8:1-15.

Swan J, Grist TM, Korosec FR, Kennell T, Hoch J, Heisey D. MR Angiography of the Aorto-iliac Arteries During a Breath-hold Using Gadoinium-enhanced 3D TOF with k-space Zero-filling and a Contrast Timing Scan. The International Society of Magnetic Resonance in Medicine, 1996.

Image Analysis Techniques

Carroll TJ, Korosec FR, Swan JS, Grist TM, Frayne R, Mistretta CA. Method for rapidly determining and reconstructing the peak arterial frame from a time-resolved CE-MRA exam. Magn Reson Med 2000;44:817-820.

Davis CP, Hany TF, Wildermuth S, Schmidt M, Debatin JF. Postprocessing techniques for gadolinium-enhanced three-dimensional MR angiography. Radiographics 1997; 17:1061-1077.

Davis CP, Ladd ME, Romanowski BJ, Wildermuth S, Knoblauch JF, Debatin JF. Human aorta: preliminary results with virtual endoscopy based on three-dimensional MR imaging data sets. Radiology 1996; 199:37-40.

Frayne R, Grist TM, Swan JS, Peters DS, Korosec FR, Mistretta CA. 3D MR DSA: Effects of injection protocol and image masking. J Magn Reson Imag 2000:12:476-487.

Hany TF, Schmidt M, Davis CP, Göhde SC, Debatin JF. Diagnostic impact of four post-processing techniques in evaluating of contrast-enhanced three-dimensional MR angiography. AJR Am J Roentgenol 1998; 170:907-912.

Lee VS, Flyer MA, Weinreb JC, Krinsky GA, Rofsky NM. Image subtraction in gadolinium-enhanced MR imaging. AJR Am J Roentgenol 1996; 167:1427-1432.

Leung DA, Pelkonen P, Hany TF, Zimmermann G, Pfammatter T, Debatin JF. Value of image subtraction in 3D Gd-enhanced MR angiography of the renal arteries. J Magn Reson Imaging 1998; 8:598-602.

Mezrich R. A perspective on K-space. Radiology 1995; 195:297-315.

Svensson J, Leander P, Maki JH, Stahlberg F, Olsson LE. Separation of arteries and veins using flow-induced phase effects in contrast-enhanced MRA of the lower extremities. Magn Reson Imaging. 2002 Jan;20(1):49-57.

Wang Y, Johnston DL, Breen JF, Huston J III, Jack CR, Julsrud PR, Kiely MJ, King BF, Riederer SL, Ehman RL. Dynamic MR digital subtraction angiography using contrast enhancement, fast data acquisition, and complex subtraction. Magn Reson Med 1996; 36:551-556.

Contrast Safety

Arrigo G, Cavaliere G, Scalia A, Schiavina G, D'Amico G. Radiocontrast media nephrotoxicity: clinical aspects. Contrib Nephrol 1987; 55:176-188.

Bluemke DA, Stillman AE, Bis KG, Grist TM, Baum RA, D'Agostino R, Malden ES, Pierro JA, Yucel EK. Carotid MR angiography: Phase II study of safety and efficacy for MS-325. Radiology 2001;219:114-122.

Carvlin MJ, De Simone DN, Meeks MJ. Phase II clinical trial of gadoteridol injection, a low-osmolal magnetic resonance imaging contrast agent. Invest Radiol 1992; 27:S16-S21.

Cohan RH, Leder RA, Hezberg AJ, Hedlund LW, Wheeler CT, Beam CA, Nadel SN, Dunnick NR. Extravascular toxicity of two magnetic resonance contrast agents. Preliminary experience in the rat. Invest Radiol 1991; 26:224-226.

Goldstein HA, Kashanian FK, Blumetti RF, Holyoak WL, Hugo FP, Blumenfield DM. Safety assessment of gadopentetate dimeglumine in U.S. clinical trials. Radiology 1990; 174:17-23.

Goyen M, Ruehm SG, Debatin JF. MR-Angiography: The Role of Contrast Agents Eur J Radiol 2000 ; 34: 247-256.

Harpur ES, Worah D, Hals PA, Holtz E, Furuhama K, Nomura H. Preclinical safety assessment and pharmacokinetics of gadodiamide injection, a new magnetic resonance imaging contrast agent. Invest Radiol 1993; 28:S28-S43.

Haustein J, Niendorf HP, Krestin G, Louton T, Schuhmann-Giampieri G, Clauss W, Junge W. Renal tolerance of Gd-DTPA/dimeglumine in patients with chronic renal failure. Invest Radiol 1992; 27:153-156.

Jordan RM, Mintz RD. Fatal reaction to gadopentetate dimeglumine. AJR Am J Roentgenol 1995; 164:743-744.

Katayama H, Yamaguchi K, Kozuka T, Takashima T, Seez P, Matsuura K. Adverse reactions to ionic and nonionic contrast media: a report from the Japanese Committee on the Safety of Contrast Media. Radiology 1990; 175:621-628.

Kinno Y, Odagiri K, Andoh K, Itoh Y, Tarao K. Gadopentetate dimeglumine as an alternative contrast material for use in angiography. Am J Roentgenol 1993; 160:1293-1294.

Leander P, Allard M, Caille JM, Golman K. Early effect of gadopentate and iodinated contrast media on rabbit kidneys. Invest Radiol 1992; 27:922-926.

Lufkin RB. Severe anaphylactoid reaction to Gd-DTPA [Letter to the Editor]. Radiology 1990; 176:879.

Lundby B, Berg KJ, Lien HH, Aamdal S. A double blind study to evaluate the tolerability of gadodiamide injection and its effect on renal function in patients undergoing cerebral magnetic resonance imaging. Br J Rad 1993; 66:871-876.

Nelson KL, Gifford LM, Lauber-Huber C, Gross CA, Lasser TA. Clinical safety of gadopentetate dimeglumine. Radiology 1995; 196:439-443.

Niendorf HP, Dinger JC, Haustein J, Cornelius I, Alhassan A, Clauss W. Tolerance data of Gd-DTPA: a review. Eur J Radiol 1991; 13:15-20.

Niendorf HP, Haustein J, Cornelius I, Alhassan A, Clauss W. Satety of gadolinium-DTPA: extended clinical experience. Magn Reson Med 1991; 22:222-228.

Niendorf HP, Haustein J, Louton T, Beck W, Laniado M. Safety and tolerance after intravenous administration of 0.3 mmol/kg Gd-DTPA. Results of a randomized, controlled clinical trial. Invest Radiol 1991; 26:S221-S223.

Oksendal AN, Hals PA. Biodistribution and toxicity of MR imaging contrast media. J Magn Reson Imaging 1993; 3:157-165.

Prince MR, Arnoldus C, Frisoli JK. Nephrotoxicity of high dose gadolinium compared to iodinated contrast. J Magn Reson Imaging 1996; 6:162-166.

Quinn AD, O'Hare NJ, Wallis FJ, Wilson GF. Gd-DTPA: an alternative contrast medium for CT. J Comput Assist Tomogr 1994; 18:634-636.

Reinton V, Berg JK, Svaland MG, Andrew E, Normann PT, Rootwelt K. Pharmacokinetics of gadodiamide injection in patients with moderately impaired renal function. Acad Radiol 1994; 1:S56-S61.

Rocklage SM, Worah D, Kim SH. Metal ion release from paramagnetic chelates: what is tolerable? Magn Reson Med 1991; 22:216-221.

Rofsky NM, Weinreb JC, Bosniak MA, Libes RB, Birnbaum BA. Renal lesion characterization with gadolinium-enhanced MR imaging: efficacy and safety in patients with renal insufficiency. Radiology 1991; 180:85-89.

Runge VM, Bradley WG, Brant-Zawadzki MN, Carvlin MJ, DeSimone DN, Dean BL, Dillon WP, Drayer BP, Flanders AE, Harms SE, Haughton VM, Howieson J, Joy SE, Kanal E, Kumar AJ, Liu T, Lufkin RB, Maravilla KR, Mezrich RS, Mikhael MA, Morgan FW, Nadel SN, Pollei SR, Pomeranz SJ, Price AC, Ramsey RG, Yuh W, Zelch JV. Clinical safety and efficacy of gadoteridol: a study in 411 patients with suspected intracranial and spinal disease. Radiology 1991; 181:701-709.

Santyr G, Niendorf E, Kim A. Pharmacokinetic properties of gadodiamide injection in patients with impaired renal function. In Proceedings of Society of Magnetic Resonance, 1994.

Schuhmann-Giampieri G, Krestin G. Pharmacokinetics of Gd-DTPA in patients with chronic renal failure. Invest Radiol 1991; 26:975-979.

Weinmann HJ, Brasch RC, Press WR, Wesbey GE. Characteristics of gadolinium-DTPA complex: a potential NMR contrast agent. AJR Am J Roentgenol 1984; 142:619-624.

Weinmann HJ, Laniado M, Mutzel, W. Pharmacokinetics of Gd-DTPA/dimeglumine after intravenous injection into healthy volunteers. Physiol Chem Phys Med NMR 1984; 16:167-172.

Weiss KL. Severe anaphylactoid reaction after i.v. Gd-DPTA. Magn Reson Imaging 1990; 8:817-818.

Blood Pool Contrast Agents

Adzamli K, Haar JP Jr, Hynes MR, Miller DB, Polta JA, Wallace RA, Woulfe SR, Adams MD. Development of a novel nonaromatic small-molecule MR contrast agent for the blood pool. Acad Radiol 1998; 5:S210-S213.

Bjornerud A, Wendland MF, Johansson L, Ahlstrom HK, Higgins CB, Oksendal A. Use of intravascular contrast agents in MRI. Acad Radiol 1998; 5:S223-S225.

Bluemke DA, Stillman AE, Bis KG, Grist TM, Baum RA, D'Agostino R, Malden ES, Pierro JA, Yucel EK. Carotid MR angiography: phase II study of safety and efficacy for MS-325. Radiology. 2001;219(1):114-22.

Grist TM, Korosec FR, Peters DC, Witte S, Walovitch RC, Dolan RP, Bridson WE, Yucel EK, Mistretta CA. Steady-state and dynamic MR angiography with MS-325: initial experience in humans. Radiology 1998; 207:539-44.

Hofman MB, Adzamli K, Allen JS, Fischer SE, Brown JJ, Adams MD, Wickline SA, Lorenz CH. Kinetics of a novel blood pool agent (MP-2269) with persistent high relaxivity for MR angiography. Acad Radiol 1998; 5:S206-S209; discussion S226-S227.

Lauffer RB, Parmelee DJ, Dunham SU, Ouellet HS, Dolan RP, Witte S, McMurry TJ, Walovitch RC. MS-325: albumin-targeted contrast agent for MR angiography. Radiology 1998; 207:529-538.

Lauffer RB, Parmelee DJ, Ouellet HS, Dolan RP, Sajiki H, Scott DM, Bernard PJ, Buchanan EM, Ong KY, Tyeklar Z, Midelfort KS, McMurry TJ, Walovitch RC. MS-325: a small-molecule vascular imaging agent for magnetic resonance imaging. Acad Radiol 1996; 3:S356-S358.

Lin W, Abendschein DR, Celik A, Dolan RP, Lauffer RB, Walovitch RC, Haacke EM. Intravascular contrast agent improves magnetic resonance angiography of carotid arteries in minipigs. J Magn Reson Imaging 1997; 7:963-971.

Nolte-Ernsting C, Adam G, Bucker A, Berges S, Bjornerud A, Gunther RW. Abdominal MR angiography performed using blood pool contrast agents: comparison of a new superparamagnetic iron oxide nanoparticle and a linear gadolinium polymer. AJR Am J Roentgenol 1998; 171:107-113.

Prasad PV, Cannillo J, Chavez DR, Li W, Pinchasin ES, Dolan RP, Walovitch R, Edelman RR. Contrast-enhanced MR angiography and first-pass renal perfusion imaging using MS-325, an intravascular contrast agent. Acad Radiol 1998; 5:S219-S222; discussion S226-S227.

Schwickert HC, Stiskal M, van Dijke CF, Roberts TP, Mann JS, Demsar F, Brasch RC. Tumor angiography using high-resolution, three-dimensional magnetic resonance imaging: comparison of gadopentetate dimeglumine and a macromolecular blood-pool contrast agent. Acad Radiol 1995; 2:851-858.

Shibata DK, Schmiedl UP, Yuan C, Nelson JA. Two prototype blood-pool agents for contrast-enhanced magnetic resonance angiography of the portal vein in pigs. Acad Radiol 1995; 2:705-708.

Pulmonary MRA Bibliography

Bongartz G, Boos M, Scheffler K, Steinbrich W. Pulmonary circulation. Eur Radiol 1998; 46(3):280-286.

Eisenhauer MD, Kinney JB Jr, Ho VB, Sahn DJ, Braxton M, Peake J. Preoperative gadolinium-enhanced magnetic resonance pulmonary venography in an adolescent with atrial septal defect [published erratum appears in Mil Med 1997; 162:preceding 643]. Mil Med 1997; 162:640-642.

Ferrari VA, Scott CH, Holland GA, Axel L, Sutton MS. Ultrafast three-dimensional contrast-enhanced magnetic resonance angiography and imaging in the diagnosis of partial anomalous pulmonary venous drainage. J Am Coll Cardiol 2001;37(4):1120-8.

Gefter WB, Hatabu H, Holland GA, Gupta KB, Henschke CI, Palevsky HI. Pulmonary thromboembolism: recent developments in diagnosis with CT and MR imaging. Radiology 1995; 197:561-574.

Godart F, Willoteaux S, Rey C, Cocheteux B, Francart C, Beregi JP. Contrast enhanced magnetic resonance angiography and pulmonary venous anomalies. Heart. 2001 Dec;86(6):705.

Goyen M, Laub G, Ladd ME, Debatin JF, Barkhausen J, Truemmler KH, Bosk S, Ruehm SG. Dynamic 3D MR angiography of the pulmonary arteries in under four seconds. J Magn Reson Imaging 2001 Mar;13(3):372-7.

Goyen M, Jagenburg A, Barkhausen J, Ruehm SG, Kroger K, Debatin JF. Pulmonary Arteriovenous Malformation: Characterization with Time-Resolved Ultrafast 3D MR Angiography. J Magn Reson Imaging 2001; 13: 358-360.

Grist TM, Sostman HD, MacFall JR, Foo TK, Spritzer CE, Witty L, Newman GE, Debatin JF, Tapson V, Saltzman HA. Pulmonary angiography with MR imaging: preliminary clinical experience. Radiology 1993; 189:523.

Gupta A, Frazer CK, Ferguson JM, Kumar AB, Davis SJ, Fallon MJ, Morris IT, Drury PJ, Cala LA. Acute pulmonary embolism: diagnosis with MR angiography. Radiology 1999 Feb;210(2):353-9.

Hany TF, Schmidt M, Steiner P, Debatin JF. Optimization of contrast dosage for gadolinium-enhanced 3D MRA of the pulmonary and renal arteries. Magn Reson Imaging 1998 (in press).

Hatabu H. MR pulmonary angiography and perfusion imaging: recent advances. Semin Ultrasound CT MR 1997; 18:349-61.

Hatabu H, Gaa J, Kim D, Li W, Prasad PV, Edelman RR. Pulmonary perfusion and angiography: evaluation with breath-hold enhanced three-dimensional fast imaging steady-state precession MR imaging with short TR and TE. AJR Am J Roentgenol 1996; 167:653-655.

Hudson ER, Smith TP, McDermott VG, Newman GE, Suhocki PV, Payne CS, Stackhouse DJ. Pulmonary angiography performed with iopamidol: complications in 1,434 patients. Radiology 1996; 198:61-65.

Isoda H, Ushimi T, Masui T, Mochizuki T, Goto S, Suzuki K, Shirakawa T, Ohta A, Takahashe M, Kaneko M. Clinical evaluation of pulmonary 3-D time-of-flight MRA with breath holding using contrast media. J Comput Assist Tomogr 1995; 19:911-919.

Ito T, Takahashi H, Ida M, Kato H. [Evaluation of hilar pulmonary vessels using magnetic resonance angiography (MRA)]. Journal of the Japanese Association for Thoracic Surgery 1998; 46(3):280-286.

Kacl GM, Follath F, Salomon F, Debatin JF. Primary angiosarcoma of the pulmonary arteries: dynamic contrast-enhanced MRI. J Comput Assist Tomogr 1998 (in press).

Khalil A, Farres MT, Mangiapan G, Tassart M, Bigot JM, Carette MF. Pulmonary arteriovenous malformations. Chest 2000; 117:1399-1403.

Kondo C, Takada K, Yokoyama U, Nakajima Y, Momma K, Sakai F. Comparison of three-dimensional contrast-enhanced magnetic resonance angiography and axial radiographic angiography for diagnosing congenital stenoses in small pulmonary arteries. Am J Cardiol 2001 Feb 15;87(4):420-4.

Kreitner KF, Ley S, Kauczor HU, Kalden P, Pitton MB, Mayer E, Laub G, Thelen M. Contrast media enhanced three dimensional MR angiography of the pulmonary arteries in patients with chronic recurrent pulmonary embolism – comparison with selective intra-arterial DSA. Rofo Fortschr Geb Rontgenstr Neuen Bildgeb Verfahr 2000;172(2):122-8.

Kruger S, Haage P, Hoffmann R, Breuer C, Bucker A, Hanrath P, Gunther RW. Diagnosis of pulmonary arterial hypertension and pulmonary embolism with magnetic resonance angiography. Chest 2001;120: 1556-1561.

Ladd ME, Goehde SC, Steiner P, Pfamatter T, McKinnon GC, Debatin JF. Virtual MR angioscopy of the pulmonary tree. J Comput Assist Tomogr 1996, 20:782-785.

MacFall JR, Sostman HD, Foo TK. Thick-section, single breath-hold magnetic resonance pulmonary angiography. Invest Radiol 1992; 27:318-322.

Maki DD, Siegelman ES, Roberts DA, Baum RA, Gefter WB. Pulmonary arteriovenous malformations: Three-dimensional gadolinium-enhanced MR angiography-initial experience. Radiology. 2001;219:243-246.

Meaney JF, Weg JG, Chenevert TL, Stafford-Johnson D, Hamilton BH, Prince MR. Diagnosis of pulmonary embolism with magnetic resonance angiography [see comments]. NEJM 1997; 336:1422-1427.

Ohno Y, Hatabu H, Takenaka D, Adachi S, Hirota S, Sugimura K. Contrast-enhanced MR perfusion imaging and MR angiography: utility for management of pulmonary arteriovenous malformations for embolotherapy. Eur J Radiol 2002;41(2):136-146.

Ohno Y, Adachi S, Motoyama A, Kusumoto M, Hatabu H, Sugimura K, Kono M. Multiphase ECG-triggered 3D contrast-enhanced MR angiography: utility for evaluation of hilar and mediastinal invasion of bronchogenic carcinoma. J Magn Reson Imaging 2001;13: 215-24.

Rafal RB, Nichols JN, Markisz JA. Pulmonary artery sarcoma: diagnosis and postoperative follow-up with gadolinium-diethylenetriamine pentaacetic acid-enhanced magnetic resonance imaging. Mayo Clin Proc 1995; 70:173-176.

Steiner P, McKinnon GC, Romanowski BJ, Goehde SC, Hany TF, Debatin JF. Contrast-enhanced, ultrafast 3D pulmonary MR angiography in a single breathhold: initial assessment of imaging performance. J Magn Reson Imaging, 1997; 7:177-182.

Wolff K, Bergin CJ, King MA, Ghadishah E, Sung DW, Clopton P, Bookstein JJ, Auger WR, Moser KM. Accuracy of contrast-enhanced magnetic resonance angiography in chronic thromboembolic disease. Acad Radiol 1996; 3(1):10-17.

Thoracic Aorta

Amah G, Milliez P, Blacher J, Girerd X, Couetil JP, Safar ME. Delayed diagnosis of aortic coarctation : the third medical visit. Circulation 1999;100(11):e51-2.

Arpasi PJ, Bis KG, Shetty AN, White RD, Simonetti OP. MR angiography of the thoracic aorta with an electrocardiographically triggered breath-hold contrast-enhanced sequence. Radiographics. 2000 Jan-Feb;20(1):107-20.

Boehm DH, Wintersperger BJ, Reichenspurner H, Gulbins H, Detter C, Kur F, Meiser B, Reichart B. Contrast-enhanced magnetic resonance angiography for control of minimally invasive coronary artery bypass conduits (MIDCAB/OPCAB). Heart Surg Forum 1999;2(3):222-5.

Brenner P, Wintersperger B, von Smekal A, Agirov V, Bohm D, Kreuzer E, Reiser M, Reichart B. Detection of coronary artery bypass graft patency by contrast enhanced magnetic resonance angiography. Eur J Cardiothorac Surg 1999;15(4):389-93.

Carpenter JP, Holland GA, Golden MA, Barker CF, Lexa FJ, Gilfeather M, Schnall MD. Magnetic resonance angiography of the aortic arch. J Vasc Surg 1997; 25:145-151.

Cesare ED, Giordano AV, Cerone G, De Remigis F, Deusanio G, Masciocchi C. Comparative evaluation of TEE, conventional MRI and contrast-enhanced 3D breath-hold MRA in the post-operative follow-up of aneurysms. Int J Card Imaging. 2000 Jun;16(3):135-47.

Choe YH, Kim DK, Koh EM, Do YS, Lee WR. Takayasu arteritis: diagnosis with MR imaging and MR angiography in acute and chronic active stages. J Magn Reson Imaging. 1999 Nov;10(5):751-7.

Choudhary SK, Bhan A, Talwar S, Goyal M, Sharma S, Venugopal P. Tubercular pseudoaneurysms of aorta. Ann Thorac Surg. 2001 Oct;72(4):1239-44.

Cosottini M, Zampa V, Petruzzi P, Ortori S, Cioni R, Bartolozzi C. Contrast-enhanced three-dimensional MR angiography in the assessment of subclavian artery diseases. Eur Radiol. 2000;10(11):1737-44.

Czum JM, Ho VB. MR of the thoracic aorta: a pulse sequence approach to discrete feature analysis. Crit Rev Diagn Imaging. 1999 Apr;40(1):23-61.

Dymarkowski S, Bosmans H, Marchal G, Bogaert J. Three-dimensional MR angiography in the evaluation of thoracic outlet syndrome. AJR Am J Roentgenol 1999;173(4):1005-8.

Engelmann MG, Knez A, von Smekal A, Wintersperger BJ, Huehns TY, Hofling B, Reiser MF, Steinbeck G. Non-invasive coronary bypass graft imaging after multivessel revascularisation. Int J Cardiol 2000;76(1):65-74.

Fellner FA, Fellner C, Wutke R, Lang W, Laub G, Schmidt M, Janka R, Denzel C, Bautz W. Fluoroscopically triggered contrast-enhanced 3D MR DSA and 3D time-of-flight turbo MRA of the carotid arteries: first clinical experiences in correlation with ultrasound, x-ray angiography, and endarterectomy findings. Magn Reson Imaging 2000;18(5):575-85.

Flamm SD, VanDyke CW, White RD. MR Imaging of the thoracic aorta. MRI Clin N Am 1996; 4:217-235.

Gaubert JY, Moulin G, Mesana T, Chagnaud C, Caus T, Delannoy L, Blin D, Bartoli JM, Kasbarian M. Type A dissection of the thoracic aorta: use of MR imaging for long term follow-up. Radiology 1995; 196:363-369.

Gilkeson RC, Clampitt MS, Stewart RM, Laden NS. Pseudoaneurysm of aortic cannulation site after coronary artery bypass grafting: evaluation with gadolinium-enhanced MR angiography. AJR Am J Roentgenol 1999;172(3):843-4.

Hartnell GG, Finn JP, Zenni M, Cohen MC, Dupuy DE, Wheeler HG, Longmaid HE 3rd. MR imaging of the thoracic aorta: comparison of spin-echo, angiographic and breath-hold techniques. Radiology 1994; 191:697-704.

Ho VB, Prince MR. Thoracic MR aortography: imaging techniques and strategies. Radiographics 1998; 18:287-309.

Holland AE, Barentsz JO, Skotnicki S, Ruijs SH, Goldfarb JW. Preoperative MRA assessment of the coronary arteries in an ascending aortic aneurysm. J Magn Reson Imaging 2000;11(3):324-6.

Holland AE, Barentsz JO, Heijstraten FM, Skotnicki S, Pruszczynski MS, Verheugt FW, Goldfarb JW. Images in cardiovascular medicine. Aortic dissection at the coronary artery sinus: magnetic resonance angiography findings. Circulation 2000; 102(5):597.

Holmqvist C, Larsson E-M, Stahlberg F, Laurin S. Contrast-enhanced thoracic 3D-MR angiography in infants and children. Acta Radiol. 2001 Jan;42(1):50-8.

Ingu A, Ando M, Okita Y, Yamada N, Kitamura S. Redo operation for thoracoaortic aneurysm after entire aortic replacement. Ann Thorac Surg 2001;72(5):1766-7.

Kreitner KF, Kunz RP, Kalden P, Kauczor HU, Schmitt S, Kuroczynski W, Mohr-Kahaly

S, Voigtlander T, Krummenauer F, Laub G, Thelen M. Contrast-enhanced three-dimensional MR angiography of the thoracic aorta: experiences after 118 examinations with a standard dosecontrast administration and different injection protocols. Eur Radiol. 2001;11(8):1355-63.

Krinsky GA, Freedberg R, Lee VS, Rockman C, Tunick PA. Innominate artery atheroma: a lesion seen with gadolinium-enhanced MR angiography and often missed by transesophageal echocardiography. Clin Imaging. 2001 Jul-Aug;25(4):251-7.

Krinsky GA, Reuss PM, Lee VS, Carbognin G, Rofsky NM. Thoracic aorta: comparison of single-dose breath-hold and double-dose non-breath-hold gadolinium-enhanced three-dimensional MR angiography. AJR Am J Roentgenol. 1999 Jul;173(1):145-50.

Krinsky G, Maya M, Rofsky N, Lebowitz J, Nelson PK, Ambrosino M, Kaminer E, Earls J, Masters L, Giangola G, Litt A, Weinreb J. Gadolinium-enhanced 3D MRA of the aortic arch vessels in the detection of atherosclerotic cerebrovascular occlusive disease. J Comput Assist Tomogr 1998; 22:167-178.

Krinsky G, Rofsky NM. MR angiography of the aortic arch vessels and upper extremities. MRI Clin N Am 1998; 6:269-292.

Krinsky GA, Rofsky NM, DeCorato DR, Weinreb JC, Earls JP, Flyer MA, Galloway AC, Colvin SB. Thoracic aorta: comparison of gadolinium-enhanced three-dimensional MR angiography with conventional MR imaging. Radiology 1997; 202:183-193.

Krinsky G, Rofsky N, Flyer M, Giangola G, Maya M, DeCoroto D, Earls J, Weinreb J. Gadolinium-enhanced three-dimensional MR angiography of acquired arch vessel disease. AJR Am J Roentgenol 1996;167:981-987.

Krinsky G, Weinreb J. Gadolinium-enhanced three-dimensional MR angiography of the thoracoabdominal aorta. Semin Ultrasound CT MR 1996; 17:280-303.

Kumar S, Gupta S, Gujral R. Aneurysmal form of aortoarteritis with aberrant right subclavian artery: diagnosis by Magnetic Resonance Angiography. Minerva Cardioangiol. 1995 Sep;43(9):375-8.

Kutz SM, Lee VS, Tunick PA, Krinsky GA, Kronzon I. Atheromas of the thoracic aorta: A comparison of transesophageal echocardiography and breath-hold gadolinium-enhanced 3-dimensional magnetic resonance angiography. Am Soc Echocardiogr. 1999 Oct;12(10):853-8.

Lam WW, Chan JH, Hui Y, Chan F. Non-breath-hold gadolinium-enhanced MR angiography of the thoracoabdominal aorta: experience in 18 children. AJR Am J Roentgenol 1998; 170:478-480.

Lankipalli RS, Pellecchia M, Burke JF. Magnetic resonance angiography in the evaluation of aortic pseudoaneurysm. Heart 2002;87(2):157.

Leung DA, Debatin JF. Three-dimensional contrast-enhanced magnetic resonance angiography of the thoracic vasculature. Eur Radiol 1997; 7:981-989.

Leiner T, Elenbaas TW, Kaandorp DW, Ho KY, de Haan MW, van Engelshoven JM. Magnetic resonance angiography of an aortic dissection. Circulation 2001;103(14):E76-8.

Loubeyre P, Delignette A, Bonefoy L, Douek P, Amiel M, Revel D. Magnetic resonance imaging evaluation of the ascending aorta after graft-inclusion surgery: comparison between an ultrafast contrast-enhanced MR sequence and conventional cine-MRI. J Magn Reson Imaging. 1996 May-Jun;6(3):478-83.

Maspes F, Gandini R, Pocek M, Mazzoleni C, Fiaschetti V, Marchetti Ascoli, Pistolese GR, Simonetti G. Breath-hold gadolinium enhanced tree-dimensional MR angiography: personal experience in the thoracic-abdominal area. Radiol Med (Torino) 1999;98(4):275-82.

Molinari G, Sardanelli F, Zandrino F, Balbi M, Masperone MA. Value of navigator echo magnetic resonance angiography in detecting occlusion/patency of arterial and venous, single and sequential coronary bypass grafts. Int J Card Imaging 2000;16(3):149-60.

Neimatallah MA, Ho VB, Dong Q, Williams D, Patel S, Song JH, Prince MR. Gadolinium-enhanced 3D magnetic resonance angiography of the thoracic vessels. J Magn Reson Imaging. 1999 Nov;10(5):758-70.

Neimatallah MA, Chenevert TL, Carlos RC, Londy FJ, Dong Q, Prince MR, Kim HM. Subclavian MR arteriography: reduction of susceptibility artifact with short echo time and dilute gadopentetate dimeglumine. Radiology. 2000 Nov;217(2):581-6.

O'Connor AR, Moody AR, Ludman CN. Images in cardiology. Aortic coarctation diagnosed by magnetic resonance angiography. Heart 1999;81(6):671.

de Paiva Magalhaes E, Fernandes SR, Zanardi VA, Furtado Medeiros CA, Midori RY, Sachetto Z, Samara AM. Ehlers-Danlos syndrome type IV and multiple aortic aneurysms-a case report. Angiology 2001;52(3):223-8.

Prince MR, Narasimham DL, Jacoby WT, Williams DM, Cho KJ, Marx MV, Deeb GM. Three-dimensional gadolinium-enhanced MR angiography of the thoracic aorta. AJR Am J Roentgenol 1996; 166:1387-1397.

Revel D, Loubeyre P, Delignette A, Douek P, Amiel M. Contrast-enhanced magnetic resonance tomoangiography: a new imaging technique for studying thoracic great vessels. Magn Reson Imaging 1993; 11:1101-1105.

Roche KJ, Krinsky G, Lee VS, Rofsky N, Genieser NB. Interrupted aortic arch: diagnosis with gadolinium-enhanced 3D MRA. J Comput Assist Tomogr 1999;23(2):197-202.

Stables RH, Mohiaddin R, Panting J, Pennell DJ, Pepper J, Sigwart U. Images in cardiovascular medicine. Exclusion of an aneurysmal segment of the thoracic aorta with covered stents. Circulation. 2000;101(15):1888-9.

Stone JA, Mukherji SK, Semelka R, Kelekis N, Neelon B, Castillo M. Contrast-enhanced 3D FISP MR angiography of the aortic arch ostia: preliminary results. J Comput Assist Tomogr 2000;24:369-74.

Van Grimberge F, Dymarkowski S, Budts W, Bogaert J. Role of magnetic resonance in the diagnosis of subclavian steal syndrome. J Magn Reson Imaging 2000;12(2):339-42.

Vetter HO, Driever R, Mertens H, Kempkes U, Cramer BM. Contrast-enhanced magnetic resonance angiography of mammary artery grafts after minimally invasive coronary bypass surgery. Ann Thorac Surg 2001;71(4):1229-32.

Vogt FM, Goyen M, Debatin JF: Modern diagnostic concepts in dissection and aortic occlusion. Radiologe 2001; 41: 640-652.

von Smekal A, Knez A, Seelos KC, Haberl R, Spiegl F, Reichart B, Steinbeck G, Reiser M. A comparison of ultrafast computed tomography, magnetic resonance angiography and selective angiography for the detection of coronary bypass patency. Rofo Fortschr Geb Rontgenstr Neuen Bildgeb Verfahr 1997;166(3):185-91.

Wintersperger BJ, Huber A, Preissler G, Holzknecht N, Helmberger T, Petsch R, Billing A, Scheidler J, Reiser M. MR angiography of the supraaortic vessels. Radiologe 2000;40(9):785-91.

Wintersperger BJ, Engelmann MG, von Smekal A, Knez A, Penzkofer HV, Hofling B, Laub G, Reiser MF. Patency of coronary bypass grafts: assessment with breath-hold contrast-enhanced MR angiography – value of a non-electrocardiographically triggered technique. Radiology 1998;208(2):345-51.

Wintersperger BJ, von Smekal A, Engelmann MG, Knez A, Penzkofer HV, Laub G, Reiser M. Contrast media enhanced magnetic resonance angiography for determining patency of a coronary bypass. A comparison with coronary angiography. Rofo Fortschr Geb Rontgenstr Neuen Bildgeb Verfahr 1997;167(6):572-8.

Yamada I, Nakagawa T, Himeno Y, Kobayashi Y, Numano F, Shibuya H. Takayasu arteritis: diagnosis with breath-hold contrast-enhanced three-dimensional MR angiography. J Magn Reson Imaging 2000;11(5):481-7.

Yamada N, Takamiya M, Kuribayashi S, Okita Y, Minatoya K, Tanaka R. MRA of the Adamkiewicz artery: a preoperative study for thoracic aortic aneurysm. J Comput Assist Tomogr. 2000;24(3):362-8.

Abdominal Aorta

Arlart IP, Gerlach A, Kolb M, Erpenbach S, Wurstlin S. MR angiography using Gd-DTPA in staging of abdominal aortic aneurysm: a correlation with DSA and CT. Rofo Fortschr Geb Rontgenstr Neuen Bildgeb Verfahr 1997;167(3):257-63.

Atkinson DJ, Vu B, Chen DY, Duerinckx A, Bradley WG. First pass MRA of the abdomen: ultrafast, non-breath-hold time-of-flight imaging using Gd-DTPA bolus. J Magn Reson Imaging 1997; 7:1159-1162.

Di Cesare E, Cerone G, Giordano AV, Marsili L, Barile A, Michelini O, Spartera C, Masciocchi C. Magnetic resonance angiography with contrast media bolus in the evaluation of aneurysms of the abdominal aorta. Radiol Med (Torino) 2000;100(3):126-32.

Gaa J, Bohm C, Richter A, Trede M, Georgi M. Aortocaval fistula complicating abdominal aortic aneurysm: diagnosis with gadolinium-enhanced three-dimensional MR angiography. Eur Radiol 1999;9(7):1438-40.

Gilfeather M, Holland GA, Siegelman ES, Schnall MD, Axel L, Carpenter JP, Golden MA. Gadolinium-enhanced ultrafast three-dimensional spoiled gradient-echo MR imaging of the abdominal aorta and visceral and iliac vessels [published erratum appears in Radiographics 1997; 17:804]. Radiographics 1997; 17:423-432.

Grist TM. MRA of the abdominal aorta and lower extremities. J Magn Reson Imag 2000;11:32-43.

Hany TF, Debatin JF, Leung DA, Pfammatter T. Evaluation of the aortoiliac and renal arteries: comparison of breath-hold, contrast-enhanced, three-dimensional MR angiography with conventional catheter angiography. Radiology 1997;204(2):357-62.

Hany TF, Pfammatter T, Schmidt M, Leung DA, Debatin JF. [Ultrafast contrast-enhanced 3D MR angiography of the aorta and renal arteries in apnea]. [German] Rofo 1997; 166:397-405.

Kaufman JA, Geller SC, Petersen MJ, Cambria RP, Prince MR, Waltman AC. MR imaging (including MR angiography) of abdominal aortic aneurysms: comparison with conventional angiography. AJR Am J Roentgenol 1994; 163:203-210.

Kelekis NL, Semelka RC, Worawattanakul S, Molina PL, Mauro MA. Magnetic resonance imaging of the abdominal aorta and iliac vessels using combined 3-D gadolinium-enhanced MRA and gadolinium-enhanced fat-suppressed spoiled gradient echo sequences. Magn Reson Imaging 1999;17(5):641-51.

Kelekis NL, Semelka RC, Molina PL, Warshauer DM, Sharp TJ, Detterbeck FC. Immediate postgadolinium spoiled gradient-echo MRI for evaluating the abdominal aorta in the setting of abdominal MR examination. J Magn Reson Imaging 1997; 7:652-656.

Laissy JP, Soyer P, Tebboune D, Tiah D, Hvass V, Menu Y. Abdominal aortic aneurysms: assessment with gadolinium-enhanced time-of-flight coronal MR angiography (MRA). Eur J Radiol 1995; 20:1-8.

Leung DA, Hany TF, Debatin JF. Three dimensional contrast-enhanced MR angiography of the abdominal arterial system. Cardiovasc Intervent Radiol 1998; 21:1-10.

Maspes F, Gandini R, Pocek M, Mazzoleni C, Fiaschetti V, Marchetti Ascoli, Pistolese

GR, Simonetti G. Breath-hold gadolinium enhanced tree-dimensional MR angiography: personal experience in the thoracic-abdominal area. Radiol Med (Torino) 1999;98(4):275-82.

Petersen MJ, Cambria RP, Kaufman JA, LaMuraglia GM, Gertler JP, Brewster DC, Geller SC, Waltman AC, L'Italien GJ, Abbott WM. Magnetic resonance angiography in the preoperative evaluation of abdominal aortic aneurysms. J Vasc Surg 1995; 21:891-898; discussion 899.

Prince MR, Narasimham DL, Stanley JC, Wakefield TW, Messina LM, Zelenock GB, Jacoby WT, Marx MV, Williams DM, Cho KJ. Gadolinium-enhanced magnetic resonance angiography of abdominal aortic aneurysms. J Vasc Surg 1995;21(4):656-69.

Prince MR, Narasimham DL, Stanley JC, Chenevert TL, Williams DM, Marx MV, Cho KJ. Breath-hold gadolinium-enhanced MR angiography of the abdominal aorta and its major branches. Radiology 1995; 197:785-792.

Prince MR, Narasimham DL, Stanley JC, Wakefield TW, Messina LM, Zelenock GB, Jacoby WT, Marx MV, Williams DM, Cho KJ. Gadolinium-enhanced magnetic resonance angiography of abdominal aortic aneurysms. J Vasc Surg 1995; 21:656-669.

Schoenberg SO, Essig M, Hallscheidt P, Sharafuddin MJ, Stolpen AH, Knopp MV, Yuh WT. Multiphase magnetic resonance angiography of the abdominal and pelvic arteries: results of a bicenter multireader analysis. Invest Radiol. 2002 Jan;37(1):20-8.

Shetty AN, Shirkhoda A, Bis KG, Alcantara A. Contrast-enhanced three dimensional MR angiography in a single breath-hold: a novel technique. AJR Am J Roentgenol 1995; 165:1290-1292.

Sivananthan UM, Ridgway JP, Bann K, Verma SP, Cullingworth J, Ward J, Rees MR. Fast magnetic resonance angiography using turbo-FLASH sequences in advanced aortoiliac disease. Br J Radiol 1993; 66:1103-1110.

Snidow JJ, Johnson MS, Harris VJ, Margosian PM, Aisen AM, Lalka SG, Cikrit DF, Trerotola SO. Three-dimensional gadolinium-enhanced MR angiography for aortoiliac inflow assessment plus renal artery screening in a single breath hold. Radiology 1996; 198:725-732.

Torigian DA, Carpenter JP, Roberts DA. Mycotic aortocaval fistula: efficient evaluation by bolus-chase MR angiography. J Magn Reson Imaging 2002;15(2):195-8.

Walter F, Blum A, Quirin-Cosmidis I, Bauer P, Pinelli G, Roland J. An aortocaval fistula diagnosed with 1.5-T magnetic resonance angiography. J Cardiovasc Magn Reson 2000;2(3):213-6.

Yucel EK. MR angiography for evaluation of abdominal aortic aneurysm: has the time come? Radiology 1994; 192:321-323.

Renal Arteries

Bakker J, Ligtenberg G, Beek FJ, van Reedt Dortland RW, Hene RJ. Preoperative evaluation of living renal donors with gadolinium-enhanced magnetic resonance angiography. Transplantation 1999;67(8):1167-72.

Bakker J, Beek FJ, Beutler JJ, Hene RJ, de Kort GA, de Lange EE, Moons KG, Mali WP. Renal artery stenosis and accessory renal arteries: accuracy of detection and visualization with gadolinium-enhanced breath-hold MR angiography. Radiology 1998; 207:497-504.

Baskaran V, Pereles FS, Nemcek AA Jr, Carr JC, Miller FH, Ly J, Krupinski E, Finn JP. Gadolinium-enhanced 3D MR angiography of renal artery stenosis: a pilot comparison of maximum intensity projection, multiplanar reformatting, and 3D volume-rendering postprocessing algorithms. Acad Radiol 2002;9(1):50-9.

Bass JC, Prince MR, Londy FJ, Chenevert TL. Effect of gadolinium on phase-contrast MR angiography of the renal arteries. AJR Am J Roentgenol 1997; 168:261-266.

Becker BN, Odorico JS, Becker YT, Leverson G, McDermott JC, Grist T, Sproat I, Heisey DM, Collins BH, D'Alessandro AM, Knechtle SJ, Pirsch JD, Sollinger HW. Peripheral vascular disease and renal transplant artery stenosis: A reappraisal of transplant renovascular disease. Clin Transplantation 1999; 13:349-355.

Buzzas GR, Shield CF III, Pay NT, Neuman MJ, Smith JL. Use of gadolinium-enhanced, ultrafast, three-dimensional, spoiled gradient-echo magnetic resonance angiography in the preoperative evaluation of living renal allograft donors. Transplantation 1997; 64:1734-1737.

Carlos RC, Dong Q, Stanley JC, Prince MR. MR angiography after renal revascularization: spectrum of expected anatomic results and postintervention complications. Radiographics. 1999;19(6):1555-68.

Chan YL, Leung CB, Yu SC, Yeung DK, Li PK. Comparison of non-breath-hold high resolution gadolinium-enhanced MRA with digital subtraction angiography in the evaluation on allograft renal artery stenosis. Clin Radiol 2001;56(2):127-32.

Choyke PL, Walther MM, Wagner JR, Rayford W, Lyne JC, Linehan WM. Renal cancer: preoperative evaluation with dual-phase three-dimensional MR angiography. Radiology 1997; 205:767-771.

De Cobelli F, Venturini M, Vanzulli A, Sironi S, Salvioni M, Angeli E, Scifo P, Garancini MP, Quartagno R, Bianchi G, Del Maschio A. Renal arterial stenosis: prospective comparison of color Doppler US and breath-hold, three-dimensional, dynamic, gadolinium-enhanced MR angiography. Radiology 2000;214(2):373-80.

De Cobelli F, Vanzulli A, Sironi S, Mellone R, Angeli E, Venturini M, Garancini MP, Quartagno R, Bianchi G,

Debatin JF, Ting RH, Wegmüller H, Sommer FG, Fredrickson JO, Brosnan TJ, Bowman BS, Myers BD, Herfkens RJ, Pelc NJ. Renal artery blood flow: quantitation with phase-contrast MR imaging with and without breath holding. Radiology 1994; 190:371-378.

Debatin JF, Sostman HD, Knelson M, Argabright M, Spritzer CE. Renal magnetic resonance angiography in the preoperative detection of supernumerary renal arteries in potential kidney donors. Invest Radiol 1993; 28:882-889.

Debatin JF, Spritzer CE, Grist TM, Beam C, Svetkey LP, Newman GE, Sostman HD. Imaging of the renal arteries: value of MR angiography. AJR Am J Roentgenol 1991; 157:981-990.

Del Maschio A. Renal artery stenosis: evaluation with breath-hold, three-dimensional, dynamic, gadolinium-enhanced versus three-dimensional, phase-contrast MR angiography. Radiology 1997; 205:689-95.

Fain SB, King BF, Breen JF, Kruger DG, Riederer SJ. High-spatial-resolution contrast-enhanced MR angiography of the renal arteries: a prospective comparison with digital subtraction angiography. Radiology 2001;218(2):481-90.

Ferreiros J, Mendez R, Jorquera M, Gallego J, Lezana A, Prats D, Pedrosa CS. Using gadolinium-enhanced three-dimensional MR angiography to assess arterial inflow stenosis after kidney transplantation. AJR Am J Roentgenol 1999;172(3):751-7.

Gibson M, Cook G, Gedroyc WM. Case report: renal transplant artery stenosis–three cases where magnetic resonance angiography was superior to conventional arteriography. Br J Radiol 1995; 68:89-92.

Grist TM, Sproat IA, Kennel TW, Korosec FR, Swan JS. MR angiography of the renal arteries during a breath-hold using gadolinium-enhanced 3D TOF with k-space zero-filling and a contrast timing scan. Proceedings of the ISMRM 4th Scientific Meeting and Exhibition. New York, NY: International Society for Magnetic Resonance in Medicine,1996; 63.

Grist TM. Magnetic resonance angiography of renal artery stenosis. Am J Kidney Dis 1994; 24:700-712.

Hahn U, Miller S, Nagele T, Schick F, Erdtmann B, Duda S, Claussen CD. Renal MR angiography at 1.0 T: three-dimensional (3D) phase-contrast techniques versus gadolinium-enhanced 3D fast low-angle shot breath-hold imaging. AJR Am J Roentgenol 1999;172(6):1501-8.

Hany TF, Leung DA, Pfammatter T, Debatin JF. Contrast-enhanced magnetic resonance angiography of the renal arteries. Original investigation. Invest Radiol 1998;33(9):653-9.

Hany TF, Pfammatter T, Schmidt M, Leung DA, Debatin JF. Value of contrast-enhanced 3D magnetic resonance angiography of the renal arteries. Radiologe 1997;37(7):547-53.

Hany TF, Debatin JF, Leung DA, Pfammatter T. Evaluation of the aortoiliac and renal arteries: comparison of breath-hold, contrast-enhanced, three-dimensional MR angiography with conventional catheter angiography. Radiology 1997; 204:357-362.

Hany TF, Pfammatter T, Schmidt M, Leung DA, Debatin JF. [Ultrafast contrast-enhanced 3D MR angiography of the aorta and renal arteries in apnea]. Fortschritte auf dem Gebiete der Rontgenstrahlen und der Neuen Bildgebenden Verfahren. [German] Rofo 1997; 166:397-405.

Holland GA, Dougherty L, Carpenter JP, Golden MA, Gilfeather M, Slossman F, Schnall MD, Axel L. Breath-hold ultrafast three-dimensional gadolinium-enhanced MR angiography of the aorta and the renal and other visceral abdominal arteries. AJR Am J Roentgenol 1996;166(4):971-81.

Hood MN, Ho VB, Corse WR. Three-dimensional phase-contrast magnetic resonance angiography: a useful clinical adjunct to gadolinium-enhanced three-dimensional renal magnetic resonance angiography? Mil Med 2002;167(4):343-9.

Huber A, Heuck A, Scheidler J, Holzknecht N, Baur A, Stangl M, Theodorakis J, Illner WD, Land W, Reiser M. Contrast-enhanced MR angiography in patients after kidney transplantation. Eur Radiol 2001;11(12):2488-95.

Jha RC, Korangy SJ, Ascher SM, Takahama J, Kuo PC, Johnson LB. MR angiography and preoperative evaluation for laparoscopic donor nephrectomy. AJR Am J Roentgenol 2002;178(6):1489-95.

Johnson DB, Lerner CA, Prince MR, Kazanjian SN, Narasimham DL, Leichtman AB Cho KJ. Gadolinium-enhanced magnetic resonance angiography of renal transplants. Magn Reson Imaging 1997; 15:13-20.

Kaufman JA, Waltman AC, Rivitz SM, Geller SG. Anatomical observations on the renal veins and inferior vena cava at magnetic resonance angiography. Cardiovasc Intervent Radiol 1995; 18:153-157.

Korst MB, Joosten FB, Postma CT, Jager GJ, Krabbe JK, Barentsz JO. Accuracy of normal-dose contrast-enhanced MR angiography in assessing renal artery stenosis and accessory renal arteries. AJR Am J Roentgenol 2000;174(3):629-34.

Krebs TL, Daly B, Wong JJ, Chow CC, Bartlett ST. Vascular complications of pancreatic transplantation: MR evaluation. Radiology 1995;196(3):793-8.

Leung DA, Hoffmann U, Pfammatter T, Hany TF, Rainoni L, Milfiker P, Schneider E, Debatin JF. Renovascular disease: a prospective comparison of 3D MR angiography, duplex sonography and conventional angiography. Hypertension 1998 (in press).

Leung DA, Pelkonen P, Hany TF, Zimmermann G, Pfammatter T, Debatin JF. Value of image Ssubtraction in 3D Gd-enhanced MR-angiography of the renal arteries. J Magn Reson Imaging 1998; 8:598-602

Loubeyre P, Trolliet P, Cahen R, Grozel F, Labeeuw M, Minh VA. MR angiography of renal artery stenosis: value of the combination of three-dimensional time-of flight and three-dimensional phase-contrast MR angiography sequences. Am J Roentgenol 1996; 167:489-494.

Low RN, Martinez AG, Steinberg SM, Alzate GD, Kortman KE, Bower BB, Dwyer WJ, Prince SK. Potential renal transplant donors: evaluation with gadolinium-enhanced MR angiography and MR urography. Radiology 1998; 207:165-172.

Meyers SP, Talagala SL, Totterman S, Azodo MV, Kwok E, Shapiro L, Shapiro R, Pabico RC, Applegate GR. Evaluation of the renal arteries in kidney donors: value of three-dimensional phase-contrast MR angiography with maximum-intensity-projection or surface rendering. AJR Am J Roentgenol 1995; 164:117-121.

Mitty HA, Shapiro RS, Parsons RB, Silberzweig JE. Renovascular hypertension. Radiol Clin North Am 1996; 34:1017-1036.

Nelson HA, Gilfeather M, Holman JM, Nelson EW, Yoon HC. Gadolinium-enhanced breathhold three-dimensional time-of-flight renal MR angiography in the evaluation of potential renal donors. J Vasc Interv Radiol 1999;10(2 Pt 1):175-81.

Omary RA, Baden JG, Becker BN, Odorico JS, Grist TM. Impact of MR angiography on the diagnosis and management of renal transplant dysfunction. JVIR 2000;11:991-996.

Omary RA, Henseler KP, Salem R, McDermott JC, Sproat I, Wojtowycz M, Becker BN, Acher CW, Chrisman HB, Saker MB, Grist TM. Effect of MR angiography on the diagnosis and treatment of patients with suspected renovascular disease. JVIR 2001;12(10):1179-1183.

Omary RA, Henseler KP, Unal O, Maciolek LJ, Finn P, Li D, Nemcek AA, Vogelzang RL, Grist TM. Comparison of intra-arterial and intravenous gadolinium-enhanced MR angiography with X-ray digital subtraction angiography for the detection of renal artery stenosis. Am J Roentgenol 2002;178:119-123.

Petersen MJ, Cambria RP, Kaufman JA, LaMuraglia GM, Gertler JP, Brewster DC, Geller SC, Waltman AC, L'Italien GJ, Abbott WM. Magnetic resonance angiography in the preoperative evaluation of abdominal aortic aneurysms. J Vasc Surg 1995;21(6):891-8.

Prince MR, Schoenberg SO, Ward JS, Londy FJ, Wakefield TW, Stanley JC. Hemodynamically significant atherosclerotic renal artery stenosis: MR angiographic features. Radiology 1997; 205:128-136.

Prince MR, Narasimham DL, Stanley JC, Chenevert TL, Williams DM, Marx MV, Cho KJ. Breath-hold gadolinium-enhanced MR angiography of the abdominal aorta and its major branches. Radiology 1995; 197:785-792.

Rankin SC, Jan W, Koffman CG. Noninvasive imaging of living related kidney donors: evaluation with CT angiography and gadolinium-enhanced MR angiography. 94: AJR Am J Roentgenol 2001;177(2):349-55.

Rieumont MJ, Kaufman JA, Geller SC, Yucel EK, Cambria RP, Fang LS, Bazari H, Waltman AC. Evaluation of renal artery stenosis with dynamic gadolinium-enhanced MR angiography. AJR Am J Roentgenol 1997; 169:39-44.

Ros PR, Gauger J, Stoupis C, Burton S, Mao J, Wilcox C, Rosenberg EB, Briggs RW. Diagnosis of renal artery stenosis:feasibility of combining MR angiography, MR renography, and gadopentetate - based measurements of glomerular filtration rate. AJR Am J Roentgenol 1995; 165:1447-1451.

Sawicki PT, Kaiser S, Heinemann L, Frenzel H, Berger M. Prevalence of renal artery stenosis in diabetes mellitus-an autopsy study. J Intern Med 1991; 229:489-492.

Schoenberg SO, Knopp MV, Londy F, Krishnan S, Zuna I, Lang N, Essig M, Hawighorst H, Maki JH, Stafford-Johnson D, Kallinowski F, Chenevert TL, Prince MR. Morphologic and functional magnetic resonance imaging of renal artery stenosis: a multireader tricenter study. J Am Soc Nephrol 2002;13(1):158-69.

Schoenberg SO, Prince MR, Knopp MV, Allenberg JR. Renal MR angiography. MRI Clin N Am 1998; 6:351-370.

Schoenberg SO, Knopp MV, Bock M, Kallinowski F, Just A, Essig M, Hawighorst H, Schad LR, van Kaick G. Renal artery stenosis: grading of hemodynamic changes with cine phase contrast MR blood flow measurements. Radiology 1997; 203:45-53.

Schoenberg SO, Knopp MV, Londy F, Krishnan S, Zuna I, Lang N, Essig M, Hawighorst H, Maki JH, Stafford-Johnson D, Kallinowski F, Chenevert TL, Prince MR. Morphologic and functional magnetic resonance imaging of renal artery stenosis: a multireader tricenter study. J Am Soc Nephrol. 2002 Jan;13(1):158-69.

Servois V, Laissy JP, Feger C, Sibert A, Delahousse M, Baleynaud S, Mery JP, Meny Y. Two-dimensional time-of-flight magnetic resonance angiography of renal arteries without maximum intensity projection: a prospective comparison with angiography in 21 patients screened for renovascular hypertension. Cardiovasc Intervent Radiol 1994; 17:138-142.

Shetty AN, Bis KG, Kirsch M, Weintraub J, Laub G. Contrast-enhanced breath-hold three-dimensional magnetic resonance angiography in the evaluation of renal arteries: optimization of technique and pitfalls. J Magn Reson Imaging 2000;12(6):912-23.

Siegelman ES, Gilfeather M, Holland GA, Carpenter JP, Golden MA, Townsend RR, Schnall MD. Breath-hold ultrafast three-dimensional gadolinium-enhanced MR angiography of the renovascular system. AJR Am J Roentgenol 1997; 168:1035-1040.

Smith, HJ, Bakke SJ. MR angiography of in situ and transplanted renal arteries. Early experience using a three-dimensional time-of-flight technique. Acta Radiol 1993; 34:150-155.

Snidow JJ, Johnson MS, Harris VJ, Margosian PM, Aisen AM, Lalka SG, Cikrit DF, Trerotola SO. Three-dimensional gadolinium-enhanced MR angiography for aortoiliac inflow assessment plus renal artery screening in a single breath hold. Radiology 1996; 198:725-732.

Stafford-Johnson DB, Lerner CA, Prince MR, Kazanjian SN, Narasimham DL, Leichtman AB, Cho KJ. Gadolinium-enhanced magnetic resonance angiography of renal transplants. Magn Reson Imaging 1997; 15:13-20.

Steffens JC, Link J, Grassner J, Mueller-Huelsbeck S, Brinkmann G, Reuter M, Heller M. Contrast-enhanced, k-space-centered, breath-hold MR angiography of the renal arteries and the abdominal aorta. J Magn Reson Imaging 1997; 7:617-722.

Steinborn M, Wintersperger BJ, Heck A, Theodorakis J, Waggershauser T, Hillebrand GF, Reiser M. Contrast enhanced MR angiography in the preoperative evaluation of living kidney donors. Rofo Fortschr Geb Rontgenstr Neuen Bildgeb Verfahr 1999;171(4):313-8.

Tello R, Thomson KR, Witte D, Becker GJ, Tress BM. Standard dose Gd-DTPA dynamic MR of renal arteries. J Magn Reson Imaging 1998; 8:421-426.

Thornton J, O'Callaghan J, Walshe J, O'Brien E, Varghese JC, Lee MJ. Comparison of digital subtraction angiography with gadolinium-enhanced magnetic resonance angiography in the diagnosis of renal artery stenosis. Eur Radiol 1999;9(5):930-4.

Thornton MJ, Thornton F, O'Callaghan J, Varghese JC, O'Brien E, Walshe J, Lee MJ. Evaluation of dynamic gadolinium-enhanced breath-hold MR angiography in the diagnosis of renal artery stenosis. AJR Am J Roentgenol 1999;173(5):1279-83.

Voiculescu A, Hofer M, Hetzel GR, Malms J, Modder U, Grabensee B, Hollenbeck M. Noninvasive investigation for renal artery stenosis: contrast-enhanced magnetic resonance angiography and color Doppler sonography as compared to digital subtraction angiography. Clin Exp Hypertens 2001;23(7):521-31.

Volk M, Strotzer M, Lenhart M, Manke C, Nitz WR, Seitz J, Feuerbach S, Link J. Time-resolved contrast-enhanced MR angiography of renal artery stenosis: diagnostic accuracy and interobserver variability. AJR Am J Roentgenol 2000;174(6):1583-8.

Walsh P Rofsky NM, Krinsky GA, Weinreb JC. Asymmetric signal intensity of the renal collecting systems as a sign of unilateral renal artery stenosis following administration of gadolpentetate dimeglumine. J Comput Assist Tomogr 1996; 20:812-814.

Winterer JT, Strey C, Wolffram C, Paul G, Einert A, Altehoefer C, Uhrmeister P, Kirste G, Laubenberger J. Preoperative examination of potential kidney transplantation donors: value of gadolinium-enhanced 3D MR angiography in comparison with DSA and urography. Rofo Fortschr Geb Rontgenstr Neuen Bildgeb Verfahr 2000;172(5):449-57.

Mesenteric Arteries

Baden JG, Racy DJ, Grist TM. Contrast-enhanced three-dimensional magnetic resonance angiography of the mesenteric vasculature. J Magn Reson Imag 1999;10:369-375.

Carlos RC, Stanley JC, Stafford-Johnson D, Prince MR. Interobserver variability in the evaluation of chronic mesenteric ischemia with gadolinium-enhanced MR angiography. Acad Radiol 2001;8(9):879-87.

Choyke PL, Yim P, Marcos H, Ho VB, Mullick R, Summers RM. Hepatic MR angiography: a multiobserver comparison of visualization methods. Am J Roentgenol. 2001 Feb;176(2):465-70.

Gaa J, Laub G, Edelman RR, Georgi M. First clinical results of ultrafast, contrast-enhanced 2-phase 3D-angiography of the abdomen. Rofo Fortschr Geb Rontgenstr Neuen Bildgeb Verfahr 1998;169(2):135-9.

Glockner JF, Forauer AR, Solomon H, Varma CR, Perman WH. Three-dimensional gadolinium-enhanced MR angiography of vascular complications after liver transplantation. AJR Am J Roentgenol 2000;174(5):1447-53.

Hahn U, Miller S, Nagele T, Schick F, Erdtmann B, Duda S, Claussen CD. Renal MR angiography at 1.0 T: three-dimensional (3D) phase-contrast techniques versus gadolinium-enhanced 3D fast low-angle shot breath-hold imaging. AJR Am J Roentgenol 1999;172(6):1501-8.

Haliloglu M, Hoffer FA, Gronemeyer SA, Furman WL, Shochat SJ. 3D gadolinium-enhanced MRA: evaluation of hepatic vasculature in children with hepatoblastoma. J Magn Reson Imaging 2000;11(1):65-8.

Hany TF, Schmidt M, Schoenenberger A, Debatin JF. Contrast-enhanced 3D MRA of the splanchnic vasculature before and after caloric stimulation. Invest Radiol 1998 (in press).

Holland GA, Dougherty L, Carpenter JP, Golden MA, Gilfeather M, Slossman F, Schnall MD, Axel L. Breath-hold ultrafast three-dimensional gadolinium-enhanced MR angiography of the aorta and the renal and other visceral abdominal arteries. AJR Am J Roentgenol 1996;166(4):971-81.

Kopka L, Rodenwaldt J, Vosshenrich R, Fischer U, Renner B, Lorf T, Graessner J, Ringe B, Grabbe E. Hepatic blood supply: comparison of optimized dual phase contrast-enhanced three-dimensional MR angiography and digital subtraction angiography. Radiology 1999;211(1):51-8.

Lavelle MT, Lee VS, Rofsky NM, Krinsky GA, Weinreb JC. Dynamic contrast-enhanced three-dimensional MR imaging of liver parenchyma: source images and angiographic reconstructions to define hepatic arterial anatomy. Radiology 2001;218(2):389-94.

Li KC, Wright GA, Pelc LR, Dalman RL, Brittain JH, Wegmuller H, Lin DT, Song CK.

Oxygen saturation of blood within the superior mesenteric vein: in vivo verification of MR imaging measurements in a canine model. Radiology 1995; 194:321-325.

Li KC, Whitney WS, McDonnell CH, Fredrickson JO, Pelc NJ, Dalman RL, Jeffrey RB Jr. Chronic mesenteric ischemia: evaluation with phase-contrast cine MR imaging. Radiology 1994; 190:175-179.

Meaney JF, Prince MR, Nostrant TT, Stanley JC. Gadolinium-enhanced MR angiography of visceral arteries in patients with suspected chronic mesenteric ischemia. J Magn Reson Imaging 1997; 7:171-176.

Oberholzer K, Kreitner KF, Kalden P, Pitton M, Requardt M. Contrast-enhanced MR angiography of abdominal vessels using a 1.0 T system. Rofo Fortschr Geb Rontgenstr Neuen Bildgeb Verfahr 2000;172(2):134-8.

Shirkhoda A, Konez O, Shetty AN, Bis KG, Ellwood RA, Kirsch MJ. Mesenteric circulation: three-dimensional MR angiography with a gadolinium-enhanced multiecho gradient-echo technique. Radiology 1997; 202:257-261.

Wasser MN, Geelkerken RH, Kouwenhoven M, van Bockel J, Hermans J, Schultze Kool LJ, de Roos A. Systolically gated phase-contrast MRA of mesenteric arteries in suspected mesenteric ischemia. J Comput Assist Tomogr 1996;20:262-268.

Zeh H, Choyke PL, Alexander HR, Bartlett DL, Libutti SK, Chang R, Summers RM. Gadolinium-enhanced 3D MRA prior to isolated hepatic perfusion for metastases. J Comput Assist Tomogr 1999;23(5):664-9.

Portal Vein

Balci NC, Semelka RC, Sandhu JS. Intrahepatic arterioportal fistula: gadolinium-enhanced 3D magnetic resonance angiography findings and angiographic embolization with steel coils. Magn Reson Imaging 1999;17(3):475-8.

Butts K, Riederer SJ, Ehman RL. The effect of respiration on the contrast and sharpness of liver lesions in MRI. Magn Reson Med 1995; 33:1-7.

Cheng YF, Chen CL, Huang TL, Chen TY, Lee TY, Chen YS, Wang CC, de Villa V, Goto S, Chiang YC, Eng HL, Jawan B, Cheung HK. Single imaging modality evaluation of living donors in liver transplantation: magnetic resonance imaging. Transplantation 2001;72(9):1527-33.

Ernst O, Asnar V, Sergent G, Lederman E, Nicol L, Paris JC, L'Hermine C. Comparing contrast-enhanced breath-hold MR angiography and conventional angiography in the evaluation of mesenteric circulation. AJR Am J Roentgenol 2000;174(2):433-9.

Glockner JF, Forauer AR, Solomon H, Varma CR, Perman WH. Three-dimensional gadolinium-enhanced MR angiography of vascular complications after liver transplantation. AJR Am J Roentgenol 2000;174(5):1447-53.

Goyen M, Ruehm SG, Barkhausen J, Testa G, Malago M, Debatin JF: Right-lobe living related liver transplantation: Evaluation of a comprehensive magnetic resonance imaging protocol for assessing potential donors. Liver Transpl 2002; 8: 241-250

Haliloglu M, Hoffer FA, Gronemeyer SA, Furman WL, Shochat SJ. 3D gadolinium-enhanced MRA: evaluation of hepatic vasculature in children with hepatoblastoma. J Magn Reson Imaging 2000;11(1):65-8.

Kopka L, Rodenwaldt J, Vosshenrich R, Fischer U, Renner B, Lorf T, Graessner J, Ringe B, Grabbe E. Hepatic blood supply: comparison of optimized dual phase contrast-enhanced three-dimensional MR angiography and digital subtraction angiography. Radiology 1999;211(1):51-8.

Kreft B, Strunk H, Flacke S, Wolff M, Conrad R, Gieseke J, Pauleit D, Bachmann R, Hirner A, Schild HH. Detection of thrombosis in the portal venous system: comparison of contrast-enhanced MR angiography with intraarterial digital subtraction angiography. Radiology 2000;216(1):86-92.

Kroencke TJ, Taupitz M, Arnold R, Fritsche L, Hamm B. Three-dimensional gadolinium-enhanced magnetic resonance venography in suspected thrombo-occlusive disease of the central chest veins. Chest 2001;120(5):1570-6

Murakami T, Kim T, Oi H, Nakamura H, Igarashi H, Matsushita M, Okamura J, Kozuka T. Detectability of hypervascular hepatocellular carcinoma by arterial phase images of MR and spiral CT. Acta Radiologica 1995; 36:372-376.

Pavone P, Guiliani S, Cardone G, Occhiato R, Di Renzi P, Petroni GA, Buoni C, Passariello R. Intraarterial portography with gadopentetate dimeglumine: improved liver-to-lesion contrast in MR imaging. Radiology 1991; 179:693-697.

Rodgers PM, Ward J, Baudouin CJ, Ridgway JP, Robinson PJ. Dynamic contrast enhanced MR imaging of the portal venous system: comparison with X-ray angiography. Radiology 1994; 191:741-745.

Shinde TS, Lee VS, Rofsky NM, Krinsky GA, Weinreb JC. Three-dimensional gadolinium-enhanced MR venographic evaluation of patency of central veins in the thorax: initial experience. Radiology 1999;213(2):555-60.

Squillaci E, Mazzoleni C, Sodani G, Fanucci E, Masala S, Romagnoli A, Sergiacomi G, Simonetti G. Magnetic resonance angiography with three-dimensional dynamic technique after contrast media administration for the study of the portal system. Radiol Med (Torino) 2001;102(4):238-44.

Stafford-Johnson DB, Hamilton BH, Dong Q, Cho KJ, Turcotte JG, Fontana RJ, Prince MR. Vascular complications of liver transplantation: evaluation with gadolinium-enhanced MR angiography. Radiology 1998; 207:153-160.

Uematsu H, Yamada H, Sadato N, Hayashi N, Yamamoto K, Yonekura Y, Ishii Y. Multiple single sections Turbo FLASH MR arterial portography in the detection of hepatic neoplasms. Eur J Radiol 1998; 26:257-260.

Ward J, Spencer JA, Guthrie JA, Robinson PJ. Liver transplantation: dynamic contrast-enhanced magnetic resonance imaging of the hepatic vasculature. Clin Radiol 1996; 51:191-197.

Wilson MW, Hamilton BH, Dong Q, Stafford-Johnson DB, Kazanjian SN, Williams DM, Marx MV, Cho KJ, Prince MR. Gadolinium-enhanced magnetic resonance venography of the portal venous system prior to transjugular intrahepatic portosystemic shunts and liver transplantation. Original investigation. Invest Radiol 1998;33(9):644-52.

Yamashita Y, Mitsuzaki K, Miyazaki T, Namimoto T, Sumi S, Urata J, Abe Y, Ogata I, Takahashi M. Gadolinium-enhanced breath-hold three-dimensional MR angiography of the portal vein: value of the magnetization-prepared rapid acquisition gradient-echo sequence. Radiology 1996; 201:283-288.

Peripheral Arteries

Baum RA, Rutter CM, Sunshine JH, Blebea, JS, Blebea J, Carpenter JP, Dickey, KW, Quinn SF, Gomes AS, Grist TM, McNeil BJ. Multicenter trail to evaluate vascular magnetic resonance angiography of the lower extremity. JAMA 1995; 274:875-880

Bendib K, Berthezene Y, Croisille P, Villard J, Douek PC. Assessment of complicated arterial bypass grafts: value of contrast-enhanced subtraction magnetic resonance angiography. J Vasc Surg 1997;26(6):1036-42.

Bertschinger K, Cassina PC, Debatin JF, Ruehm SG. Surveillance of peripheral arterial bypass grafts with three-dimensional MR angiography: comparison with digital subtraction angiography. AJR Am J Roentgenol 2001;176(1):215-20.

Bourlet P, De Fraissinnette B, Garcier JM, Lipiecka E, Privat C, Ravel A, Franconi JM, Boyer L. Comparative assessment of helical CT-angiography, 2D TOF MR-angiography and 3D gadolinium enhanced MRA in aorto-iliac occlusive disease. J Radiol 2000;81(11):1619-25.

Brillet PY, Tassart M, Bazot M, Le Blanche AF, Allaire E, Boudghene F. Investigation of peripheral vascular bed in critical lower limb ischemia: comparative study between arteriography and magnetic resonance angiography. J Mal Vasc 2001;26(1):31-8.

Carriero A, Maggialetti A, Pinto D, Salcuni M, Mansour M, Petronelli S, Bonomo L. Contrast-enhanced magnetic resonance angiography MoBI-trak in the study of peripheral vascular disease. Cardiovasc Intervent Radiol 2002;25(1):42-7.

di Cesare E, Giordano AV, Santarelli B, Cariello G, Marsili L, Barile A, Ronzino L, Masciocchi C. MR-angiography with contrast bolus vs digital angiography in peripheral arterial occlusive disease of the legs. Radiol Med (Torino) 2001;102(1-2):55-61.

Dorenbeck U, Seitz J, Volk M, Strotzer M, Lenhart M, Feuerbach S, Link J. Evaluation of arterial bypass grafts of the pelvic and lower extremities with gadolinium-enhanced magnetic resonance angiography: comparison with digital subtraction angiography. Invest Radiol 2002;37(2):60-4.

Douek PC, Revel D, Chazel S, Falise B, Villard J, Amiel M. Fast MR angiography of the aortoiliac arteries and arteries of the lower extremity: value of bolus-enhanced, whole-volume subtraction technique. AJR Am J Roentgenol 1995; 165:431-437.

Du J, Carroll TJ, Wagner HJ, Vigen K, Fain SB, Block WF, Korosec F, Grist TM, Mistretta CA. Time-resolved, undersampled projection reconstruction imaging with vessel segmentation for high resolution CE-MR of the peripheral vasculature. Magn Reson Med, accepted 2002.

Erel H, Prince MR, Rajagopalan S. Images in vascular medicine. An unusual case of claudication. Vasc Med. 2002;7(1):55.

Goyen M, Ruehm SG, Barkhausen J, Kroger K, Ladd ME, Truemmler K-H, Bosk S, Debatin JF: Improved Multi-Station Peripheral MR Angiography with a Dedicated Vascular Coil. J Magn Res Imaging 2001; 13: 475-480

Goyen M, Debatin JF, Ruehm SG: Peripheral MR-Angiography Top Magn Res Imaging 2001; 12: 327-335

Goyen M, Ruehm SG, Debatin JF: Magnetic Resonance Angiography for Assessment of Peripheral Vascular Disease Radiol Clin North Am 2002; 40(4): 835-846

Hany TF, Carroll TJ, Omary RA, Esparza-Coss E, Korosec FR, Mistretta CA, Grist TM. Aorta and runoff vessels: single-injection MR angiography with automated table movement compared with multiinjection time-resolved MR angiography - initial results. Radiology 2001;221:266-272.

Hany TF, Debatin JF, Leung DA, Pfammatter T. Evaluation of the aortoiliac and renal arteries: comparison of breath-hold, contrast-enhanced, three-dimensional MR angiography with conventional catheter angiography. Radiology 1997; 204:357-362.

Ho KY, de Haan MW, Kessels AG, Kitslaar PJ, van Engelshoven JM. Peripheral vascular tree stenoses: detection with subtracted and nonsubtracted MR angiography. Radiology 1998; 206:673-681.

Ho KY, Leiner T, de Haan MW, Kessels AG, Kitslaar PJ, van Engelshoven JM. Peripheral vascular tree stenoses: evaluation with moving-bed infusion-tracking MR angiography. Radiology 1998; 206:683-69.

Huber A, Heuck A, Baur A, Helmberger T, Waggershauser T, Billing A, Heiss M, Petsch R, Reiser M. Dynamic contrast-enhanced MR angiography from the distal aorta to the ankle joint with a step-by-step technique. AJR Am J Roentgenol 2000;175(5):1291-8.

Khilnani NM, Winchester PA, Prince MR, Vidan E, Trost DW, Bush HL Jr, Watts R, Wang Y. Peripheral vascular disease: combined 3D bolus chase and dynamic 2D MR angiography compared with x-ray angiography for treatment planning. Radiology 2002;224(1):63-74.

Krinsky G, Jacobowitz G, Rofsky N. Gadolinium-enhanced MR angiography of extraanatomic arterial bypass grafts. AJR Am J Roentgenol 1998; 170:735-741.

Lam WW, Tam PK, Ai VH, Chan KL, Cheng W, Chan FL, Leong L. Gadolinium-infusion magnetic resonance angiogram: a new, noninvasive, and accurate method of pre-operative localization of impalpable undescended testes. J Pediatr Surg 1998; 33:123-126.

Lenhart M, Herold T, Volk M, Seitz J, Manke C, Zorger N, Dorenbeck U, Requardt M, Nitz WR, Kasprzak P, Feuerbach S, Link J. Contrast media-enhanced MR angiography of the lower extremity arteries using a dedicated peripheral vascular coil system. First clinical results. Rofo Fortschr Geb Rontgenstr Neuen Bildgeb Verfahr 2000;172(12):992-9.

Lenhart M, Djavidani B, Volk M, Strotzer M, Manke C, Requardt M, Nitz WR, Kasprzak P, Feuerbach S, Link J. Contrast medium-enhanced MR angiography of the pelvic and leg vessels with an automated table-feed technique. Rofo Fortschr Geb Rontgenstr Neuen Bildgeb Verfahr 1999;171(6):442-9.

Link J, Steffens JC, Brossmann J, Graessner J, Hackethal S, Heller M. Iliofemoral arterial occlusive disease: contrast-enhanced MR angiography for preinterventional evaluation and follow-up after stent placement. Radiology 1999;212(2):371-7.

Loewe C, Cejna M, Lammer J, Thurnher SA. Contrast-enhanced magnetic resonance angiography in the evaluation of peripheral bypass grafts. Eur Radiol 2000;10(5):725-32.

Lundin P, Svensson A, Henriksen E, Jonason T, Forssell C, Backbro B, Bodlund M, Ringqvist I. Imaging of aortoiliac arterial disease. Duplex ultrasound and MR angiography versus digital subtraction angiography. Acta Radiol 2000;41(2):125-32.

Meaney JF, Ridgway JP, Chakraverty S, Robertson I, Kessel D, Radjenovic A, Kouwenhoven M, Kassner A, Smith MA. Stepping-table gadolinium-enhanced digital subtraction MR angiography of the aorta and lower extremity arteries: preliminary experience. Radiology 1999;211(1):59-67.

Mitsuzaki K, Yamashita Y, Sakaguchi T, Ogata I, Takahashi M, Hiai Y. Abdomen, pelvis, and extremities: diagnostic accuracy of dynamic contrast-enhanced turbo MR angiography compared with conventional angiography-initial experience. Radiology 2000;216(3):909-15.

Perrier E, Dubayle P, Boyer B, Mousseaux E, Larroque P, Vergos M, Fiessinger JN. Comparison of magnetic resonance angiography with injection of gadolinium and conventional arteriography of the ilio-femoral arteries. J Radiol 1998;79(12):1493-8.

Poon E, Yucel EK, Pagan-Marin H, Kayne H. Iliac artery stenosis measurements: comparison of two-dimensional time-of-flight and three-dimensional dynamic gadolinium-enhanced MR angiography. AJR Am J Roentgenol 1997; 169:1139-1144.

Prince MR. Peripheral vascular MR angiography: the time has come. Radiology 1998; 206:592-593.

Prince MR, Chabra SG, Watts R, Chen CZ, Winchester PA, Khilnani NM, Trost D, Bush HA, Kent KC, Wang Y. Contrast material travel times in patients undergoing peripheral MR angiography. Radiology. 2002 Jul;224(1):55-61.

Oberholzer K, Kreitner KF, Kalden P, Requardt M, Pitton M, Mildenberger P, Thelen M. MR angiography of peripheral vessels with automatic tracking table technique at 1.0 in comparison with intra-arterial digital subtraction angiography. Rofo Fortschr Geb Rontgenstr Neuen Bildgeb Verfahr 1999 Sep;171(3):240-3

Quinn SF, Sheley RC, Semonsen KG, Leonardo VJ, Kojima K, Szumowski J. Aortic and lower-extremity arterial disease: evaluation with MR angiography versus conventional angiography. Radiology 1998; 206:693-701.

Reid SK, Pagan-Marin HR, Menzoian JO, Woodson J, Yucel EK. Contrast-enhanced moving-table MR angiography: prospective comparison to catheter arteriography for treatment planning in peripheral arterial occlusive disease. J Vasc Interv Radiol 2001;12(1):45-53.

Rofsky NM. MR angiography of the aortoiliac and femoropopliteal vessels. MRI Clin N Am 1998; 6:371-384.

Rofsky NM, Johnson G, Adelman MA, Rosen RJ, Krinsky GA, Weinreb JC. Peripheral vascular disease evaluated with reduced-dose gadolinium-enhanced MR angiography. Radiology 1997;205(1):163-9.

Rofsky NM, Purdy DE, Johnson G, DeCorato DR, Earls JP, Krinsky G, Weinreb JC. Suppression of venous signal in time-of-flight MR angiography of the lower extremities after administration of gadopentetate dimeglumine. Radiology 1997; 202:177-182.

Rofsky NM, Johnson G, Adelman MA, Rosen RJ, Krinsky GA, Weinreb JC. Peripheral vascular disease evaluated with reduced-dose gadolinium-enhanced MR angiography. Radiology 1997; 205:163-169.

Ruehm SG, Goyen M, Barkhausen J, Kroger K, Bosk S, Ladd ME, Debatin JF. Rapid magnetic resonance angiography for detection of atherosclerosis. Lancet 2001;357(9262):1086-91.

Ruehm SG, Nanz D, Baumann A, Schmid M, Debatin JF. 3D contrast-enhanced MR angiography of the run-off vessels: value of image subtraction. J Magn Reson Imaging 2001;13(3):402-11.

Ruehm SG, Hany TF, Pfammatter T, Schneider E, Ladd M, Debatin JF. Pelvic and lower extremity arterial imaging: diagnostic performance of three-dimensional contrast-enhanced MR angiography. AJR Am J Roentgenol 2000;174(4):1127-35.

Saeed M, Wendland MF, Engelbrecht M, Sakuma H, Higgins CB. Contrast-enhanced magnetic resonance angiography in the coronary and peripheral arteries. Acad Radiol 1998; 5:S108-S112.

Shetty AN, Shirkhoda A, Bis KG, Ellwood R, Li D. 3D breath-hold contrast-enhanced MRA: a preliminary experience in aorta and iliac vascular disease. J Comput Assist Tomogr 1998; 22:179-185.

Schoenberg SO, Essig M, Hallscheidt P, Sharafuddin MJ, Stolpen AH, Knopp MV, Yuh WT. Multiphase magnetic resonance angiography of the abdominal and pelvic arteries: results of a bicenter multireader analysis. Invest Radiol 2002;37(1):20-8.

Snidow JJ, Johnson MS, Harris VJ, Margosian PM, Aisen AM, Lalka SG, Cikrit DF, Trerotola SO. Three-dimensional gadolinium-enhanced MR angiography for aortoiliac inflow assessment plus renal artery screening in a single breath hold. Radiology 1996; 198:725-732.

Snidow JJ, Aisen AM, Harris VJ, Trerotola SD, Johnson MS, Sawchuk AP, Dalsing MC. Iliac artery MR angiography: comparison of three-dimensional gadolinium-enhanced and two-dimensional time-of-flight techniques. Radiology 1995; 196:371-378.

Stehling MK, Liu L, Laub G, Fleischmann K, Rohde U. Gadolinium-enhanced magnetic resonance angiography of the pelvis in patients with erectile impotence. Magma 1997; 5:247-254.

Sueyoshi E, Sakamoto I, Matsuoka Y, Hayashi H, Hayashi K. Symptomatic peripheral vascular tree stenosis. Comparison of subtracted and nonsubtracted 3D contrast-enhanced MR angiography with fat suppression. Acta Radiol 2000;41(2):133-8.

Swan JS, Kennell TW, Acher CW, Heisey DM, Grist TM, Korosec FR, Hagenauer ME. Magnetic resonance angiography of aorto-iliac disease. Am J Surg 2000;180(1):6-12.

Swan JS, Carroll TJ, Kennell TW, Heisey DM, Korosec FR, Frayne R, Mistretta CA, Grist TM. Time-resolved 3D contrast-enhanced MRA of the peripheral vessels. Radiology, accepted 2001.

Wang Y, Winchester PA, Khilnani NM, Lee HM, Watts R, Trost DW, Bush HL Jr, Kent KC, Prince MR. Contrast-enhanced peripheral MR angiography from the abdominal aorta to the pedal arteries: combined dynamic two-dimensional and bolus-chase three-dimensional acquisitions. Invest Radiol. 2001;36(3):170-7.

Wang Y, Lee HM, Avakian R, Winchester PA, Khilnani NM, Trost D. Timing algorithm for bolus chase MR digital subtraction angiography. Magn Reson Med 1998; 39:691-696.

Wang Y, Lee HM, Khilnani NM, Trost DW, Jagust MB, Winchester PA, Bush HL, Sos TA, Sostman HD. Bolus-chase MR digital subtraction angiography in the lower extremity. Radiology 1998; 207:263-269.

Wang Y, Chen CZ, Chabra SG, Winchester PA, Khilnani NM, Watts R, Bush HL Jr, Craig Kent K, Prince MR. Bolus arterial-venous transit in the lower extremity and venous contamination in bolus chase three-dimensional magnetic resonance angiography. Invest Radiol. 2002 Aug;37(8):458-63.

Watanabe Y, Dohke M, Okumura A, Amoh Y, Ishimori T, Oda K, Dodo Y. Dynamic subtraction MR angiography: first-pass imaging of the main arteries of the lower body. AJR Am J Roentgenol 1998; 170:357-360.

Wikstrom J, Holmberg A, Johansson L, Lofberg AM, Smedby O, Karacagil S, Ahlstrom H. Gadolinium-enhanced magnetic resonance angiography, digital subtraction angiography and duplex of the iliac arteries compared with intra-arterial pressure gradient measurements. Eur J Vasc Endovasc Surg 2000;19(5):516-23.

Winterer JT, Schaefer O, Uhrmeister P, Zimmermann-Paul G, Lehnhardt S, Altehoefer C, Laubenberger J. Contrast enhanced MR angiography in the assessment of relevant stenoses in occlusive disease of the pelvic and lower limb arteries: diagnostic value of a two-step examination protocol in comparison to conventional DSA. Eur J Radiol 2002;41(2):153-60.

Yamashita Y, Mitsuzaki K, Ogata I, Takahashi M, Hiai Y. Three-dimensional high-resolution dynamic contrast-enhanced MR angiography of the pelvis and lower extremities with use of a phased array coil and subtraction: diagnostic accuracy. J Magn Reson Imaging 1998;8(5):1066-72.

Yamashita Y, Mitsuzaki K, Tang Y, Namimoto T, Takahashi M. Gadolinium-enhanced breath-hold three-dimensional time-of-flight MR angiography of the abdominal and pelvic vessels: the value of ultrafast MP-RAGE sequences. J Magn Reson Imaging 1997; 7:623-628.

Carotid Arteries

Barbier C, Lefevre F, Bui P, Denny P, Aiouaz C, Becker S. Contrast-enhanced MRA of the carotid arteries using 0.5 Tesla: comparison with selective digital angiography. J Radiol 2001;82(3 Pt 1):245-9.

Carroll TJ, Korosec FR, Petermann GM, Grist TM, Turski PA. Carotid bifurcation: Evaluation of time-resolved three-dimensional contrast-enhanced MR angiography. Radiology 2001;220:525-532.

Catalano C, Laghi A, Pediconi F, Fraioli F, Napoli A, Passariello R. Magnetic resonance angiography with contrast media in the study of carotid arteries. Radiol Med (Torino) 2001;101(1-2):54-9.

Chakeres DW, Schmalbrock P, Brogam M, Yuan C, Cohen L. Normal venous anatomy of the brain: demonstration with gadopentetate dimeglumine in enhanced 3-D MR angiography. AJR Am J Roentgenol 1991; 156:161-172.

Cloft HJ, Murphy KJ, Prince MR, Brunberg JA. 3D gadolinium-enhanced MR angiography of the carotid arteries. Magn Reson Imaging 1996; 14:593-600.

Creasy JL, Price RR, Presbrey T, Goins D, Partain CL, Kessler RM. Gadolinium-enhanced MR angiography. Radiology 1990; 175:280-283.

Executive Committee for the Asymptomatic Carotid Atherosclerosis Study. Endarterectomy for asymptomatic carotid artery stenosis. JAMA 1995; 273:1421-1428.

Fellner FA, Fellner C, Wutke R, Lang W, Laub G, Schmidt M, Janka R, Denzel C, Bautz W. Fluoroscopically triggered contrast-enhanced 3D MR DSA and 3D time-of-flight turbo MRA of the carotid arteries: first clinical experiences in correlation with ultrasound, x-ray angiography, and endarterectomy findings. Magn Reson Imaging 2000;18(5):575-85.

Huston J 3rd, Fain SB, Riederer SJ, Wilman AH, Bernstein MA, Busse RF. Carotid arteries: maximizing arterial to venous contrast in fluoroscopically triggered contrast-enhanced MR angiography with elliptic centric view ordering. Radiology 1999 Apr;211(1):265-73.

Huston J 3rd, Fain SB, Wald JT, Luetmer PH, Rydberg CH, Covarrubias DJ, Riederer SJ, Bernstein MA, Brown RD, Meyer FB, Bower TC, Schleck CD. Carotid artery: elliptic centric contrast-enhanced MR angiography compared with conventional angiography. Radiology 2001;218(1):138-43.

Kim JK, Farb RI, Wright GA. Test bolus examination in the carotid artery at dynamic gadolinium-enhanced MR angiography. Radiology 1998; 206:283-289.

Kollias SS, Binkert CA, Ruesch S, Valavanis A. Contrast-enhanced MR angiography of the supra-aortic vessels in 24 seconds: a feasibility study. Neuroradiology 1999; 41(6):391-400.

Korosec FR, Turski PA, Carroll TJ, Mistretta CA, Grist TM. Contrast-enhanced MR angiography of the carotid bifurcation. J Magn Reson Imag 1999;10:317-325.

Leclerc X, Lucas C, Godefroy O, Nicol L, Moretti A, Leys D, Pruvo JP. Preliminary experience using contrast-enhanced MR angiography to assess vertebral artery structure for the follow-up of suspected dissection. AJNR 1999;20(8):1482-90.

Levy R, Prince MR. Arterial-phase three-dimensional contrast-enhanced MR angiography of the carotid arteries. AJR Am J Roentgenol 1996; 167:211-215.

Leclerc X, Martinat P, Godefroy O, Lucas C, Giboreau F, Ares GS, Leys D, Pruvo JP. Contrast-enhanced three-dimensional fast imaging with steady-state precession (FISP) MR angiography of supraaortic vessels: preliminary results. AJNR 1998;19(8):1405-13.

Lin W, Haacke EM, Smith AS, Clampitt ME. Gadolinium-enhanced high-resolution MR angiography with adaptive vessel tracking: preliminary results in the intracranial circulation. J Magn Reson Imaging 1992; 2:277-284.

Morikawa M, Numaguchi Y, Rigamonti D, Kuroiwa T, Rothman MI, Zoarski GH, Simard JM, Eisenberg H, Amin PD. Radiosurgery for cerebral arteriovenous malformations: assessment of early phase magnetic resonance imaging and significance of gadolinium-DTPA enhancement. Int J Radiat Oncol Biol Phys 1996; 34:663-675.

NASCET. Beneficial effect of carotid endarterectomy in symptomatic patients with high-grade carotid stenosis. NEJM 1991; 325:445-453.

Oberholzer K, Kreitner KF, Kalden P, Pitton M, Requardt M, Thelen M. Contrast-enhanced three-dimensional MR angiography of the carotid artery at 1.0 Tesla compared to i.a. DSA: is the method suitable for the diagnosis of carotid stenosis? Rofo Fortschr Geb Rontgenstr Neuen Bildgeb Verfahr. 2001 Apr;173(4):350-5.

Phan T, Huston J 3rd, Bernstein MA, Riederer SJ, Brown RD Jr. Contrast-enhanced magnetic resonance angiography of the cervical vessels: experience with 422 patients. Stroke. 2001;32(10):2282-6.

Randoux B, Marro B, Koskas F, Duyme M, Sahel M, Zouaoui A, Marsault C. Carotid artery stenosis: prospective comparison of CT, three-dimensional gadolinium-enhanced MR, and conventional angiography. Radiology 2001;220(1):179-85.

Remonda L, Senn P, Barth A, Arnold M, Lovblad KO, Schroth G. Contrast-enhanced 3D MR angiography of the carotid artery: comparison with conventional digital subtraction angiography. AJNR 2002;23(2):213-9.

Remonda L, Senn P, Barth A, Arnold M, Lovblad KO, Schroth G. Contrast-enhanced 3D MR angiography of the carotid artery: comparison with conventional digital subtraction angiography. AJNR 2002;23(2):213-9.

Remonda L, Heid O, Schroth G. Carotid artery stenosis, occlusion, and pseudo-occlusion: first-pass, gadolinium-enhanced, three-dimensional MR angiography--preliminary study. Radiology 1998;209(1):95-102.

Sardanelli F, Zandrino F, Parodi RC, De Caro G. MR angiography of internal carotid arteries: breath-hold Gd-enhanced 3D fast imaging with steady-state precession versus unenhanced 2D and 3D time-of-flight techniques. J Comput Assist Tomogr 1999; 23:208 –215.

Scarabino T, Carriero A, Giannatempo GM, Marano R, De Matthaeis P, Bonomo L, Salvolini U. Contrast-enhanced MR angiography (CE MRA) in the study of the carotid stenosis: comparison with digital subtraction angiography (DSA). J Neuroradiol 1999 Jun;26(2):87-91.

Serfaty JM, Chirossel P, Chevallier JM, Ecochard R, Froment JC, Douek PC. Accuracy of three-dimensional gadolinium-enhanced MR angiography in the assessment of extracranial carotid artery disease. AJR 2000;175:455-463.

Slosman F, Stolpen AH, Lexa FJ, Schnall MD, Langlotz CP, Carpenter JP, Goldberg HI. Extracranial atherosclerotic carotid artery disease: evaluation of non-breath-hold three-dimensional gadolinium-enhanced MR angiography. AJR 1998;170(2):489-95.

Turski PA, Korosec FR, Carroll TJ, Willig D, Grist TM, Mistretta CA. Contrast-enhanced magnetic resonance angiography of the carotid bifurcation using the time-resolved imaging of contrast kinetics (TRICKS) technique. Topics in Magn Reson Imag, 2001;12(3):175-181.

Van Grimberge F, Dymarkowski S, Budts W, Bogaert J. Role of magnetic resonance in the diagnosis of subclavian steal syndrome. J Magn Reson Imaging 2000; 12(2):339-42.

Watts R, Wang Y, Redd B, Winchester PA, Kent KC, Bush HL, Prince MR. Recessed elliptical-centric view-ordering for contrast-enhanced 3D MR angiography of the carotid arteries. Magn Reson Med. 2002;48(3):419-24.

Wintersperger BJ, Huber A, Preissler G, Holzknecht N, Helmberger T, Petsch R, Billing A, Scheidler J, Reiser M. MR angiography of the supraaortic vessels. Radiologe 2000;40(9):785-91.

Gadolinium-Enhanced MR Venography

Aslam Sohaib SA, Teh J, Nargund VH, Lumley JS, Hendry WF, Reznek RH. Assessment of tumor invasion of the vena caval wall in renal cell carcinoma cases by magnetic resonance imaging. J Urol 2002;167(3):1271-5.

Cheng YF, Chen CL, Huang TL, Chen TY, Lee TY, Chen YS, Wang CC, de Villa V, Goto S, Chiang YC, Eng HL, Jawan B, Cheung HK. Single imaging modality evaluation of living donors in liver transplantation: magnetic resonance imaging. Transplantation 2001;72(9):1527-33.

Diaz-Candamio MJ, Lee VS, Golimbu CN, Scholes JV, Rofsky NM. Intrafibular varix: MR diagnosis. J Comput Assist Tomogr 1999;23(2):328-30.

Erel H, Erkan D, Lehman TJ, Prince MR. Diagnostic usefulness of 3 dimensional gadolinium enhanced magnetic resonance venography in antiphospholipid syndrome. J Rheumatol. 2002 Jun;29(6):1338-9.

Fitoz S, Atasoy C, Yagmurlu A, Erden I, Akyar S. Gadolinium-enhanced three-dimensional MR angiography in jugular phlebectasia and aneurysm. Clin Imaging 2001;25(5):323-6.

Ernst O, Asnar V, Sergent G, Lederman E, Nicol L, Paris JC, L'Hermine C. Comparing contrast-enhanced breath-hold MR angiography and conventional angiography in the evaluation of mesenteric circulation. AJR Am J Roentgenol 2000;174(2):433-9.

Goyen M, Barkhausen J, Kröger K, Bosk S, Ladd ME, Debatin JF. Whole Body 3D MRA: 5 Steps And a Single Injection in 72 s. LANCET 2001; 357: 1086-1091.

Grau AJ, Schoenberg SO, Lichy C, Buggle F, Bock M, Hacke W. Lack of evidence for pulmonary venous thrombosis in cryptogenic stroke: a magnetic resonance angiography study. Stroke. 2002 May;33(5):1416-9.

Hoshi T, Hachiya T, Kanauchi T, Hando Y, Homma T. Gd-enhanced subtraction MR venography. Nippon Igaku Hoshasen Gakkai Zasshi 1999;59(12):674-8.

Jha RC, Korangy SJ, Ascher SM, Takahama J, Kuo PC, Johnson LB. MR angiography and preoperative evaluation for laparoscopic donor nephrectomy. AJR Am J Roentgenol 2002;178(6):1489-95.

Kaufman JA, Waltman AC, Rivitz SM, Geller SG. Anatomical observations on the renal veins and inferior vena cava at magnetic resonance angiography. Cardiovasc Intervent Radiol 1995; 18:153-157.

Konig CW, Kaiser WA. [MR venography of the deep leg veins: signal enhancement by volume infusion]. Fortschritte auf dem Gebiete der Rontgenstrahlen und der Neuen Bildgebenden Verfahren. [German] Rofo. 1997; 166:206-209.

Kroencke TJ, Taupitz M, Arnold R, Fritsche L, Hamm B.Three-dimensional gadolinium-enhanced magnetic resonance venography in suspected thrombo-occlusive disease of the central chest veins. Chest 2001;120(5):1570-6.

Lebowitz JA, Rofsky NM, Krinsky GA, Weinreb JC. Gadolinium-enhanced body MR venography with subtraction technique. AJR Am J Roentgenol 1997; 169:755-758.

Menegazzo D, Laissy JP, Durrbach A, Debray MP, Messin B, Delmas V, Mignon F, Schouman-Claeys E. Hemodialysis access fistula creation: preoperative assessment with MR venography and comparison with conventional venography. Radiology 1998;209(3):723-8.

Ruehm SG, Wiesner W, Debatin JF. Pelvic and lower extremity veins: contrast-enhanced three-dimensional MR venography with a dedicated vascular coil-initial experience. Radiology 2000;215(2):421-7.

Ruehm SG, Zimny K, Debatin JF: Direct contrast-enhanced 3D MR venography. Eur Radiol 2001;11: 102-112.

Stafford-Johnson DB, Hamilton BH, Dong Q, Cho KJ, Turcotte JG, Fontana RJ, Prince MR. Vascular complications of liver transplantation: evaluation with gadolinium-enhanced MR angiography. Radiology 1998;207(1):153-60.

Shinde TS, Lee VS, Rofsky NM, Krinsky GA, Weinreb JC. Three-dimensional gadolinium-enhanced MR venographic evaluation of patency of central veins in the thorax: initial experience. Radiology 1999;213(2):555-60.

Thornton MJ, Ryan R, Varghese JC, Farrell MA, Lucey B, Lee MJ. A three-dimensional gadolinium-enhanced MR venography technique for imaging central veins. AJR Am J Roentgenol 1999;173(4):999-1003.

Subject Index